Professional Studies for Midwifery Practice

For Churchill Livingstone:

Publishing Manager: Inta Ozols
Project Development Manager: Valerie Dearing
Project Manager: Derek Robertson
Design Direction: George Ajayi

Professional Studies for Midwifery Practice

Edited by

Diane Fraser PhD MPhil BEd MTD RM RN

Head of the Academic Division of Midwifery,
School of Human Development, University of Nottingham, Nottingham, UK

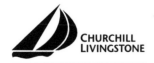
CHURCHILL
LIVINGSTONE

EDINBURGH LONDON NEW YORK PHILADELPHIA ST LOUIS SYDNEY TORONTO 2000

CHURCHILL LIVINGSTONE
An imprint of Harcourt Publishers Limited

© Harcourt Publishers Limited 2000

First published 2000

ISBN 0443 06114 9

British Library Cataloguing in Publication Data
A catalogue record for this book is available from the British
Library

Library of Congress Cataloging in Publication Data
A catalog record for this book is available from the Library
of Congress

Note
Medical knowledge is constantly changing. As new
information becomes available, changes in treatment,
procedures, equipment and the use of drugs become
necessary. The editor, contributors and the publishers
have, as far as it is possible, taken care to ensure that the
information given in this text is accurate and up to date.
However, readers are strongly advised to confirm that the
information, especially with regard to drug usage, complies
with the latest legislation and standards of practice.

The
publisher's
policy is to use
**paper manufactured
from sustainable forests**

Printed in China

Contents

Contributors

E Rosemary Buckley BSc RGN RM
Rosemary Buckley has worked for 8 years as a Senior Midwife in quality and audit at Nottingham City Hospital. She is the author of the book *Delivering Quality in Midwifery*.

Janet L Charity BSc(Hons) CertEd ADM RM RN
Janet Charity is a Midwife Teacher at the University of Nottingham, within the Academic Division of Midwifery. She is involved in all aspects of the curriculum for pre-registration midwifery and is also involved with post-registration midwifery. Janet has particular interest and experience in the subject of ethics; she is currently undertaking an MPhil investigating the ethico-legal interface of informed consent in midwifery practice.

Penny Church MEd ADM PGCEA RN RM
Penny Church is a Midwife Teacher in the Academic Division of Midwifery at the University of Nottingham. She obtained her MEd in Human Relations from the School of Education at the University of Nottingham.

Iris G Cooper RN RM
Iris Cooper completed her nursing training in 1962 and her midwifery training in 1969. From 1979 until 1998, when she retired, she was a Senior Midwifery Officer at Queens Medical Centre, Nottingham. She qualified as a Supervisor of Midwives in 1978 and held the post of Trent Regional Supervisor of Midwives from 1986 to 1996. From 1994 to 1998 Iris was a Senior Midwifery Adviser to the Confidential Enquiry into Maternal Deaths Committee.

Colleen Drury MA DipEd CertEd ADM MTD RN RM
Colleen Drury is a midwifery education coordinator and Supervisor of Midwives within the Academic Division of Midwifery, University of Nottingham. She is involved in both pre- and post-registration midwifery programmes. Colleen has undertaken the role of Supervisor of Midwives within the South Derbyshire Health District for the past four years. She has a particular interest in the management of midwifery services and staff development. In 1998, Colleen achieved an MA in Sociolegal Studies (Children) at Nottingham Trent University.

Nicola J Dunn MA ADM CertEd RGN RM
Nicola Dunn has been a midwifery tutor for 9 years and is currently working at the University of Hull where she is undertaking a MPhil/PhD in the Department of Medicine.

Diane M Fraser PhD MPhil BEd MTD RM RN
Diane Fraser is Reader in Midwifery at the University of Nottingham. She is Head of the Academic Division of Midwifery in the School of Human Development. This school arose as a unique merger of the academic units of Child Health, Midwifery, and Obstetrics and Gynaecology. Diane's doctoral study is entitled Action Research for Curriculum Improvement in Pre-Registration Midwifery Programmes. Commissioned research has included an outcome evaluation of pre-registration midwifery and the role of the teacher/lecturer in practice. Both studies were published in 1998 by the English

National Board for Nursing, Midwifery and Health Visiting.

Nicki Hastie MA
Nicki Hastie has an MA from the English Department at Leicester University. She is a lesbian with a cultural studies research background and has published on women's health and lesbian cultural production. Since 1996 she has worked as Information Officer at Self Help Nottingham, a development agency which provides information about and support for self-help groups.

Chris Johnson BSc(Hons) DipN MTD RN RM
Chris Johnson is a Midwife Teacher in the Academic Division of Midwifery at the University of Nottingham.

Sarah Kirkwood MSc RGN RM
Sarah Kirkwood is currently a Locality Manager of Clinical Midwifery, Community Nursing and Health Visiting within Nottingham Community Health NHS Trust. She is also a Supervisor of Midwives. Sarah has recently completed a Master's degree with the University of Nottingham for which she undertook research into parent education – the focus of her dissertation.

Jayne E Marshall MA ADM PGCEA RGN RM
An experienced Midwife Teacher, Jayne Marshall is currently undertaking a major research study for an MPhil/PhD examining informed consent during intrapartum care through ethnographic participant observation. Jayne has also carried out research into shared learning between pre-registration diploma in midwifery and nursing students as part of her Master's degree at Loughborough University, and has a particular interest in the complexities surrounding law and ethics relating to midwifery practice.

Ransolina Morgan BA(Hons) SRN SCM MTD
Ransolina Morgan is a Midwife Teacher at the University of Nottingham, School of Human Development, Academic Division of Midwifery. She obtained her BA(Hons) in Social Policy and Administration at the University of Nottingham in 1993. She is co-module writer and teacher to the sociology modules and has responsibility for in-service and continuing education. As an AP(E)L adviser, she is involved in supporting midwives making claims for academic credits. She is an external examiner for the return to midwifery refresher course at Hull University, and is currently undertaking an MPhil degree.

Carol Newton BSc(Hons) PGDL ADM RM RN
Carol Newton is a Midwife Researcher at Nottingham City Hospital NHS Trust.

Beverley A Ord BSc(Hons) PGDip ADM RN RM
Beverley Ord is a Midwife Teacher at the University of Nottingham, within the Academic Division of Midwifery. She is involved in all aspects of the curriculum for pre-registration midwifery and is also involved with post-registration midwifery. She obtained a degree in health studies which incorporated the subject of ethics.

Maureen D Raynor MA ADM PGCEA RMN RGN RM
Maureen D Raynor is a Midwife Teacher at the University of Nottingham, School of Human Development, Academic Division of Midwifery. She obtained an MA from the Women and Gender Studies Department of the University of Warwick. She is interested in women's health issues, particularly those of minority groups.

Wendy Stanton BA DipLib ALA
Wendy Stanton is Assistant Librarian at the Greenfield Medical Library, University of Nottingham, responsible for the provision of subject services to the Faculty of Medicine and Health Sciences. She has a special interest in the teaching of information handling skills and the design and delivery of user education programmes to students. She was recently a member of a project team set up to develop a computer assisted learning program, CALIBRE, funded by Enterprise in Higher Education.

Margaret Staples MSc ADM MTD CertEd RN RSCN RM
Margaret Staples trained as a general and Registered Sick Children's Nurse prior to embarking on her career in midwifery. She gained 10 years' valuable experience working in an African mission hospital before training to be a Midwife Teacher. From 1980 Margaret worked at King's Mill Hospital, Sutton in Asfield, as a Midwife Teacher and, in 1996, she became Supervisor of Midwives. In 1998 she achieved an MSc in the Practice of Education from the University of Surrey.

Preface

The overall purpose of this book has been to bring together those key areas of practice identified by midwives and students as being of concern or of difficulty for them. The emphasis on a woman-centred maternity service has inevitably raised parent's expectations and with it an increase in negligence claims. Midwives are expected to become more knowledgeable, increase their competence in new skills, base their practice on best available evidence and operate in a cost-effective, target-setting NHS. The explosion of information makes it difficult for practitioners to keep up to date, seek out relevant evidence to develop their practice and maintain a quality personal life.

Busy practitioners should be able to use this book as a reference text according to their needs at the time, as each chapter can be read independently. The chapters include information which can be easily assimilated by those who have done very little recent study as well as being thought provoking to aid reflection, stimulate critical inquiry and engender a thirst for new knowledge.

The style of each chapter varies according to focus and includes illustrations, case studies and activities as appropriate. For example, Chapter 1 guides the inexperienced library user through the complexities of undertaking a literature search or accessing the Cochrane Library. Chapter 3 confronts the dilemmas and lack of knowledge experienced by students when encountering difficult cultural practices and prejudices. A theoretical framework and case scenarios are provided in Chapter 5 to assist with ethical dilemmas arising from advanced technology and assisted reproduction. Chapter 9 describes the ways in which one NHS trust established a risk management scheme. The final chapter draws upon the views of a wide variety of different stakeholders in the maternity services to challenge the reader to become actively involved in influencing the maternity services.

All chapters are relevant to some aspect of contemporary midwifery practice and are intended to provide a springboard for the acquisition of further knowledge and professional debate with the aim of continually improving the maternity services. We hope this book answers many questions but raises many more for all those who use it as a resource.

Diane M Fraser
Nottingham, 2000

Acknowledgements

The editor would like to extend particular thanks to the following: Sue Sergeant, formerly of Nurture—Division of Reproductive Medicine, University of Nottingham and Liz Ellis, King's Mill NHS Trust for their advice on ethical dilemmas (Chapter 5); and Nicky Addison for all of her administrative and secretarial support.

1

Accessing the literature

Wendy Stanton   Diane Fraser

The aims of this chapter are to outline the process of literature searching and help you use libraries effectively. It introduces you to some of the key sources of information, both printed and electronic, that are relevant to midwifery practice. It offers practical advice on how to conduct an effective literature search using examples from some of these key sources.

It aims to introduce you to the key sources of information on clinical effectiveness. Finally, it aims to promote information-handling skills, which will assist you in your professional development

INTRODUCTION

The publication of Changing Childbirth (DoH 1993) requires midwives to base their professional practice on current research findings and relevant evidence to enable them to offer women more informed choices about their care. The range of information sources available in both printed and electronic formats, presented with different user interfaces, is growing rapidly. New periodical titles are announced almost daily, making it impossible to keep up with this growth by scanning the journals, especially as many subjects relevant to midwifery overlap with medicine, psychology, social science and nursing. Searching the literature, therefore, is an important skill, particularly at a time when health care resources are diminishing and there is a growing need to demonstrate that current practice is cost effective.

Literature searches need to be conducted in a systematic way if they are to be successful and, although it takes time to develop the skill, once mastered it may be applied to any future research you undertake. It can be a time-consuming and frustrating process; however, if you allocate sufficient time to spend in your library to get to know the resources available and approach the search in a systematic way, the process will not seem so daunting. Be prepared to be flexible and adapt your search strategy according to your findings. There are a number of reasons why it is important to do a literature search:

- to become familiar with the literature on a subject
- to follow up a subject of particular interest
- to gather ideas for a research project
- to keep up to date with research in a specialist subject area
- to avoid duplication of effort in research
- to compare opposing views and form your own opinions.

This chapter will describe some of the major resources available for midwifery research and examples of search strategies from some of the key sources will be provided. Many of the resources described are available in both print and electronic format at present and, whilst acknowledging the tremendous impact of networked information in the health care field, the authors are aware that in many maternity units the infrastructure required to support this development is not yet in place. Access to networked information may be limited, therefore, to students either pursuing courses run by institutes of higher education, where they will have automatic access to a university network, or to those with access through an Internet provider at home.

Starting off

The process of searching for information is ongoing and is best illustrated by the cycle illustrated in Fig. 1.1.

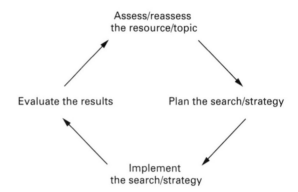

Figure 1.1   The literature-searching process.

This process may be applied to any search strategy and will help you to clarify your research statement and to identify relevant search terms. It will also help you to decide which sources of information are most appropriate for your search.

ASSESSING THE RESOURCES AVAILABLE

Before you start your literature search you will need to find out about the wide range of sources of information which are available to you and you will need to learn how to use them effectively. There may be local libraries or libraries of professional associations who you can contact by phone or there may be useful sites available over the Internet.

Libraries and librarians

Libraries

Find out which libraries you have access to, (there may be more than one) and use the checklist in Box 1.1 to assess their usefulness.

Familiarize yourself with the layout of the libraries you decide to use and find out where the different types of information are located.

The librarian

Librarians are your key resource when you need to find information. They will have specialist

Box 1.1 Checklist of services available in your local libraries

Access and Materials
- What type of library is it? (university, postgraduate, hospital)
- Is access free or is there a charge?
- Do you need proof of who you are/where you work/course of study?
- Do you need to take a photograph of yourself for your library card?
- What are the hours of opening?
- What is the telephone/fax number?
- In what format is the library catalogue (e.g. card index, computerized)?
- Are there separate collections of stock (e.g. short loan, reference)?
- What are the loan periods?
- Is there a separate collection of recent journals?
- Which printed indexing and abstracting services are available?
- Which databases are available electronically? (e.g. the Cochrane Library)
- Do you need a username/password to access electronic information?
- Does the library offer an online searching facility?
- Does the library offer information skills sessions to users?
- Does the library produce any publicity material e.g. library guides or handouts?

Services
Loans:
- How many books are you allowed to borrow at any one time?
- How long is the normal loan period?
- Is it possible to renew books on loan?
- May books be renewed by telephone or must you do this in person?
- Can books be requested by telephone or letter?
- How do you reserve a book which is already on loan to another reader?

Interlibrary loans:
- Does the library offer an interlibrary loan service?
- Is there a limit on the number of requests you may make?
- Is a charge made for each interlibrary loan request?

Photocopying:
- Is a photocopier provided for use within the library?
- Is it a coin- or card-operated machine?
- What is the cost of a photocopy?
- Can you request photocopies of articles to be posted to you?

subject knowledge and will be able to suggest the most appropriate sources of information, databases, statistics, etc. which may be relevant to your search. They will also be aware of the nuances of the system of indexing articles in each database and will help you to adapt your search strategy to each one. More importantly, they will help you construct your search strategy to ensure that you find as much relevant information as possible. You will find it helpful to attend any induction sessions offered to staff.

Professional associations

Consider also the services offered by professional associations, who may provide a literature-searching service, or they may be prepared to send photocopies of journal articles through the post; a charge is usually made for these services. A list of professional associations and their addresses are included at the end of the chapter.

Personal computers

Personal computers (PCs) feature in the lives of most people today, either at work or at home; a PC can help you to produce and update the information required for your professional development report; it can also help you to organize your thoughts and ideas for your research project.

As you conduct your review of the literature it is important to keep full and accurate records of the sources of information you have used and the references you have found. These can be stored on a PC and incorporated into programs such as Endnote or Reference manager, which are examples of database management programs, designed to help you keep track of your references, import references directly from databases such as Medline and produce bibliographies. Alternatively, you may want to create your own database of references, which will be easier to update on a PC, and which can be used to create your own bibliography. It also helps to keep a record of each database or individual issues of the indexing and abstracting publications you are going to use and to keep a record of which titles you have already consulted as your search progresses.

PCs with CDROM (compact disk read only memory) drives will enable you to access the wide range of high quality multimedia programs which are published today. If you have a modem and relevant communications software you will be able to link to the Internet and access some of the databases available via the World Wide Web which are described in this chapter.

PLANNING A SEARCH STRATEGY

Assessing the topics for study

Before you begin any research project it is necessary to conduct a literature search to establish which subjects would be suitable topics to study. A literature search may:

- help to clarify search terms
- reveal which aspects of a topic have already been investigated
- suggest new approaches to the subject
- indicate a problem that requires solving
- produce unanswered questions
- identify instruments already developed and tested
- highlight methods of data analysis.

Refining your topic

The next stage in the process is to define the nature of the subject which you are choosing to study. The key element of any research project is the research question. Sindhu (1997) p. 40 states that: 'A clearly defined research question is vital in maintaining the direction of all aspects of the review'. Initial statements of a problem can be either too broad or too vague; therefore it is helpful if you can convert the topic into a problem statement such as that in the following example:

'What factors influence success when breast feeding the preterm infant?'

Identify each individual concept expressed in the statement and think of any alternative words or synonyms which describe each topic; a general or medical/nursing thesaurus may help you. Then list these terms, bearing in mind Americanisms and American spelling, variable endings of terms and differences in the meaning of words, which can change over time. It

helps if you begin by searching for each concept separately, starting with the broader terms first and then gradually narrow your search to retrieve the most relevant results.

The following list of terms could be identified from the example given above:

Topic 1: breast feeding   breast milk
lactation   infant feeding   nutrition.

Topic 2: preterm infant   infant
neonate(s)   premature infant   newborn.

Topic 3: factors   birth weight   weight gain
support.

Activity 1.1 will help you to practise identifying keywords; the more you can identify, the more complete your search will be.

Activity 1.1

Make a list of all the keywords you would have to consider when finding articles on:

The role of the midwife in the prevention of sudden infant death.

Limiting your search

You may be unable to define the limits of your search when you start and you may find that any limits you apply may change as the search progresses. The extent of your search may be limited by the time available to you, for example, or the subject itself may be self-limiting. As a general rule, however, a 5 year search of the literature is acceptable. There are other reasons why you may need to consider limiting your search:

- you may be faced with too much information or too little
- you may be interested in specific age groups
- you may be interested in a specific type of information e.g. a systematic review
- there may be geographical boundaries, which influence your search.

Identifying your search terms

The next stage is to use your list of keywords to find articles in the periodical literature. Most periodicals articles are listed by subject in indexing and abstracting publications; some may also be available on CDROM. CDROMs are capable of storing large amounts of data which may be searched using a computer and offer more flexible methods of searching across a number of years, using natural language, subject headings, journal titles and authors and search terms, for example. This is a quick and easy method of searching, once you have learnt some basic commands, and your results may be viewed, printed out or downloaded onto disk.

An increasing number of databases are becoming available via the Internet; some databases, such as Medline, are offered free of charge e.g. PubMed and Internet Grateful Med, however, these services, whilst supporting natural language searching, offer limited options for comprehensive searching of the medical literature (Anagnostelis & Cooke 1997).

The strategies you need to use to identify articles relevant to your subject, are the same for all of these databases. Most indexing and abstracting services list periodical articles by subject using a standard set of terms, called 'thesaurus terms' or 'subject headings'. A thesaurus is a controlled vocabulary which a particular indexing publication has decided to use to index periodical articles. You will need to check the list of keywords you have produced, using the guidelines above, against the subject headings or thesaurus terms used by each publication. For example, articles written on the subject of pre-conception care may be indexed using several similar terms, some of which may be hyphenated:

prenatal care   pre-conception care
preconception care.

Be aware, also, that some words may be used incorrectly, for example the word 'pre-conceptual' may be used instead of 'pre-conception'.

The most important and comprehensive thesaurus of terms published is Medical Subject Headings, often abbreviated to MeSH headings, which are used to index articles in Index Medicus. MeSH headings are becoming recognized as the standard for most databases and are also used to index information in the Cochrane Library and the National Research Register (NRR). The subject headings used by the International Nursing Index and Cumulative Index to Nursing and Allied Health Literature (CINAHL), are also based on the MeSH thesaurus; however, they contain additional nursing and midwifery-related terms. MeSH headings are naturally biased towards the medical literature and do not always reflect midwifery practice; therefore a comprehensive search for information on midwifery would require a search using the following terms:

midwifery   nurse-midwifery   obstetrical
nursing   obstetrics.

Different indexes produce their own list of subject headings or thesaurus of terms, which is designed to help you find all relevant subject terms on a topic. They provide links to other similar search terms by adding 'see' and 'see related headings'. The date when a term was first introduced is frequently given. The CINAHL subject headings apply the following sub headings, which can help you to refine your search:

Age groups: in infancy and childhood
in adolescence   in pregnancy   in utero.

Topical: education   methods   nursing
psychological factors   rehabilitation.

Document Types: care plans   case studies
protocols   questionnaires   research.

The example given in Box 1.2 shows how MeSH headings interpret the terms 'breast feeding' and 'breast milk'. 'See' means use instead of, i.e. use 'milk, human' not 'Breast Milk', because Index Medicus also includes many animal studies. *See related* and *XR* terms help you to broaden your search by suggesting similar, related terms.

The CINAHL thesaurus entry for breast feeding and associated terms is slightly different, offering more relevant alternatives (see Box 1.3).

When using any thesaurus of terms it is usual to start by looking in the alphabetical list of subject terms; however, not all of the terms

---

Box 1.2 Example from the MeSH thesaurus

breast feeding
G6.696.259.750.500
see related
    bottle feeding
XR lactation
XR milk, human
breast milk see milk, human

Box 1.3 Example from the CINAHL subject headings

breast feeding
\$E2421.416.177 + G6.696.750.500

see also INEFFECTIVE BREASTFEEDING (NANDA); INTERRUPTED BREASTFEEDING (NANDA); MILK HUMAN

XX LACTATION
XX MILK, HUMAN

breast feeding consultants see LACTATION CONSULTANTS

---

relevant to your subject will be listed next to each other. Therefore two further tools have been designed to help you to find related terms in MeSH headings and the list of CINAHL subject headings.

The first is the 'permuted list of terms', published with the list of CINAHL subject headings, which brings together every heading or phrase which contains the same term, e.g. breast:

- breast diseases
- breast feeding
- breast self-examination
- fibrocystic diseases of breast.

The second is the 'tree structures', published with both the CINAHL and MeSH headings, which arrange the subject headings in a subject classification, or hierarchy of terms. You may have noticed that the MeSH term 'breast feeding' in Box 1.3 was followed by the number G6.696.259.750.500. This number refers to the position of the term within the tree structures, G6 being the top of the BIOCHEMICAL PHENOMENA, METABOLISM, NUTRITION tree.

NUTRITION is further subdivided into more specific nutritional term (see Box 1.4).

Box 1.4 MeSH tree structure

nutrition	G6.696
animal nutrition	G6.696. 116
child nutrition	G6.696.259
adolescent nutrition	G6.696.259.500
infant nutrition	G6.696.259.750
breast feeding	G6.696.259.750.500
weaning	G6.696.259.750.750

Thesaurus terms, therefore, differ from keywords in the following ways:
Keywords are:

- non standard terms used by authors in a title or abstract
- dependent on an agreed terminology and the vagaries of the English language
- very specific where there is accepted terminology
- difficult to use for very general subject areas
- not specific to any databases
- may be truncated, e.g. neonat* will retrieve neonate, neonates, and neonatal.

(Be careful when using truncation; for example, infant* would retrieve not only infant and infants, but also infantile and infanticide.)
Thesaurus terms are:

- standard terms set by databases providers
- accurate/more precise than keywords
- helpful for searching broad subject areas
- specific to individual databases e.g. British Nursing Index, CINAHL, Medline.

When searching for information over many years in several disciplines, it may be more effective and efficient for you to search the computerized databases, which offer greater flexibility for searching, for example for both keyword and thesaurus terms, authors and ranges of years.

If, however, you cannot find any equivalent thesaurus term to describe your subject, you may need to search using both keyword and thesaurus terms in combination to increase your chances of finding relevant references. The example in

Activity 1.2 will help you to find thesaurus terms in two indexes using a list of identified keywords.

Activity 1.2

Using the keywords identified in Activity 1.1, find and compare the equivalent thesaurus terms listed in:

1. Cumulative Index to Nursing and Allied Health Literature
2. British Nursing Index

Having identified and refined your search terms, the next stage is to compare the list of terms you have produced with the equivalents in the indexing and abstracting publications available, to help you develop your search strategy. You need to decide which of these sources of information you are going to use.

Linking search terms

Once you have made a list of all the keywords or thesaurus terms relevant to your research topic, you will need to decide how they relate to each other before you can link them together, particularly if you are searching electronic databases. A few possibilities are listed as follows:

Phrases. You may search for phrases; in most cases they may be typed in with spaces between the component words:

e.g. breast feeding   postnatal care.

OR. This retrieves references containing either or both terms specified in a record, which may be useful if you are having difficulty finding information on a subject.

AND. This retrieves only those references which contain both words in the record and will, therefore, reduce the number of references retrieved. (see examples in Box 1.5)

Creating complex searches

To create a detailed search strategy for use on an electronic database, you may need to search groups of terms linked by 'AND' or 'OR' statements.

Box 1.5   **Examples of linking search terms**

Example 1 OR: Searching for information on the preterm infant OR newborn infants OR neonates would retrieve references containing either of the terms

A = all articles on preterm infant
B = all articles on newborn infants
C = all articles on either preterm infants **or** newborn infants (shaded area)

Example 2 AND: Searching for information on health promotion AND breast feeding would retrieve references containing both terms; this operation narrows your search to include only those references which include all of your search terms.

A = all articles on health promotion
B = all articles on breast feeding
C = articles only about health promotion **and** breast feeding

---

Example

(HIV infection OR Human Immunodeficiency OR virus transmission OR HIV-1 seropositive) AND (Breastfeeding OR Breast Milk OR Lactation AND Morbidity OR Prognosis)

The strategy is to search for each concept separately then combine each one using the 'AND' and 'OR' statements as described above.

IMPLEMENTING THE SEARCH STRATEGY

The following section provides a brief description of the sources you might use as part of your search strategy. Before you begin any research project, it is important to establish whether your topic has been the subject of previous research to avoid duplication, therefore you will need to find out about what research is ongoing and also conduct a thorough search of the literature. New research ideas are often communicated by word of mouth at conferences and study days and this can be a useful way of meeting researchers with similar interests.

Joining mailing lists and discussion groups is another way of becoming aware of new research interests; these are described further in the section on the World Wide Web (p. 18). Box 1.6 highlights some of the databases and their formats available to you. Descriptions of the most common follow.

Box 1.6	Examples of research sources of information

Type of Information	Examples
Research	Word of mouth
	Mailing lists
	ASLIB's Index to Theses
	Current Research in
	Britain
	MIRIAD
	RCN Steinberg Collection
	of Nursing Research
	National Research
	Register
Abstracts and Indexes	Applied Social Science
	Index and Abstracts
	(ASSIA)
	British Nursing Index
	Cumulative Index to
	Nursing and Allied
	Health Literature
	(CINAHL)
	Index Medicus
	MIDIRS
	MIRIAD
Electronic databases	ASSIA
	BIDS
	British Nursing Index
	CINAHL
	Cochrane Library
	Medline
	Psychlit

The reference collection

It may be necessary to read around a subject to help you decide on the precise nature of the topic and to help you refine it. Begin your search in the reference section of the library and use dictionaries and encyclopaedias to help you define search terms, particularly if you are unfamiliar with a topic.

Library catalogues

Although books are not as up to date as the periodical literature, they can be a useful starting point for providing background information on a topic. Books will help you to clarify terminology, will often describe classic articles on a subject and will provide citations to key references, particularly if the book is a review of a particular subject. If a book is unavailable in your local library, it may be possible to search the catalogues of other libraries. Most UK universities make available their libraries' OPACs (Online Public Access Catalogues) via the Internet.

There are several sources of information, which will help you to identify current research in your field.

Current Research in Britain

Published annually by the British Library, Current Research in Britain is the major source of on going research published. It appears in three volumes: Physical sciences, Biological sciences and Social sciences: the Social sciences volume includes research being conducted in nursing and midwifery.

National Research Register

The National Research Register consists of a set of databases of current research and development projects in the (National Health Service) NHS, and work funded by the Scottish and Welsh Offices and the Department of Health (DoH). It will expand to include work funded through the research and development levy within NHS providers towards the end of 1998. The main register includes for each record: details of the title of the research project, the main research question, lead researcher, primary location of the research and methodology. Medical subject headings (MeSH) are used to index each record. In addition to the register itself, the CDROM also includes the following databases:

- *MRC clinical trials directory*—details of clinical trials in receipt of a grant from the Medical Research Council
- *Register of registers*—information about other registers which hold similar information to the research and development projects

- *Reviews in progress*—the database of research reviews in progress produced by the NHS Centre for Reviews and Dissemination
- *Health research at York*—information about ongoing research produced within the Centre for Health Economics and the NHS Centre for Reviews and Dissemination.

Theses

Theses submitted for higher degrees are listed in a publication called ASLIB's Index to Theses. All academic libraries should hold copies of this publication, which has a subject and author index and includes a summary of the research to help you to assess the relevance of the research. It may be possible for you to request copies of theses from the British Library through your local library. The British Library holds only the abstracts and contents pages of theses and will request the original from the university library where the degree was awarded and will supply a copy on microfilm, for reference only. It is sometimes possible to borrow theses from overseas, you will need to ask at your local library.

RCN Steinberg Collection of Nursing Research

The Steinberg Collection of Nursing Research is the most comprehensive collection of theses and dissertations by nurses and midwives submitted for degrees at masters and doctoral level in the United Kingdom. This unique collection, covering nursing, midwifery and health-related topics, was set up in 1974 to provide a central resource to benefit students and researchers. The collection, which is housed in the Royal College of Nursing Library, is only available for reference, therefore access is limited to members of the Royal College of Nursing on presentation of their membership card; non-members must obtain permission from the deputy librarian. A catalogue listing the theses by author and subject has been published to enable readers to request items from the British Library or directly from university libraries.

Reviews

Reviews bring together the results of work published over a period of time in a specialized subject area. They are compiled by acknowledged experts in the field, who summarize and critically review the information. From time to time review papers are published in periodicals; however, certain periodicals contain only review papers and can be identified by the following words in their titles: 'Advances in ...', 'Annual reviews in ...', 'Progress in ...', or 'Recent advances in ...'.

Some reviews are published as books in a series, e.g. 'Recent advances in ...', 'Current opinion in ...', and the 'Midwifery practice' series edited by Alexander, Levy and Roth (for example, Alexander J, Levy V, Roth C 1990 Midwifery practice: antenatal care. Macmillan, London; Alexander J, Levy V, Roth C 1997 Midwifery practice: core topics 1. Macmillan, London).

Periodical articles will present the most up-to-date information on a subject. Use these before you begin a search to get a general overview of a subject and to identify key authors in the field. As review articles highlight areas of progress in a subject and advances in practice, they may be long and will include extensive bibliographies of the literature.

Midwives Information and Resource Services (MIDIRS)

MIDIRS: midwifery digest offers several services to midwives. A midwifery digest, which scans over 550 English language journals from around the world, is published, covering midwifery, pregnancy, childbirth, the neonate and maternity services. The database consists of over 46 000 records, with abstracts, and the type of literature covered includes statistics, government and official reports, books, conference proceedings, newspaper articles and consumer health information leaflets. They offer an enquiry service and will provide lists of references on any topic. Books and videos may be ordered by mail and a midwifery portfolio, to help midwives keep a record of their professional development, is available.

The Midwifery Research Database (MIRIAD)

The MIRIAD database receives funding from the National Research Register (NRR) and is the only source of information about midwifery research in the UK; it is, consequently, the most important publication you will need to use. First published in 1988, it aims to provide information about both published and unpublished, completed and ongoing research in the field of midwifery. The database includes studies in clinical practice, midwifery education, the organization of midwifery services and the history of midwifery. The following criteria apply for entry onto the MIRIAD database:

- the studies must be carried out in the UK
- the study must be related to midwifery, however, the researchers need not be midwives
- studies are not usually included if they were completed as part of a first degree, except in exceptional cases.

From March 1999, MIRIAD was no longer responsible for the collection and dissemination of midwifery research, it will be incorporated into the NRR instead. The studies which have been registered with MIRIAD will appear on the University of Leeds mother and infant research unit website.

Indexing and abstracting publications

The rapid growth in the periodical literature has led to the development of new methods of searching databases electronically, either on CDROM, or via the World Wide Web. All of the major databases in the health care field are available electronically and these are designed to be searched by the end user and include on-screen help. Software providers, such as Silver Platter and OVID, who produce both CDROM and World Wide Web versions of Medline, based on Index Medicus and CINAHL, the electronic equivalent of the Cumulative Index to Nursing and Allied Health Literature, are just two examples. Electronic media, whether available on CDROM or via the Internet, are more up to date than their printed equivalents, and offer more options for searching (e.g. by periodical title, author, keyword or subject heading) because the indexing of articles is more thorough.

British Nursing Index (BNI)

BNI was first published in 1997 as a result of the merger of Nursing Bibliography, which ceased in 1995, and Nursing and midwifery index, which was published 1991–1996. The database is available monthly in printed format, quarterly on CDROM and over the World Wide Web. The printed index is one of the most up to date published in the field of nursing and midwifery and, because it is a British index, the articles indexed are more likely to be held in your local library.

Cumulative Index to Nursing and Allied Health Literature (CINAHL)

CINAHL is one of the major indexes published covering nursing, midwifery and allied health literature. Although this index is available in printed form, many libraries provide access to the database via the Internet, a networked or a stand-alone PC. CINAHL is produced and compiled in America and contains references from over 650 journals and is updated monthly on CDROM and bimonthly in printed form. Many British journals are included in the database; however some are only partially indexed. References are organized according to a detailed thesaurus of terms or CINAHL subject headings, which is structured in a similar way to the MeSH headings used with Index Medicus/Medline. CINAHL is also available via the World Wide Web with links to full text journals.

Medline

The main source of medical information available in most health care libraries is Medline, produced by the National Library of Medicine in the United States. It indexes over 3800 journals, including the key nursing and midwifery related titles and is searchable using the list of thesaurus terms called MeSH, or Medical Subject Headings (see p. 5). These same headings are used to index the reviews, which are held on the database of the Cochrane Library, thus easing the transfer of search strategies from one database to another. The Medline database is compiled from the same data which is used to produce Index Medicus and the International Nursing Index, both of which are available in printed format; the database may also be searched electronically either online, on CDROM, or via the Internet. The electronic versions allow several different methods of searching (e.g. keyword, author or journal title). There are several versions of Medline which are freely available via the World Wide Web, such as PubMed and GratefulMed. There is also a new OVID version of Medline available via the World Wide Web, which provides links to some full text journals.

Midwifery Index

Midwifery Index, produced by the Royal College of Midwives, is an invaluable source of information for retrospective searching of midwifery and related topics. It is published in two volumes, the first covering the period 1980–1986, with selective coverage of 1976–1979, and the second covering 1987–1991 (Ayres 1987, 1992).

Applied Social Science Index and Abstracts (ASSIA)

Applied Social Science Index and Abstracts is a British database which focuses on the sociological and psychological aspects of health and welfare service rather than clinical issues, which are already covered by CINAHL and BNI. It includes brief abstracts from over 550 international English language journals from 1987 onwards and you are more likely to be able to get hold of the articles from your local library.

Psychological abstracts

Psychological Abstracts is published by the American Psychological Association and would be useful for finding information on psychological aspects of health care, for example postnatal depression or mother–infant bonding.

Evidence-based literature

What is evidence-based literature?

Sackett et al (1997, p. 2) provides the following definition of evidence-based medicine, which could be applied to any aspect of evidence-based practice: 'The practice of evidence-based medicine means integrating individual clinical expertise with the best available external clinical evidence from systematic research'.

In order to find the best clinical evidence to support clinical practice you need to be aware of the following different types of evidence-based literature published:

- systematic reviews of the literature
- guidelines and protocols which take the reviews further and indicate how to put research into practice
- major trials (i.e. randomized controlled trials (RCTs).

These are described in more detail below.

Why is it important?

The rate at which primary literature in medicine and related subjects is growing is such that it is impossible to read all the primary sources that have been published. Medline includes approximately 8 million records from 1966 to the present. Most of the records are primary research articles; however they also include reviews of the literature, that is, articles with narrative reviews offering the author's personal opinion on a subject.

According to Dickersin, Sherer & Lefebvre (1994), searching the Medline database retrieves only half of the clinical trials published; it is, therefore, necessary to complete a hand search of all the current literature to pick up additional trials to avoid bias (Sackett et al 1997, p. 15).

The Cochrane Library is a database, which contains the work of the Cochrane Collaboration.

The Collaboration identifies all primary research in the form of clinical trials. It then carries out systematic reviews of the primary research using review methods developed by the Collaboration. As researchers, you need access to the best evidence available, the gold standard literature, which reviews the primary sources of information for you. According to Lefebvre (1994, p. 235), 'Reviews are necessary because of the continuing explosion in the primary literature and the difficulty of accessing some primary material. In addition reviews can create new evidence'.

Glanville, Haines & Auston (1998) also refer to the proliferation of collections of systematic reviews and critical appraisals of primary research, which are creating their own information explosion.

Systematic reviews are, therefore, becoming an increasingly important source of evidence about the effects of health care interventions because:

- they help to overcome the sheer volume of literature published by summarizing it
- they provide new information which may not be apparent from individual studies where the effects under investigation are small
- they provide more reliable results by aiming to present all the evidence on a given topic.

What is a systematic review?

Single studies rarely provide definitive answers to research questions or particularly health interventions; systematic reviews of the literature combine and analyse the results of several single studies and they provide conclusions which cannot be drawn from smaller, individual studies. Systematic reviews are important because they promote a scientific rather than a subjective approach to summarizing what is already known and they also provide more reliable evidence. Follow Activity 1.3 to find an example of a systematic review. Systematic reviews therefore reduce the number of inaccuracies resulting from bias, and replicability is enhanced. The NHS Centre for Reviews and Dissemination at York aims to promote the use of and access to research-based knowledge in health care by carrying out systematic reviews and making

Activity 1.3

This reference is an example of a good systematic review of the literature on a midwifery-related topic. Find a copy of the article in your local medical library and list the key features of the review. How does it differ from a typical research article?

Lucassen P L B J, Assendelft W J J, Gubbels J W, van Eijk T M, van Geldrop W J, Knuistingh Neven A 1998 Effectiveness of a treatment for infantile colic; systematic review. British Medical Journal 316(7144): 1563–1569

them available via DARE, the database of abstracts of reviews of effectiveness, which is available via both the World Wide Web and the Cochrane Library.

Sources of evidence-based literature

A number of groups in the United Kingdom are actively involved in the dissemination of research findings, notably the Cochrane Library and the NHS Centre for Reviews and Dissemination. Much of this work is based on what is commonly referred to as the 'gold standard' for research, the RCT. There are several new initiatives in print form which act as signposts to the increasing number of sources of effectiveness information published across a broad range of evidence types and subject areas. Some are subject based such as the Health Evidence Bulletins–Wales, which include information from RCTs if available; if they are not available, high quality evidence has been sought from observational and other studies. The Bulletin for Maternal and Early Child Health covers maternal health and the health of the child from pre-conception through the perinatal period.

The information contained in this and all the bulletins is likely to be valid for about a year, by which time significant new research evidence may have become available. Examples of similar digests of information are Bandolier, and the Journal of Clinical Effectiveness and Evidence Based Medicine Journal. Some are article based, like ACP Journal Club and the UK equivalent

Evidence Based Medicine. You may also come across guidelines which attempt to interpret the evidence and evaluate the cost effectiveness and implications of the evidence for practice (e.g. the Wessex DEC (Development and Evaluation Committee) reports and the Trent Institute Working Group on Acute Purchasing guidance notes).

There are also several 'new' databases such as DARE, Best Evidence, TRIP (Turning Research Into Practice) and IDEA (Internet Database of Evidence Abstracts and Articles) which gather together and disseminate the 'good' evidence published in the primary sources, such as Medline and Embase. However, at present there is no single comprehensive index to all the material available.

Several sources of evidence-based literature are also available via the World Wide Web. These have been assembled and described on a very useful site produced by Anthony Booth, Director of Information Resources at the School of Health and Related Research (ShaRR), Sheffield. The site is called 'Netting the Evidence' at http://panizzi.shef.ac.uk/auracle/links.html. Some examples are listed in Appendix. II, p. 20.

The Cochrane Library

The Cochrane Library is a major source of information on clinical effectiveness in healthcare, the library is named after Archie Cochrane who, in the 1970s, identified the need for greater awareness of the effects of health care and for improved access to the evidence available. He highlighted the need to identify RCTs in all medical specialities which could be used to assess the effectiveness of treatments. There are several subject specific Cochrane Collaboration groups worldwide who have volunteers who produce reviews of the literature. Most areas of health care are covered by the library; however, some subjects areas, such as pregnancy and childbirth, are further developed than others.

The library consists of the following databases:

- regularly updated systematic reviews, maintained by the Cochrane Collaboration

- Database of abstracts of reviews of effectiveness of treatment (DARE), which is produced by the Centre for Dissemination of Reviews of Effectiveness at York University, and includes abstracts and references of systematic reviews derived from databases such as Medline and Embase; structured abstracts are included for the best reviews and all the reviews are quality assessed
- a register of RCTs, which also includes ongoing trials
- contact details for collaborative review groups and Cochrane Centres
- a bibliography on the science of reviewing.

The Library is designed so that when you conduct a search the databases listing the best sources of evidence are given first (i.e. the Cochrane database of systematic reviews), therefore, when you begin your search, look for a Cochrane review, then try and find a review in progress; if these aren't available, look for a good quality recent review on the DARE database, then search for a RCT.

The Cochrane Library is currently produced on CDROM and should be available from your local library; if you have access to the Internet, the DARE database is also available via the World Wide Web. The whole Library is also available via this network on subscription.

The Cochrane Library includes the following types of information:

- the original full text systematic review and meta-analysis, including graphs
- regularly updated reviews
- odds ratio diagrams to give a clear visual representation of the results
- critical appraisals of high quality reviews published elsewhere
- the information included is quality assessed
- RCTs.

As the Cochrane Library involves mainly research undertaken by the medical profession, you might be asking how it differs from Medline. Medline includes approximately 8 million records from 1966 to the present. Most of the records are primary research articles; however, they also include reviews of the literature (i.e. articles which discuss the results of two or more publications on a subject). The Cochrane Library, however, is a smaller database which attempts to identify all the systematic reviews on a subject and applies a rigorous set of criteria to each study before adding them to the database. Cochrane also includes 200 000 clinical controlled trials.

Searching the database. This section describes a simple search using the example of 'breast feeding the preterm infant'. A detailed guide to using the Cochrane Library on CDROM can be downloaded from Oxford and Anglia Web site at:

http://www.libr.jr2.ox.ac.uk/nhserdd/aordd/evidence/clibtrng.htm://www

Free access to the abstracts of Cochrane reviews are available at both the UK Cochrane Collaboration site at: http://www.cochrane.co.uk and at the NHS Centre for Reviews and Dissemination Web site as part of the online version of the DARE database at:

http://nhscrd.york.ac.uk/welcome.html

The Cochrane Library opening screen lists the databases against which all searches are run, as shown in Fig. 1.2.

The four databases are listed in the index window at the top of the screen and whenever you search the database the number of results for each are displayed in this window.

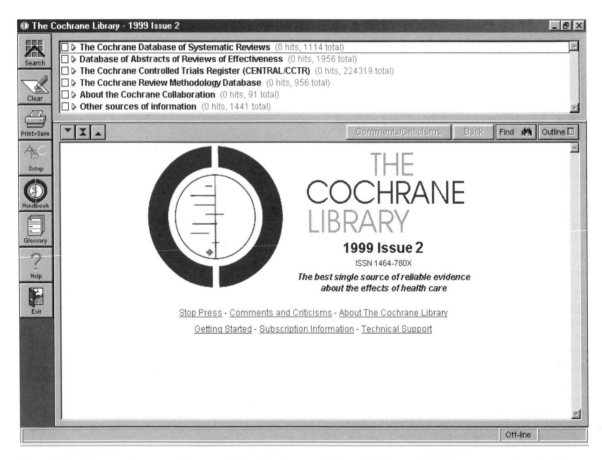

Figure 1.2 Cochrane Library opening screen (From the Cochrane Library database on CDROM 1998, reproduced with permission of Update Software).

The icons on the left hand margin allow you to search the database, print the results or copy text, or ask for help.

The database supports searching by subject using both textwords and MeSH headings, which means that any search strategies which you may have already created for use with Medline should easily transfer to this database. The options for searching by subject are shown in Fig. 1.3.

1. Simple searching

To perform a simple search, click on the button at the top left corner of the screen and the simple search option is automatically displayed.

Position the cursor in the box at the top of the screen and key in the search terms; several search terms may be entered at once and the database will search for references containing both words. This is the same as using the AND function in many databases.

e.g. breast feeding preterm infants

will retrieve references on breast feeding the preterm infant. Search terms can also be truncated using an *. Simple searching supports textwords or phrase searches.

2. Advanced searching

To perform an advanced search, click on the search button at the top left of the opening screen, this time, click on the advanced search option, which is displayed next to the simple search feature.

The advanced search option offers textword and phrase searching and allows you to develop a search strategy by combining several search statements using the AND/OR/NOT buttons at the right hand side of the screen. Search strategies are then displayed on the screen as you search, and the terms used may be recombined to produce different sets of results.

The advanced search option allows searching of specific fields within the database, and a range of dates may also be specified.

3. Searching using MeSH Headings

If you are having difficulty finding references using keywords, try clicking on the MeSH option at the top of the search screen. Position

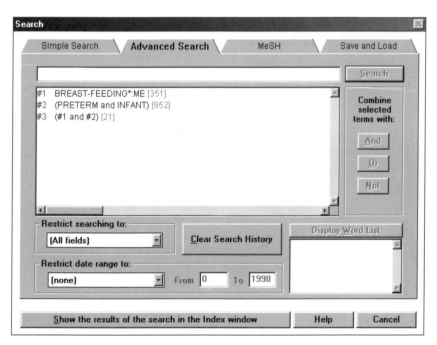

Figure 1.3   Cochrane Library search screen (From the Cochrane Library database on CDROM 1998, reproduced with permission of Update Software).

the cursor in the box at the top of the search screen, and key in your search term (e.g. breast feeding) then click on the button marked 'thesaurus' to the right of the search screen. The same list of thesaurus terms which appear when you search Medline will be displayed, e.g.:

breast
breast cysts see fibrocystic disease of breast
breast feeding
breast implants

Click on breast feeding and the tree for infant nutrition will be displayed. Highlight the term 'breast feeding' and click on the button marked 'search this term'. The results will be displayed in the document window.

Viewing the references. Click on the long button at the bottom of the screen labelled 'show the results of the search in the Index window' (Fig. 1.3) and you will return to the opening screen of the database. Your search results will be displayed in the index window in the top portion of the screen. Figure 1.4 shows how the results of the search are displayed individually for each database.

The results of the search in each database are displayed in layers. To view the results of each search, click on the name of the database and the individual results are displayed in the document window (see Fig. 1.4).

Click on the title of the review you want to view and this time, the complete review will appear in the document window (see Fig. 1.5).

Selecting the 'print' button on the left margin will allow you to print or save your results to disk. To print any references you want to keep click on the print button on the left hand side of the screen. The options for printing are:

- current item only
- selected items; using this option you may print out all your references or only those which you have marked with a tick in the check boxes next to each reference title in the index window
- output of multiple items; if you want to print more than one reference you will need

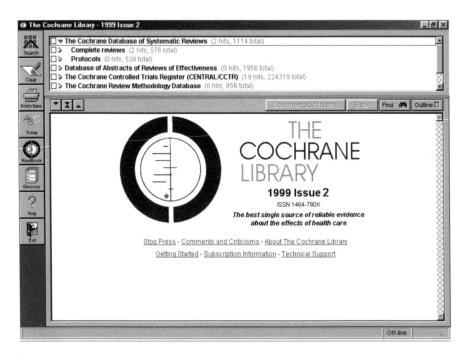

Figure 1.4 Cochrane Library—search results in the index window (From the Cochrane Library database on CDROM 1998, reproduced with permission of Update Software).

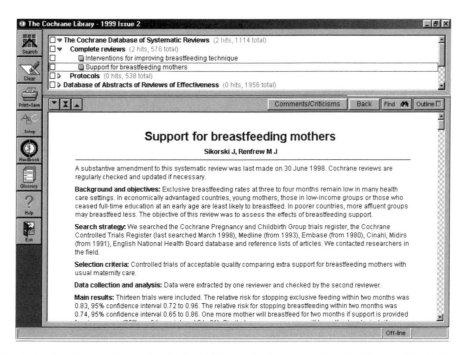

Figure 1.5 Displaying the document (From the Cochrane Library database on CDROM 1998, reproduced with permission of Update Software).

to specify the format for the print out; choosing 'exactly as they appear in the index' will give you just the title of the reference; 'short document, short reference' will print a truncated version of the full reference, therefore choose 'full document, complete reference' if you want the whole reference.

When you are ready to print, click the 'print' button at the bottom of the window.

Follow these instructions to find a clinical trial, as described in Activity 1.4.

The Odds Ratio Diagram. Odds ratio diagrams are used to summarize the results of several

Activity 1.4

Use the Cochrane Library to find a clinical trial on the effect of breast-feeding techniques and the duration of breast feeding, researcher: Mary Renfrew.

systematic reviews of the literature. With practice it is possible to interpret the symbols used in the diagrams fairly quickly. Interpreting the diagrams is described more fully in the training material available from the Oxford and Anglia site referred to earlier. The diagram presented in Fig. 1.6 is reproduced from the training material with permission (McKinnel & Elliott 1997).

Some of the symbols used to represent the results of systematic reviews in odds ratio diagrams are presented below: an example of how to interpret these diagrams is included in Fig. 1.6.

■ A blue box represents each individual trial. The smaller the trial, the smaller the box.

━■━ The line through the box represents the confidence interval. The longer the line, the greater is the degree of uncertainty.

◆ A black diamond represents the meta-analysis result. The wider the diamond, the greater is the confidence interval.

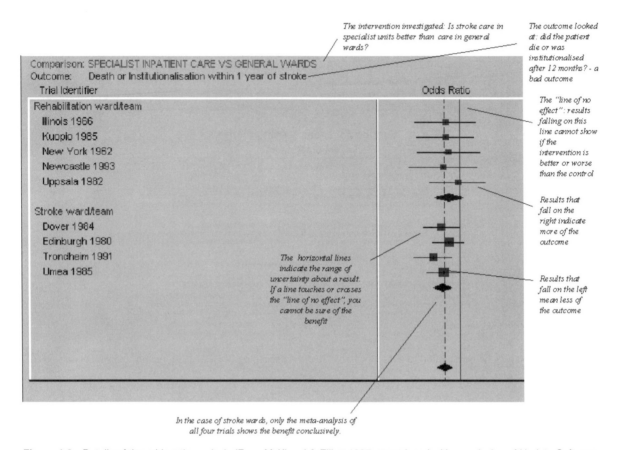

The intervention investigated: Is stroke care in specialist units better than care in general wards?

The outcome looked at: did the patient die or was institutionalised after 12 months? - a bad outcome

Comparison: SPECIALIST INPATIENT CARE VS GENERAL WARDS
Outcome: Death or Institutionalisation within 1 year of stroke
Trial Identifier

Odds Ratio

The "line of no effect": results falling on this line cannot show if the intervention is better or worse than the control

Rehabilitation ward/team
Illinois 1966
Kuopio 1985
New York 1962
Newcastle 1993
Uppsala 1982

Results that fall on the right indicate more of the outcome

Stroke ward/team
Dover 1964
Edinburgh 1980
Trondheim 1991
Umea 1985

The horizontal lines indicate the range of uncertainty about a result. If a line touches or crosses the "line of no effect", you cannot be sure of the benefit

Results that fall on the left mean less of the outcome

In the case of stroke wards, only the meta-analysis of all four trials shows the benefit conclusively.

Figure 1.6 Details of the odds ratio analysis (From McKinnel & Elliott 1997, reproduced with permission of Update Software and NHS Executive, Anglia and Oxford Region).

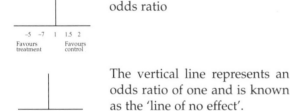

The horizontal axis shows the odds ratio

The vertical line represents an odds ratio of one and is known as the 'line of no effect'.

If the horizontal line, or confidence interval, crosses the vertical line of no effect, the results represented by the black diamond are inconclusive. If the horizontal line is longer to the left of the centre this means that there is more of an outcome, if the line is to the right this means there is less of an outcome. Each review needs to be interpreted according to the interventions being investigated; for example, results identifying less of an outcome may be favourable if fewer patients died as a result of a specific treatment.

Searching the World Wide Web

The Internet is a global network of independent computer networks, which are linked together to form one large network of networks. Programs called internet protocols allow communication between computers anywhere in the world. The Internet provides access to textual, graphical and moving images, which may be downloaded to a PC with the necessary software to receive them. This means that you could download magnetic resonance imaging (MRI) images of a baby's heart and a heartbeat onto your PC.

World Wide Web sites (WWW)

The World Wide Web allows access to sites available via the Internet by providing hypertext links to other documents within a document.

Midwifery sites on the Internet are not as numerous as those developed for physicians; however, the Internet is gradually being acknowledged as an important medium for education and professional development both within the higher education sector and in the NHS. Access to databases such as Medline and Embase over the World Wide Web for NHS staff is a major development. Some of the information available via the Web includes access to databases, electronic journals, university web sites and their catalogues, the DoH site, including access to full text copies of major reports, and patient information.

The WWW provide the following types of services:

E-mail. E-mail allows you to send and receive messages quickly with anyone else who has an e-mail address and access to an Internet account. It is possible to send attachments to your messages as well as the message itself.

Mailing Lists. Mailing lists are discussion groups, which are set up by people sharing an interest in a particular subject, who then communicate their ideas within the group. Joining a mailing list is a good way to make contact with researchers interested in a similar field; however, be selective about which ones you join and ensure that they are managed by a list moderator to ensure that your mailbox does not overflow with junk mail.

Lists are managed by list servers; Mailbase is the largest UK list server, based at Newcastle. To join, send a message to:
mailbase@mailbase.ac.uk and search the alphabetical or subject guide to the lists available.

Search engines. These allow you to search the Internet by subject, but they are not always very accurate. The following search engines offer some of the best results:

- Yahoo
  midwifery index and search page

http://www.yahoo.com/Health/Nursing/midwifery
- Altavista
  http://www.altavista.digital.com/

A list of useful World Wide Web sites is included in Appendix II, p. 20.

EVALUATING THE RESULTS

The final stage in the process is to evaluate the sources of information used and the results of your search. You should ask the following questions:

- are the references you retrieved relevant?
- have you retrieved enough information?
- are there any gaps?
- do you need to revise your strategy?
- do you need to update your search?

According to your answers to these questions, you may need to reassess the subject and the search terms you have used and start your search again. However, if after a thorough search you have identified few articles on your subject, you may be breaking new ground.

Summary

To complete a literature review successfully you need to allow yourself adequate time to conduct the search and follow the process outlined in this chapter.

Assess the resources in terms of the people you may need to consult, libraries to visit and the bibliographical resources available to you.

Plan your search carefully, take a systematic approach to searching the literature and your technique will improve with practice.

Implement your search strategy, be flexible and refine it as your search progresses.

Evaluate the results of your search, libraries used, articles retrieved. Are the references relevant to your topic? If not, revise your search strategy.

APPENDIX I: GLOSSARY

Interpreting the odds ratio diagram:

- *randomization*—allocation (not selection) of individuals/patients to control and intervention groups purely determined by chance. It will therefore minimize bias, which might influence the results (outcome)

- *randomized controlled trial (RCT)*—a trial of, for example, an intervention or therapy which has a control group and an experimental group, both being allocated randomly
- *risk*—the probability that something (bad outcome) will happen (e.g. 17 out of 1000 pregnancies will be ectopic). *Risk is a ratio of bad outcomes over total outcomes*
- *relative risk (risk ratio)*—risk in the treatment group/risk in the control group
- *risk difference*—risk in the treatment group − risk in control group
- *odds*—the ratio of bad outcomes over good outcomes; it is usually described as odds in the experimental group and odds in the control group
- *odds ratio*—the ratio of odds in the experimental group (those who received a treatment or an intervention) and the odds in the control group (those who did not receive that treatment or intervention).

APPENDIX II: MAJOR HEALTH GATEWAYS

There are several subject specific gateways which have been developed in the field of health care information, which offer more systematic methods of searching.

- Department of Health site
  http://www.open.gov.uk/doh/dhhome.htm
- English National Board site http://www.enb.org.uk
- NHS Centre for Reviews and Dissemination
  http://nhscrd.york.ac.uk/welcome.html
- Nursing and Health Care Resources on the Net
  http://www.shef.ac.uk/~nhcon
- Nursing and Midwifery Links
  http://www.hsj.macmillan.com/102/links/section/
  nursingandmidwifery-f.html
- OMNI (Organising Medical Networked Information)
  http://omni.ac.uk
- Online Birth Center
  http://www.efn.org/~djz/birth/birthindex.html#topics
- Ovid http://gateway.ovid.com/
- Royal College of Nursing
  http://www.rcn.org.uk
- SOSIG (Social Sciences Information Gateway)
  http://sosig.ac.uk
- UK Cochrane Collaboration site
  http://www.cochrane.co.uk
- UKCC http://www.ukcc.org.uk/
- World Health Organization http://www.who.ch/

Evidence-based literature

Journals

- ACP Journal Club
  http://www.acponline.org/journals/acpj/jcmenu.htm
- Bandolier http://ww.jr2.ox.ac.uk/bandolier/
- BMJ http://www.bmj.com/
- Lancet
  http://www.thelancet.com

Evidence-based practice sites

- Centre for Reviews and Dissemination
  http://www.york.ac.uk
- IDEA (Internet database of evidence abstracts and articles)
  http://www.ohsu.edu/bicc-informatics/ebm/
  ebm_topics.htm
- Netting the evidence
  http://www.shef.ac.uk/uni/academic/R–Z/Scharr/
  ir/netting.html
- TRIP (Turning Research Into Practice)
  http://www.gwent.nhs.gov.uk/trip/

Guides to using nursing and medical libraries

There are many types of libraries which you may be able to use: college, hospital, university and public libraries as well as special libraries run by health information units and those belonging to professional associations. The following guides will help you to identify these:

- Dale P 1995 Guide to libraries and information sources in medicine and health care. London, British Library.
- Library Association 1994 Directory of Medical and Health Care Libraries in the United Kingdom and Republic of Ireland. London, Library Association.

If you have difficulty getting hold of any literature locally you should be able to request items from the British Library, which provides a document supply and loan service, through your local library service.

The address is: British Library, Document Supply Centre, Boston Spa, Wetherby, West Yorkshire, LS23 7BQ

List of key professional associations

Association of Radical Midwives, 62 Greetby Hill, Ormskirk, Lancashire, L39 2DT
Tel: 01695 572776

Publications: Midwifery Matters, quarterly

Association of Supervisors of Midwives, c/o Maternity Unit, James Paget Hospital, Lowestoft Road, Gorleston, Great Yarmouth, NR31 6LA
Tel: 01493 600611 ext 269; fax: 01493 452819

Publications: Annual report

Midwives Information and Resource Services (MIDIRS), 9 Elmdale Road, Clifton, Bristol, BS8 1SL
Tel: 0800 581009; e-mail: midirs@dial.pipex.com;
Web site: http://www.gn.apc.org/midirs

MIRIAD
Mother and Infant Research Unit, University of Leeds, 22 Hyde Terrace, Leeds, LS2 9LN
Tel: (0113)233 6886; fax: (0113)233 6872
Royal College of Midwives, 15 Mansfield Street, London, W1M 0BE
Tel: (0171)872 5100; fax: (0171)872 5101

Royal College of Nursing, 20 Cavendish Square, London, W1M 0AB
Tel: (0171)409 3333; fax: (0171)491 3859

Royal College of Obstetricians and Gynaecologists, 27 Sussex Place, Regents Park, London, NW1 4RG
Tel: (0171)262 5424; fax: (0171)723 0575

REFERENCES

Anagnostelis B, Cooke A 1997 Evaluation criteria for different versions of the same database—a comparison of Medline services available via the World Wide Web. Internet WWW page at: ⟨http://omni.ac.uk/agec/iolim97/⟩. (accessed 20.3.98, created 13.3.98)

DoH (Department of Health) 1993 Changing childbirth part 1: report of the Expert Maternity Group. HMSO, London

Dickersin K, Sherer R, Lefebvre C 1994 Identifying relevant studies for systemic reviews. British Medical Journal: 309:1286–1287

Glanville J, Haines M, Auston I 1998 Getting research findings into practice: finding information on clinical effectiveness. British Medical Journal 317:200–203

Lefebvre C 1994 The Cochrane Collaboration: the role of the UK Cochrane Centre in identifying the evidence. Health Libraries Review 11:235–242

Sackett D L, Scott Richardson W, Rosenberg W, Hayes R B 1997 Evidence based medicine: how to practice and teach evidence based medicine. Churchill Livingstone, New York, Introduction, pp. 2, 5

Sindhu F 1997 Literature searching for systematic reviews. Nursing Standard 11(41):40–42

McKinnel I, Elliott J 1997 Stroke Unit Trialists' Collaboration. Specialist multidisciplinary team (stroke) care for stroke inpatients. In: Warlow C, Van Gijn J, Sandercock P, Candelise L, Langhorne P (eds) Stroke module of the Cochrane database of systematic reviews (updated 01 December 1997). Available in the Cochrane Library (database on disk and CDROM). The Cochrane collaboration 1998 Issue 1. Update Software, Oxford

PUBLISHED INFORMATION SOURCES

ASLIB (Association of Special Libraries and Information Bureaux) index to theses for higher degrees by the Universities of Great Britain and Ireland and the Council for National Academic Awards. ASLIB, London

Ayres J 1987 Midwifery index vol 1 (1976–1986). Royal College of Midwives, London

Ayres J 1992 Midwifery index vol 2 (1987–1991). Royal College of Midwives, London

British nursing index. BNI Publications, Poole

Cumulative index to nursing and allied health literature (CINAHL): including list of subject headings. Seventh-day Adventist Hospital Association, Glendale

Current research in Britain 1995 (10th edn) Social Sciences, Cartermill, London

International nursing index. Lippincott, Williams & Wilkins, Hagerstown

McCormick F, Renfrew M J 1996 The midwifery research database, MIRIAD: a sourcebook of information about research in midwifery, 2nd edn. Books for Midwives Press, Hale

MIDIRS midwifery digest. Midwives Information and Resource Service, London

NMI index of journal articles of interest to nurses, midwives and community staff. College Library Network, Poole

RCN (Royal College of Nursing) 1996 Steinberg collection of nursing research: catalogue. Royal College of Nursing, London

Simms C, McHaffie H, Renfrew M J, Ashurst H 1997 The midwifery research database MIRIAD: a sourcebook of information about research in midwifery. Books for Midwives, Hale

ELECTRONIC INFORMATION SOURCES

Applied social sciences index and abstracts. ASSIA, Bowker Saur, London

Best evidence: linking medical research to practice. American College of Physicians, Philadelphia

Cumulative index to nursing and allied health literature (CINAHL). Ovid Technologies, New York

Database of abstracts of reviews of effectiveness (DARE) http://nhscrd.york.ac.uk/cgi-bin/v1.engine?*ID= 0&*DB=ABRE

Internet database of evidence abstracts and articles (IDEA) http://www.ohsu.edu/bicc-informatics/ebm/ ebm_topics.htm

Medline/CD plus. CD Plus, New York

The Cochrane Library. BMJ Publishing Group, London

The National research register—prototype 1997. NHS Executive Headquarters, Research and Development Division, Leeds

Psychological abstracts. American Psychological Association, Washington

Turning research into practice (TRIP) http://www.gwent.nhs.gov.uk/trip/

2

Reflection and articulating intuition

Penny Church   Maureen D Raynor

This chapter aims to explore the notions of intuition and reflection. It seeks to explore how reflection can be used as a tool to develop intuitive knowledge in midwifery practice. Different dimensions of knowledge are used by experienced and skilful practitioners and this chapter seeks to identify them and provide useful ideas and examples to enable these dimensions to be developed and utilized effectively in midwifery practice.

INTRODUCTION

This chapter aims to explore the different dimensions of knowledge that are used by experienced and skilful practitioners and to provide useful ideas and examples to enable the process of reflection to occur and be effective in developing new learning for midwives.

In recent years, schools of midwifery have amalgamated and then merged with institutions of higher education, necessitating the need to develop and deepen the theoretical base from which midwifery is practised. Midwifery curricula are now designed to enable midwifery students to study to diploma or degree levels, or both. The move into higher education and increased academic requirements have highlighted the need for research and evidence-based practice. However, the drive towards academic excellence has become a source of anxiety for both educationalists and practitioners who worry that experience and expertise in practice will become undervalued and eventually would not be recognized as a valid type of knowledge in relation to academic credits in the future. There is the danger that the balance between theoretical knowledge and practice knowledge will be lost, depending on the view that the midwife has of academia: 'Midwifery is an art as well as a science, an art which is in danger of being lost as we seek constantly to predict the unpredictable and quantify the unquantifiable' (Muirhead, cited by Duff 1997). Practice will inevitably involve elements that cannot be researched to provide empirical knowledge. These areas of practice rely on experiential knowledge and a type of knowing that is often labelled as 'instinct' or 'intuition', but because there is no easy way of articulating this dimension of knowing it may be denied altogether. This chapter is an attempt to explore these particular dimensions of knowledge, because although they are not categorized as rational or evidence based, they are valid and form important constituents of competent and responsive midwifery care. However, it is not the intention to undervalue rational or evidence-based practice. All dimensions of knowledge are needed.

There is a growing body of evidence that supports the idea that, through reflection, these other dimensions of knowledge can begin to emerge and take shape. If this is the case, then attention needs to be given by educationalists, students and practitioners to develop the ability to use reflection as a learning tool to enhance and inform midwifery practice. Unfortunately, not all the dimensions of professional knowledge are easy to articulate within the traditional boundaries of 'academic' writing. This is because the use of the first person is needed to create an authentic flow in relation to experience, whereas academic tradition often requires the author to write in the third person (Webb 1992). The first person has been used liberally throughout this chapter when experiences are related in order to demonstrate how it enhances the flow in these instances.

TYPES OF KNOWLEDGE AND WAYS OF KNOWING

It has been recognized that professionals use at least two ways of knowing (Ayer 1956, Benner 1984, Eraut 1985, Jarvis 1986, Ryle 1949):

- knowing that (propositional knowledge, technical knowledge)
- knowing how (skills, practical knowledge).

Knowing that

'Knowing that' is rational and empirical and uses mainly cognitive processes; it can be articulated, demonstrated and therefore tested. This way of knowing lends itself to scholarly scrutiny and has a feel of objectivity about it. It is to do with data that either stem from research or are considered to be true, such as mathematical knowledge, which accepts that two + two = four. This type of knowing is thought to be based upon rational and logical process and is thus highly valued in Western society, which puts rationality and research above all other processes. Rational thinking and logic are considered to be objective. However, the apparent objectivity of this type of knowing may only be an illusion because the very nature of research is not totally objective (Jarvis 1984). Burnard (1989) goes as far as to say that most researchers depend to a degree on 'serendipity' or chance findings rather than on carefully planned objective knowing. There is a certain irony in this because new knowledge is generated by a process that has only a veneer of objectivity. Therefore, research must be read and interpreted intelligently.

Midwifery knowledge is dynamic and change has been brought about through the instincts of midwifery practitioners who have had the courage to explore their instincts through the research process. For example, in the early 1980s I was taught that it was better to prevent a tear happening by doing an episiotomy. This was because a tear is jagged and does not heal as well as a clean cut. This sounded logical and objective. Inherent in this belief was the idea that if a woman sustained a tear then the midwife was guilty of bad practice. In addition, I was taught that a timely episiotomy prevented the overstretching of maternal soft tissues and consequently prevented the pelvic floor muscles being weakened. The logic was that stress incontinence would be prevented by timely episiotomy. These two beliefs led to a policy of liberal episiotomy, despite many midwives sensing that this was not in the interests of womankind, until research findings proved otherwise (Sleep et al 1984, Sleep & Grant 1987). This example demonstrates how one set of objective beliefs are replaced by another through the process of exploring an instinct.

Knowing how

'Knowing how' is a more practical kind of knowledge, and essential for professional practice, but often difficult to articulate and therefore more difficult to apply objective, scholastic scrutiny. This means that this way of knowing is sometimes undervalued in the wake of striving for scientific certainties to underpin midwifery practice. Nevertheless, professional practice relies heavily on knowing how. Schön (1991) asserts that there is a hierarchy of knowledge and states that 'professional' knowledge is lower down the ranking than 'academic' knowledge. The resulting consequence is that there is the danger that some academic institutions do not pay attention to all that adds to professional knowledge and artistry. When terms such as 'art' or 'intuition' are broached, academic discussion often tends to close rather than open up. Intuition, in particular, is given a 'bad press' because it cannot easily be accounted for, is not scientific and so it is left alone by researchers (Burnard 1989).

In recent years, without losing sight of the importance that artistry plays in actual midwifery practice, midwifery education has been striving for recognition and credibility from higher education. Nevertheless, in the move towards higher education, there is the potential to foster a view of knowledge which pays selective inattention to all but the empirical dimension. The problem is, practitioners are often unable to express how their professional artistry works. This means it can be, and often is, construed as irrational and not evidence based, and this creates an uncomfortable dissonance for the practitioner. This dissonance is very real and is exacerbated by the pressure to be able to demonstrate constantly that their practice is sound and based on research type evidence. This is despite the collective sense amongst midwives that there is more to midwifery practice than the two dimensions of knowing already cited. For example, I may know the facts about how to perform an abdominal palpation, and have the skills, but if I am only using these two dimensions the artistry is missing—the fluency is not there. We can teach the theory of midwifery and demonstrate the skills but other dimensions are very difficult to articulate let alone teach. The difficulty in articulation arises because we really do not know what it is that comprises these other dimensions out of which professional 'flair' flows.

Carper's four patterns of knowing

Carper's four patterns of knowing can help identify some of the artistry in midwifery knowledge (Carper 1978). She states that science and skills are only a part of nursing knowledge, and this can be equally applied to midwifery. However, the two dimensions of 'that' and 'how' can still be identified within the four patterns (see Box 2.1). All four patterns need to be utilized in order to appreciate the whole or as she puts it 'the gestalt' of a situation.

Carper (1978) suggests that, by understanding these four fundamental patterns of knowing, there is the possibility of an increased awareness

---

Box 2.1   Carper's four patterns of knowing

1. Empirics or scientific knowledge
2. Aesthetics or the art of practice which is expressed and made visible through action rather than in written or published form
3. Personal knowledge
4. Ethics—the knowledge of morality.

of the complexity and diversity of nursing/midwifery knowledge. All are necessary and they are not mutually exclusive. The missing dimension which creates 'flair' could be implicit in Carper's 'personal knowledge'. Carper states that personal knowledge is difficult to master and teach but, ironically, it is possibly the most essential way of knowing for the practitioner. She describes it as a 'knowledge of the self'. Practitioners cannot acknowledge the uniqueness of each individual unless they know their own uniqueness. If the practitioner has this knowledge then interactions with clients will become authentic and reciprocal rather than the professional having authority over the client. This kind of knowledge cannot be described or even experienced. It can only be actualized (Carper 1978, Rose & Parker 1994).

Polanyi's tacit knowing

Polanyi (1966) describes a dimension of knowing that is very akin to Carper's 'personal knowledge' which he calls 'the tacit dimension'. He states that tacit knowledge cannot be fully described—'we know more than we can tell' (p. 4). To support this notion he makes the point that we know a face but we cannot tell how. Police often have a problem because witnesses to crimes cannot describe the perpetrator although they often say they would recognize them again. Photofits provide the police with a very useful tool to enable witnesses to articulate a description which they couldn't do before. In tacit knowing, Polanyi draws on gestalt psychology; a gestalt is a kind of completeness—a whole. In the context of knowing he describes a gestalt as: 'An active shaping of experience in the pursuit of knowledge' (Polanyi 1966 p. 6).

For Polanyi, therefore, tacit knowledge is deeply embedded in experience. This means that experience is an important teacher. How we shape that experience and internalize it, is an active process. The supposition is that experience is cast into a logic of its own—a logic of tacit thought—a tacit power of scientific and artistic genius. A gestalt, suggests Polanyi, forms a bridge to the higher creative powers of man

and draws together theory and practice in such a way that true confluence occurs.

Reflecting on the way skills develop helps the understanding of what Polanyi was trying to say. When learning a new skill, initially we are aware of its several muscular movements and it is to these movements that our attention is directed. When we become skilled, we are able to attend from the elementary movements to the achievement of the whole process of the skills. This may not occur for some time, depending on the complexity of the skill. Three good examples to illustrate this are: doing a vaginal examination, an abdominal palpation or driving a car. These are all skills that involve both 'knowing that' and 'knowing how'. Most would agree that they learnt to be skilled drivers or midwives once they had passed their assessments and when they had been left to make their own decisions. This is interesting because both the driving test and midwifery assessments measure the candidate's ability to practise their skills competently. What is it that they feel they have to learn in order to become fluent and expert in the skills? Benner (1984) suggests that expert practitioners differ from novices in as much as they are able to see the whole of a situation. The knowledge that is embedded in expertise develops when the clinician tests and refines propositions, hypotheses and principle-based expectations into the actual clinical situations. Benner draws on Heidegger's notion of experience. Heidegger implied that experience comes as a result of challenging and refining preconceived notions (Heidegger 1962). Such notions may be proven or disproved in the practice situation. Experience is therefore considered to be a prerequisite for expertise (Benner 1984).

Unfortunately, even with this understanding, it is still difficult to articulate exactly what is happening in the experiences that will shape the expertise and artistry of the practitioner which enables the utilization of tacit knowledge and an appreciation of the gestalt of a situation. This is probably because of, as Polanyi (1966) suggests, the subliminal processes at work, which affect tacit knowledge quite profoundly. The very nature of subliminal influences means that we are usually unaware of them. Polanyi, however, suggests that we can become more aware of them by silencing the conscious processes. Reflection can be a good way to achieve this, enabling us to tune in to our subliminal influences.

Tacit knowing is seen by many to be the very antithesis of science, which claims to produce objective knowledge. The aim of science is to eliminate any elements of personal knowledge. However, the whole basis of research relies upon asking the right questions. Plato, in the Meno, observes that to search for a solution to a problem is absurd for, 'either you know what you are looking for and then there is no problem; or you do not know what you are looking for, and then you cannot expect to find anything' (quoted in Polanyi 1966 p. 22).

Therefore, if all knowledge is explicit, and is capable of being clearly articulated, then we cannot know a problem or look for its answer. This paradox points to the existence of tacit knowledge. The paradox makes sense if we can admit that we can have tacit foreknowledge of yet undiscovered things, which may emerge from 'hunches' or 'felt senses'. This implies that there is something bodily about tacit knowing. Midwives talk about 'gut feelings' or feelings that are identified in other parts of the body and, furthermore, this feeling speaks to them with an authority that is akin to empirical data. They will state quite forcefully that something is wrong. If this knowing is challenged, usually the midwife will find it difficult to articulate why this should be the case. Does she *know* or does she just *believe* she knows? How does this happen? Is it intuition or a rapid processing of past experience and traditional knowledge? Could it be to do with the subliminal knowing of the normal which produces a kind of felt sense of something that does not quite fit, a feeling that there is something missing but we cannot quite put our finger on it? I can understand that it could be a rapid processing of experiences arising from tacit knowing if both the midwife and the woman are in some kind of connected proximity. However, this phenomenon also occurs when a midwife just knows that she has to go and visit someone because there is

something wrong and when she arrives the woman has been in some sort of dire circumstances? What type of knowing is this? There is something mysterious about these occurrences. Similarly, in the diagnosis of some problems the tacit dimension is combined with observable facts (Polanyi 1966).

Eraut (1985) proposes that it is important not only to think about the source of knowledge but to also consider the mode and context of use. He draws on the work of Broudy, Smith & Burnett (1964) who developed a typology to describe how knowledge acquired during schooling was used in later life. They suggest that knowledge is used in the following ways:

replication   application   interpretation association.

Replication dominates a large proportion of schooling and a significant part of higher education and is characterized by little processing or reorganization of knowledge by the user. Application occurs when the knowledge is used in different contexts to the one originally taught. Replication and application are in some way confined to technical or vocational education when a distinction is made between these and professional education. Professional education requires more. Professionals need to be able to understand and interpret situations as they occur and then make judgements. This requires an interpretive and associative application of knowledge. Therefore the interpretive use of knowledge plays some part in professional judgement to which Eraut (1985) attributes a quality of mysteriousness. However, in this context, judgement is not the same as understanding:

the brilliant political scientist or commentator does not often make a successful politician. Judgement involves practical wisdom, a sense of purpose, appropriateness and feasibility; its acquisition depends, among other things, on a wealth of professional experience. But this experience is not used in a replicative applicative mode, nor is it fully interpreted, for much practical experience accumulates with only limited time for reflection. On the one hand, we expect the wise judge to have had a sufficient range of experience to ensure a balanced perspective, to prevent over interpretation from the experience of one or two previous cases of an apparently similar nature. While on the other we expect *intuitive capacity* to digest and distil previous experience and to select from it those ideas or procedures that seem fitting and appropriate.

(Eraut 1985 p. 125)

Defining intuitive knowing

It would seem reasonable to assume that tacit knowledge *equals* intuition but there is something about intuition that is *more than* tacit knowing. Although personal and tacit knowing fit very comfortably into the notion of intuition, they probably are not an exact match. McCormack (1992) suggests that although tacit knowledge is the most closely related concept it is, however, not intuition. He identified that there are two systems functioning in tacit knowledge. First there is the part that involves perceptions of particulars and secondly there is the part that involves intuition and imagination. In fact there are many terms that may be used as surrogate terms for intuition:

- perception
- representation
- receptivity
- understanding
- will
- consciousness
- gut feeling
- sixth sense
- instinct
- reason
- feeling
- innate knowledge
- women's feelings
- cognition inference
- precognition.

All the terms listed, although associated with intuition, do not reflect the nature of the concept totally and can actually be confused with intuition. Intuition, like tacit knowledge, is a very subjective form of knowing because it often arises from deep within the person. Belesky et al (1986 p. 69) suggest that an intuitive reaction is something—'experienced, not thought out, something felt rather than actively pursued or

construed'. This was written in the context of their study of the way women know and articulate their knowledge. Throughout their work they identify a very subjective approach to knowledge, as illustrated by the following quotation from one of the women in the study:

If I read something, and if it agrees with my senses, then I believe it, I know it. If it doesn't, I'll say 'well you may be right but I can't corroborate that'. For me, proof is usually a sensory one. If you say 'water falls', yeah I believe it because I've seen it happen. If you call it gravity, then I say 'Oh, is that what you call it?' One doesn't have to be told in words. That's the point. That's the thing that's very hard for people to believe—that there are other ways of telling.   (p. 75)

If Belesky et al are right, this has implications for midwifery, because there is a predominance of women in the profession. However, it is a generalization to say that women work intuitively and that men do not, but their study does strongly indicate that there is more to knowledge than is totally rational.

Intuition is extremely hard to define scientifically. The next few paragraphs describe some of the ideas and definitions that appear in the literature. It is difficult to know where to start so I have chosen to begin with Schön (1987 p. 5) who touches on the existence of intuition when he states that, in practice, most situations are not textbook examples. In practice, the professional has to deal with these situations competently and therefore needs to improvise—to respond to a 'kind of intuitive understanding', which cannot be taught but has to develop. For example, 'we know how to teach people how to build ships but not to figure out what ships to build' (Schön 1987 p. 11). In midwifery we can teach what pain relief is available in labour and how to use it but they have to figure out the appropriate care, and the best timing, for their individual client. This requires that the midwife tap into a kind of intuitive understanding of this client's particular needs in the present situation.

An American definition quoted by Davis-Floyd & Davis (1996) says intuition is: 'the act or faculty of knowing or sensing without the use or rational processes; immediate cognition'. An older English dictionary defines intuition as

'Immediate perception by the mind without reasoning; instinctive knowledge; a truth so perceived' (New English dictionary 1932). This is interesting because both definitions accept that intuition is in fact a legitimate way of knowing and yet reason and rational processes are bypassed. Westcott (1968) highlights the variety of conceptions of intuition, which he suggests stem from a serious concern about the phenomena amongst scholars. Intuition may be the pinnacle of knowing *or* the perpetration of nonsense. He provides a useful summary of philosophical views about the notion of intuition.

Classical philosophers, for example Bergson and Spinoza (according to Westcott 1968), hold that intuition is about prime reality and is a mystical form of knowledge. It is knowledge which arises without the use of prior knowledge and without the use of reason. It is *a priori*, that is, it is foundational and therefore we can trust it. Intuited knowledge, therefore, is not knowledge of facts but knowledge of experience and is in a realm different from facts. Croce (in Westcott 1968) sees intuition as expression. There is implicit in the above three theorists, who are classical intuitionists, the notion that intuition is independent of, and opposed to, reason and intellect. Therefore the truth reached by intuition can never be reached by reason. If this is true, it means that reason can never verify, refute, describe or explain it. This way of looking at intuition places it in a different realm to Carper's (1978) personal knowledge and Benner's (1984) expert practitioner who she says will follow up their hunches but will search to verify those hunches.

However, positivist and analytical philosophers are more cautious about intuition, although essentially congenial to the notion. Their intentions were to explore the limits of its usefulness and to find a stable place for the concept in a theory of knowledge. According to Westcott, Stocks in 1939 reasserted the importance of reason but states that reason is critically dependent on intuition. Likewise, intuition is critically dependent on reason 'for it is reason which can bring an individual to the point of making intuitive judgements' (Westcott 1968 p. 17). For Stocks, intuition

of self-evident truth is direct. It is the immediate apprehension by the mind in just the way that an object presents to the sense organs is immediately and directly apprehended without mediated reasoning and without hesitation. Ewing in 1941, according to Westcott (1968), had similar ideas and felt that intuition is the immediate knowing of truth without proof and without the possibility of proof, but reason can be utilized to support intuition. Often the connections from premise to conclusions are in fact intuited connections—that is, 'Inference and intuition are linked together. Inference always presupposes intuition to provide the links in the inference, but on the other hand inference is needed to support, prepare for and develop intuition' (Westcott 1968 p. 17). Therefore, for Ewing, false intuitions can be dispelled by reason. Bahm (1960 cited by Westcott 1968) agreed that intuition is immediate apprehension and takes the position that intuition should be viewed as the truth unless other forms of evidence convince us otherwise. Also that, whatever conclusions we come to, on whatever basis, there must be an element of intuition. Both the above schools of philosophers affirm the importance and value of intuitive knowledge. However, there are equally eminent thinkers who oppose the value of intuitive knowledge. An example is Bunge (1962 cited in Westcott 1968 p. 20) who took a neopositivist viewpoint and was quite scathing about intuitionism, which he stated to be 'in the best of cases sterile … and at its worst a dangerous variety of dogmatism.'

Jung in 1923 (cited Westcott 1968), however, placed intuition into the theory of personality rather than the theory of knowledge. Intuition is a cognitive event and must be accounted for. It is not occult and not reducible to more basic activities of mind and it is one of the four mental functions constitutionally present in all people, the other three being thinking, feeling and sensation. This means that we are all capable of being intuitive to some degree or other and that intuition can be developed and used. Jung defines intuition as:

the process of perceiving immediately and unconsciously, the possibilities and potentialities of the objects which are the focus of its attention, whether external or internal. This process occurs at the expense of perceiving the details and the perceptions gained are then as truths...Intuition is a way of knowing, immediate and uncritical.

(Westcott 1968 p. 36)

The intuitive person, therefore, has a knowledge without knowing how or why they know. They just know. The function of intuition, according to Jung, within the personality, is to be non-judgemental. Intuition perceives objects as totalities at the expense of details. These perceptions are taken as truths, just as sensory details are taken as truths. Intuition is in juxtaposition to thinking. Thinking involves judgement of true or false; logical deducing; drawing inferences and is cognisant of objective fact. The function of feeling involves judgements of pleasant or unpleasant; acceptance or rejection; like and dislike. Sensation receives sensory details from the internal or external world of the person. Sensing perceives sensory details as accepted facts and makes no judgements. These four mental functions, according to Jung, encompass all the possibilities of psychological commerce and need to be balanced. In relation to knowledge, Jung describes four levels of consciousness: personal consciousness (the aware self), personal unconsciousness (subliminal), collective consciousness and collective unconsciousness. The collective consciousness appears to me to be very akin to descriptions I have heard of both intuition and instinct. Within collective consciousness are systems of symbolism, 'the knowings', typically human reactions, typically human understanding about universal hunch situations. These knowings, according to Jung, are the archetypes and they are reborn in the brain structure of each individual.

Having explored previous thinkers ideas about intuition, Westcott (1968 p. 41) offers his composite definition: 'Intuition may be described as the process of reaching a conclusion on the basis of little information which is normally reached on the basis of significantly more information.' He also states that it is interesting that for an intuitive conclusion to be classified as such requires that the thinker does not know how they reached their conclusion. Furthermore,

the conclusion does not need to be novel or unusual.

Smith (1992 cited in Rose & Parker 1994) argues that knowing is holistic and integrates threads from a variety of sources including the sciences, arts, humanities, life experiences, perceptions and reflections. The threads are drawn together by the individual and the resulting knowledge, therefore, is a reflection of the individual's personal beliefs and values. It could be that intuition is the entity that draws the threads together a bit like connective tissue holds the body together—a catalyst that brings together all the dimensions of professional knowledge and shapes the decisions made about care to fit the here and now situation. Schön suggested that this shaping will involve applied science and research-based techniques, which occupy a critically important, though limited, territory bounded on several sides by artistry. These are: an art of problem framing, an art of improvization and an art of implementation—all are necessary to mediate the use in practice of applied science and technique (Schön 1987 p. 13). In order to make sense of what Schön has written I picture the boundaries around scientific knowledge to be very solid but the boundaries around artistry to be cloud like and not so clear. Wisdom and talent are in the picture also and somehow all the facets are linked together by intuition. Intuition appears to be so moulded into the picture that of itself it has no form or structure. Because it is so *moulded in*, it is nigh on impossible to give it form or structure in words.

The importance of intuition in practice

Burnard (1989) suggests that intuition is a very important and valid way of knowing and although it will not stand on its own as a method of developing nursing and midwifery skills it needs to be acknowledged and listened to. Intuition is a very important part of human nature and therefore it can make the difference between skilled practice and skilled *human* practice. Intuition can be a vehicle to empathy and therefore is allied to the part of us that makes it possible to reach out to another person and truly care. This places intuition amongst the most fundamental ways of knowing in professional practice. It is knowledge beyond the senses and Burnard (1989) articulates it as a 'sixth sense'. Few would deny that some very important decisions both inside and outside of midwifery have been made intuitively. Some of them have been life saving. I recall in my midwifery practice a woman whom I had seen earlier that afternoon, ringing me and describing what did not sound serious. She was 37 weeks' gestation and this was her second pregnancy. What she said to me was that she had slight abdominal pain that did not feel like contractions. I didn't ask her many more questions, but I asked her to come in to labour ward where I arranged to meet her. Before she arrived I knew that something serious was happening and so did not change into uniform or even ask her to change out of her outdoor clothes before examining her. Neither did I go through the usual abdominal examination before listening to the fetal heart. I sensed that something was seriously wrong with the fetus and sure enough the fetal heart was 80 beats per minute and I quickly organized help. Her membranes then ruptured spontaneously and there was true blood-stained liquor. She was taken to theatre for an emergency caesarian section and the baby was delivered within 15 minutes of her admission, alive and in need of resuscitation but responding well. I have reflected many times on this experience and asked myself 'how did I know?' I am unable to articulate how I knew very precisely but I believe that I was drawing on at least three things: my experience of her (I knew her and had seen her regularly antenatally), my knowledge and experience of midwifery and an inner sense. All of these elements were linked into an intuitive decision. There was part of me at the time that felt irrational but the decision turned out to be life saving. There are many such stories which could be related by midwives. Unfortunately it is difficult to incorporate such skills into academic qualifications. 'You can't get a doctorate for knowing in your bones that something isn't quite right' (Flint 1995 p. 63). This is because the knowledge and skills used by midwives are often indefinable and instinctive.

In this example I had formed a relationship with the mother I was caring for and some kind of connection that allowed me to be in tune to what was happening. McCormack (1993) in his work with students noticed that, although students were not able verbally to articulate fully the concept of intuition, they did recognize that when they thought intuitively it was usually with patients that they had come to know very well. Davis-Floyd & Davis (1996) also identify the importance of knowing the client well and found that connection was an important precursor to intuition. Connection, was not only physical, but also emotional, intellectual and psychic for the midwives in their study. The connection was not only two way but more complex and involved a connection between midwife, mother, child and father in a kind of a web made up of many strands.

Benner (1984) also makes a link between familiarity and intuition and after Dreyfus and Dreyfus (1981 unpublished study cited in Benner 1984) suggests that experts are more intuitive than novices. She argues that expert practitioners learn to recognize subtle physiological changes before documental changes in vital signs are apparent. These finely tuned abilities, she suggests, come from many hours of direct observation and care. Examples of this may include knowing that a client is about to go into shock before there is evidence of bleeding. Is this intuition? Benner uses Polanyi's (1958 in Benner 1984) notion of conoisseurship to describe the perceptual recognitional ability of the expert clinician. This notion appears to be in line with Schön's ideas in relation to the reflective practitioner (Schön 1983). Case study 2.1 is a good example of an intuitive decision which could be said to have resulted from such conoisseurship. The story was told to me by a consultant obstetrician who would meet the requirements by anybody's standards to be recognized as an expert practitioner.

In contrast, Case study 2.2 is more difficult to explain.

Case study 2.1

He was looking after a woman with pre-eclampsia who had been hospitalized for rest and close monitoring of her and her baby's condition. All the scientific parameters indicated that both the mother and the baby were progressing as normally as possible. On one particular morning, the consultant had a very strong gut feeling that he should deliver the baby urgently—despite no change in any of the parameters being monitored. This gut feeling was so strong that he could not ignore it and the baby was delivered by an emergency caesarian section with an extremely low apgar score. There was no doubt in his mind that had he ignored that gut feeling the baby would have died in utero.

Although intuition as a concept is highly debated in the literature, there is agreement that it does exist and that it forms part of professional knowing. There has been research to try and define its attributes more clearly. For example, McCormack (1992) in his concept analysis identified four defining attributes of intuition:

- immediate, unjustified true belief which is not preceded by inference
- non-propositional knowledge which is holistic in nature, i.e. focuses on the whole rather than its parts
- immediate knowledge of a concept which is independent of the linear reasoning process
- represents synthesis rather than analysis.

Benner (1984) demonstrated that as nurses' level of expertise increased so did the use of intuition in their judgements. Experience is an important prerequisite for expertise. However, years of experience did not correlate with level of expertise in all instances (King & Appleton 1997). For example, a midwife may have 20 years of exposure to practice situations and not be 'experienced' in the sense that she has not reflected, challenged or redefined her propositions, hypotheses or principle-based expectations. In this instance the midwife is unlikely to become an 'expert practitioner' but may still be making intuitive judgements. There is evidence that the use of intuition is not confined to the

 Case study 2.2

A relatively newly qualified midwife on night duty, on a busy shift, received a very rapid report about the clients on the ward. The midwife had not met any of the women and asked for clarification about anything that might be a problem. She was told about a client who had suffered a primary postpartum haemorrhage on labour ward but there had been no recurrence since she had been on the ward. There was an infusion with syntocinon in place. The midwife decided that she would see this particular woman first. On examination, all the woman's physical observations were normal and her uterus was well contracted. There was no sign of abnormal lochia. The midwife, who was satisfied at this point that her client was in no danger of further haemorrhage, left the room and was half way down the corridor back to the office when she sensed that she *must go back* to this woman, so she did. When she arrived in the room, to use the midwife's own words, 'there was blood everywhere!' The woman was on the point of collapse but with the appropriate treatment, which was instigated immediately, she recovered. The midwife does not know, to this day, what made her know she had to go back but her decision to do so probably saved that client's life.

In this instance it was not a midwife who had years of experience in midwifery; however, she had been trained as a nurse and it is possible that she drew on that experience.

'expert' only. Orme & Maggs, (1993) and McCormack (1993) found that students and newly qualified nurses were also voicing intuitive concerns.

Some researchers question, however, whether intuitive knowing has any validity or authority. Davis-Floyd & Davis (1996) tried to answer this question in their research. They make the point that it is well established that there is no creativity in science, indeed, in any domain of creative activity, that does not entail intuition. Neurophysiological research has suggested that the two cerebral hemispheres are complementary in their functions. The left hemisphere is primarily associated with language production, analytical thought, and lineal and causal sequencing of events, whereas the right hemisphere mediates the production of images, gestalt or holistic thought and spatiotemporal patterning. This is probably an oversimplification of the way the brain organizes its functions and it is important to remember that the *whole* brain is involved in *all* brain functions. There is evidence that sharp functional division between the two hemispheres occurs only in people whose brains were physically split or damaged either by injury or by surgery. In the normal healthy brain, similarity and replication of function are much more common. Laughlin (1997, quoted by Davis-Floyd & Davis 1996) suggests that intuition is mediated by both lobes and that the neurocognitive processes that produce intuition are *transcendental*, that is they use both hemispheres. Laughlin's work may explain why women are often viewed as being more intuitive because the corpus callosum in the female brain is significantly larger. It can be argued, as stated by Davis-Floyd & Davis, that this part of the brain can be deliberately developed in either sex. This counteracts the general Western view of intuition which leads, as Burnard (1989) argues, to a double-edged form of sexism. 'Women's intuition' implies that women are more intuitive than men. There is the danger in our thinking that may lead to the belief that men are not intuitive and that they should not be; men should be rational.

Unfortunately in our society there is a tacit suggestion that rationality is somehow better than irrationality. This may lead to both men and women ignoring their intuition in a bid to develop their rationality. We ignore intuition at our peril. What we need to be doing is recognizing the importance and validity of intuitive decision making. It is proposed by Davis-Floyd & Davis (1996) that midwives make decisions based on a synthesis of clinical observations, theoretical knowledge, intuitive assessment and spiritual awareness. All of these components are at work to bring about competent decision making. Implicit in their proposal is the belief that intuition is valid and authoritative knowledge. However, there is a general lack of recognition of the legitimacy of intuition, regardless of its continued use by large numbers of nurses and midwives in a variety of care settings. Research evidence indicates that many feel that they should not be using intuition (Appleton 1993,

Benner & Tanner 1987, King & Appleton 1997, Orme & Maggs 1993, Pyles & Stern 1983, Schraeder & Fischer 1987). Even if intuition is devalued, it appears that practitioners will continue to use their 'gut feelings' covertly. There is a need to recognize that intuition occurs in response to knowledge, is a trigger for action or reflection, or both, and consequently has a direct bearing on the analytical processes in care (King & Appleton 1997).

However, Walsh (1997) presents a valid point in regard to professional accountability and the use of intuition. He argues that evidence-based practice, and not intuition, must be the justification in law for professional action. He claims that phenomenological perspectives, which espouse the notion that truth and knowledge are embedded in individual experience rather than any objective reality, create a subjective view of knowledge. Knowledge and meaning are embedded in the situation and are, therefore, unique to each individual practitioner. This raises the question as to which practitioner's personal theory is correct. According to Benner (1984), the consequences of this view of knowledge is the idea that there is no higher court than the expert's professional judgement. This is problematic in relation to civil law and the rules of professional practice. In civil law, judgement in negligence cases relies on the Bolam test, a precedent set through the case of *Bolam v. Friern* (1957). In that case, the judge ruled that the doctor had not been negligent because he had acted in accordance with the current, accepted practice. The accepted practice is verified by a responsible body of skilled practitioners (see Ch. 5 for further details about litigation). Walsh makes the point that it is likely that a court would require evidence to justify the practice that is brought into question. This puts intuitive decisions onto a very sticky wicket. However, if it is true that intuition is trustworthy, it is unlikely that such decisions would reach the courts of the land.

Experience and intuition

Experience is an important feature of intuitive expert practice, and many consider it to be essential. Berne (1949 in Westcott 1968 p. 38) described intuition as 'knowledge based on experience and acquired through sensory contacts without the intuiter being able to formulate to himself or others exactly how he came to his conclusion'. However, there are a few researchers who do not emphasize its importance. Instead they see intuition as preceding knowledge in order that sense can be made of experience. Experience without intuition, therefore, would consist of events which lack direction or meaning. This view, however, according to Easen & Wilcockson (1996), is in direct contrast to other researchers in this field. They come to the conclusion that there are several elements that combine to create intuition. Of primary importance is a sound knowledge base and the ability to recognize patterns in a presenting problem. Such pattern recognition, they suggest, is rooted in past decision-making and experience is essential for this linking of similar past events. But where is our locus of experiencing? Gendlin (1962) states that experience arises out of the body and all words and sentences have a 'felt' meaning located somewhere in the body. He suggests that it is this experiencing which creates meaning. Most stories that are told about intuitive decisions include the idea of 'gut' feeling, or 'a feeling in the water' or just a 'feeling'. These 'feelings' need to be listened to, but are they trustworthy? Gendlin would suggest that they are, likewise Rogers (1967, 1983). Rogers felt that one of his key learnings in life was that he could trust his experience and that as he gradually came to trust his *total* reactions more deeply that he could use them to guide his thinking and that they were more trustworthy than his intellect. Gendlin states that experience is an aspect of human living that is constant. We can trust it. Inherent in this way of thinking is the belief that the body has a wisdom of its own. Levin (1985) wrote that the authentic self cannot be realized without being in touch with the body's experience and wisdom. He seems to suggest that the body can teach the intellect and that we can integrate awareness by living well-focused in the body. Unfortunately we seem to have lost the ability to spend time in listening to the body's wisdom. Life moves at such a great pace and with the advent of the technological age, it has become very difficult to give ourselves space to reflect and tune in to what our bodies might be saying.

Gendlin (1962) asserts that the body can often guide us to move in the right direction. He uses the notion of 'hunches' to illustrate this idea. If a hunch tells us not to do something just what is it that is saying to us 'don't'? He suggests that it is not the words but an uneasy, queasy, unaccountable discomfort, a *bodily felt sense*. Instead of feeling good about the good things that are visible, you feel physically uncomfortable about the situation. (Gendlin 1993). He does recognize that some believe that things like hunches and intuition are still cognitive and in their heads rather than in their bodies but maybe we have to think differently about our bodies. If experience is of the body then the body can lead us forward but, as Rogers (1967) states, we need to learn to let the body guide. We need to be able to get in touch with our felt sense of a situation. Although the concept of intuition is difficult to grasp, it seems that Gendlin's notion of a felt sense (Gendlin 1981) is very close to it.

If the body does have a wisdom of its own, then it would be of great benefit for midwives to learn to listen to their bodily wisdom or felt senses. Reflection is a useful tool to enable this to happen. Freire (1972) made a strong connection between reflection and action and argued that bringing congruence between the two formed a kind of praxis (Jarvis 1992). (Praxis is a notion of confluence between theory and practice—the application as opposed to the theory.)

REFLECTION

The meaning of the old Anglo-Saxon word 'midwife' is 'with woman' and therefore the relationship between a midwife and a woman is very important. It has a tremendous impact upon the outcomes and effectiveness of care, as demonstrated by Flint & Poulengeris (1987). Intuition is important in midwifery, therefore, because it offers a way of perceiving another person's reality which gives scope for better interpersonal relationships to develop which enhances empathic understanding of others. However, intuition needs to be in equilibrium with other ways of knowing.

The interplay between intellect and intuition is very important (Assagioli 1974) and the ability to engage in such a subtle interplay needs to develop and be valued, otherwise midwifery care will lose its richness. Experience and reflection can provide very effective tools to enable this subtle interplay to develop. It is important that this does happen because unfortunately, over a long history, midwives have been criticized for failing to develop a critical appraisal or indeed a more systematic inquiry into their practice. (This is symptomatic of disequilibrium in favour of aesthetics and personal knowledge.) Many risked the charge of their practice being embedded in habits and dictum, which have not been closely scrutinized or challenged, but which are often accepted as given facts (Kirkham 1992). Little wonder then that in recent years increasing emphasis has been placed on the importance of reflection in midwifery practice, to such an extent that it has become one of the 'buzz' words punctuating much of the language of contemporary practice.

Reflection is, therefore, hailed as a basis for both personal and professional growth and development (Kirkham 1994). However, in the case of midwifery practice inherent difficulties and challenges posed by the concept have been explored in the quest to unleash creative ways of boosting practitioners' confidence and competence in providing effective care for mothers and babies (Kirkham 1997). Nevertheless, Murphy-Black & Faulkner (1990 p. 3) recognize the value of reflection asserting that:

if midwives want to claim their status as independent practitioners or wish to be held accountable for their practice, they should know not only what they must do and how to do it, but also why they do it. It is only by constantly questioning what is done and how it is done that midwives can build a body of knowledge on which to base their practice.

The emerging phenomenon of reflection provides a useful focus as it enables midwives to investigate the major influences which shape and guide their individual practice, which in essence may aid or hinder midwives working in partnership with women. A word of caution, however: there is no room for complacency. Reflection is not the panacea for all the ills and unrest currently affecting practitioners. Kirkham (1997) reminds us that the concept, whilst useful in cultivating insights into professional practice, leading to increased self-awareness and deeper understanding of the kinds of analysis and evaluation required to strengthen our critical skills of inquiry, is still a relatively new concept for many paradigms. But, paradigmatically, it is frequently claimed that a midwife who is self-aware and reflective is more likely to observe the effect of her actions upon the client group she serves, and adjust her actions accordingly (Kirkham 1993). This begs the question of: what is reflection? Contextually, this is what a practitioner does when he/she looks back at the practice that has occurred and reconstructs, re-enacts and/or recaptures the events, thoughts, feelings of emotions and the accomplishments of a given experience or situation (Glen, Clark & Nichol 1995). Schön (1983) provides further clarity to the term by distinguishing between two types of reflection: 'reflection on action' and 'reflection in action'.

Reflection on action

This centres around the ways in which many midwives reflect, and may be defined as the critical reflectivity or review that an individual engages in on a personal or professional level, following an event or a situation which enhances professional growth and development, and which ultimately may lead to the acquisition of new skills, as outlined in Fig. 2.1. Adults, through their socialization and education, are usually equipped to use their thought processes to interpret and learn from experience—be that good or bad. This allows for a more advanced form of thinking. Grey & Pratt (1992) claim that reflective practitioners are professionally mature, have a strong sense of self and a firm commitment to improve their practice. Additionally adult learners have the enviable quality—possessing a unique insight into their level of awareness and critiquing it—in other words 'having a mind that watches itself' (Mezirow 1990).

Reflection in action

Schön (1983) asserts that reflection in action relies on spontaneity, intuition as well as knowledge or intelligence accrued from the experiential activities midwives engage in, such as the day to day care they perform. This, Schön (1983) recognizes as the common sense approach to doing or 'knowing in action'. He uses phrases such as 'thinking on your feet; the experience of finding the groove; and the ability to keep ones wits', whilst Murphy & Atkins (1994 p. 13) acknowledge that: 'reflection in action occurs while practising, and influences the decisions made and the care given'. In illuminating the tacit day to day knowhow, the ability to reflect in action: 'offers some useful markers: firstly, by using spontaneity, intuition, knowledge and

experience' (Schön 1983 p. 54). Thus midwives are able to engage in actions, recognize events, assess and make judgements without having to think consciously about every action prior to, or during, the physical act of caring.

Secondly, midwives may use intuitive skills constantly and in so doing may not be consciously aware of learning how to cope, what to say and how to behave in certain situations, but may simply find themselves performing the task.

Reflection in action highlights the hallmark of reflective practitioners, which lies in their ability to make decisions in complex situations that are unique or involve uncertainty as well as conflicting claims and values. However, this essential feature is too often neglected.

The main purpose of reflection on action and reflection in action then, is to advance midwives' thinking regarding the conceptualization of events (Powell 1989), thus enabling practitioners to utilize the affective, cognitive and psychomotor domains depicted in Fig. 2.1.

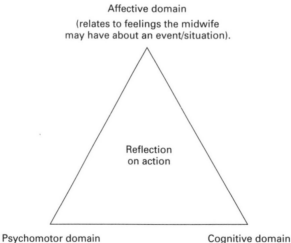

Figure 2.1 Reflection on action.

The purpose of reflection

In the ever-changing climate of the health service, the midwifery profession is required to be responsive, adaptable and flexible to meet the diverse health care needs of mothers and babies within a cross-cultural setting. Developing reflective abilities can only be advantageous as the new perspectives ultimately created will empower midwives to adjust more adeptly, and cope more efficiently with the demands and constraints and ongoing challenges placed upon her time. The UKCC (1995) embraces the notion of 'self-appraisal' to nurture professional growth and development. The aim is that practitioners will use part of their professional portfolio to document accounts regarding their reflective skills/abilities.

Naturally, this is a new way of thinking and seeing for many midwives, but there are many bonuses to be had both on a professional and personal level if the focus is right. Reflection may encourage intrinsic motivation, self-assessment, self-regulation and a questioning approach to midwifery care. This fundamentally will equip midwives on an individual level to grasp their 'window of inquiry' to develop as lifelong learners (Palmer 1997), thus contributing to practice which is competent, responsive and evidence based.

Using critical incidents

Innovation and imagination are key ingredients to harnessing midwives' reflective skills. Critical incidents are excellent tools in heightening and developing self-awareness in order that midwives can be more effective in their professional practice. A critical incident, being a rather complex and challenging occurrence, is not easy to define; a continuum of awareness is therefore vital. For simplicity a critical incident can be defined as a useful 'benchmark' relating to any event or situation which highlights or identifies a significant turning point, a shift in emphasis or a change in an individual's professional life. The intensity of the event or situation causes the midwife to pause for thought, to reflect on the experience, mull it over, learn from it, question and challenge assumptions, values beliefs and actions in relation to what they might say or do. It is important to reflect regularly but it is a skill that needs to be developed (Activity 2.1).

 Activity 2.1

Find a quiet and calm space where you feel relaxed and safe. Allocate yourself 10 minutes to think back to events which have occurred since you have been practising as a midwife. You may care to reflect on your experience during a working week, month or year. Now identify one event, situation or experience that you would like to mark out or claim as a 'critical incident'. Make a note of feelings and thoughts before you progress through the remainder of the text.

The use of examplars to aid reflection

Bulman (in Palmer, Burns & Bulman 1994 p. 152) illuminates the value of using exemplars to hone reflective skills:

exemplars are powerful, particularly in their ability to highlight a process of analytical thinking about practice and a willingness and ability to change and consider practice in relation to it...they potentially enable the practitioner to examine and act upon the actual realities of practice, in order to learn from experience.

The exemplar detailed below serves to illustrate the point of reflective writing, as well as learning from a critical incident. After reading the excerpt and reflecting on the accompanying questions, you are invited to try your skills at reflective writing by documenting your account of the critical incident marked out from Activity 2.1. Four questions identified by Palmer (1997) are useful parameters in which to work:

1. What happened?
2. What was effective?
3. What you feel?
4. What would you do differently?

Exemplar of 'what happened?'

At 37 weeks' gestation following a brisk bleed per vaginum, Sharon Davies was urgently readmitted to her local maternity unit and allocated to my team on the labour suite. I decided to become her named midwife, even though I knew from the preliminary briefing I received from colleagues that she was likely to be challenging. Sharon and her partner Robert were very well educated, questioning and determined, which for some members of staff amounted to the couple being labelled 'difficult'. Sharon had for example, at 34 weeks' gestation taken her own discharge from the unit, against medical advice, after being on the antenatal ward for 2 weeks following the diagnosis of grade IV placenta praevia. Her rationale was that her little girl, who was 4 years old at the time of the incident, was experiencing behavioural problems since Sharon's period of hospitalization. As Sharon had no further bleeding subsequent to her admission to the antenatal ward, her vulnerability and sensitivity to suggestions were particularly heightened, which strengthened her need to be at home with her family. Feeling bored, frustrated and powerless by her situation, all sense of rationality appeared to have failed Sharon. She could not understand why she needed to remain in hospital. Her perception was that none of the midwives or medical attendants could state with any certainty whether or not any further bleeding would occur. Additionally, if her condition was really as serious as the medical staff made out, the couple rightly questioned why Sharon was granted permission by her consultant to make home visits 2 days per week. She also felt that the midwifery and obstetric staff in the hospital could not guarantee her safety, in part because of the position of the antenatal bay she was in. There was only one midwife having responsibility for the care of 26 women on the mixed ante/postnatal ward to which she was admitted during the night shift. Sharon and Robert's contention was that the swift attention they have been assured may not be so readily available. This was not quite as irrational as many had thought.

Exemplar of 'what was effective?'

Trying desperately not to be influenced by the adverse remarks made by other members of the team during the report given at the beginning of the late shift, on entering the room I sensed the couple's anger and palpable tension. Therefore, on initiating our relationship, I attempted to approach Sharon in a spirit of partnership, and tried to remain open to Sharon and Robert's opinions to enhance my overall effectiveness in cultivating a therapeutic relationship. Admittedly, the first hour of our encounter was difficult as I got the distinct impression through interacting with the couple, and picking up the cues from their non-verbal communication (e.g. lack of eye contact and defensive body language) that they were wary of health care professionals. My immediate concern was to remain non-judgmental and open minded. I then employed the microskills of Egan (1994) SOLER to demonstrate my physical presence of non-verbally listening and attending, thus conveying to Sharon and Robert not just my physical presence, but conveying also that I was 'truly with them' mentally, willing to listen and connect with them mentally. Egan (1994) SOLER is an acronym which when interpreted related my congruence or genuineness in actively attending to the needs of the couple. I was able to achieve this by Sitting and facing the couple squarely, adopting an Open posture (a closed posture may have been negatively interpreted), Lean slightly forward to tell the couple non-verbally that I was listening, and perhaps more importantly that I was interested in what they have to say. This was a good method of demonstrating respect and sensitivity. Eye contact was utilized appropriately; too much intense staring may have created unease and possibly be construed as a sign of intimidation. It was important too, for me to be Relaxed in the given situation and not to try too hard to be overtly agreeable; being true in character is crucial to such encounters. I made no assumptions about the couple's background or inferences, but asked about what they already knew and what they needed to know to improve communications. (Note how the practitioner has utilized the literature to ground theory and practice in her reflective discourse.)

This approach was effective as I was later able to forge a fairly close relationship with Sharon and Robert. This helped to reduce the potential for conflict and tension. I was also able to act as their advocate when communicating with the rest of the team, and by doing so the autonomy of the couple was respected. Over the next 24 hour period all blood loss per vaginum settled and a date was discussed and agreed with the couple for a planned caesarean section. Sharon remained on the labour suite for a short period thereafter, and was later transferred to the antenatal ward.

'What did I feel?'

I felt that the anger and internal rage that Sharon was experiencing stemmed from her need to have some degree of normality restored in her life, and more poignantly to have her feelings validated. But, because she was already labelled as 'a difficult patient', I felt very conscious of the inherent dangers of making unnecessary assumptions that may have led to subjectivity and further criticisms. I felt anxious and somewhat self-conscious under the watchful gaze of the couple who appeared to be scrutinizing and assessing my every move. I also felt confusion in my emotions, believing fervently in the philosophy of woman-centred care which embraces the ubiquitous four Cs of recent government reports on the maternity service (DoH 1992, 1993). These simply translate as Sharon's right to make informed *choices* over the manner in which her pregnancy should be managed, respecting Sharon's right to dignity and *control* over the decision-making process, her right to have *continuity* of care with the same carer and finally her right to effective *communication* from the midwives and doctors involved in her care, and to have clear unbiased information communicated throughout the pregnancy continuum. Yet, achieving woman-centred care and partnership with Sharon was much more complex and challenging than I had anticipated.

'What would I do differently?

Whilst recognizing that women and their partners have to make difficult decisions in the face of controversy and confrontation, I would in future discuss problems experienced with colleagues much earlier in order to improve communication, team dynamics and efficacy. I appreciate now how crucial team work is when dealing with major conflicts and accept that it was rather naive on my part to exclude other members of the team as much as I did.

Now use the following questions in Activity 2.2 identified by Bulman (in Palmer, Burns & Bulman 1994 p. 139) to reflect on the exemplar previously outlined.

Activity 2.2

1. How much of the account detailed in the exemplar is based on description and how much is based on reflection?
2. What new insights do you think the midwife came away with, after describing and reflecting on this critical incident?
3. Can you identify any additional areas that the midwife could have expanded on, to strengthen her understanding of the situation more fully?

After answering the three questions, make a list of the ways in which the critical incident you have previously identified has contributed to your development both personally and professionally. Following completion of the exercise you may want to use this experience as a catalyst for ongoing reflection on crucial events that can be documented and filed in your personal professional portfolio.

Observational skills

Critical incidents may also enable midwives to refine and strengthen their observational skills, where they can examine and review their understanding of the dynamic forces influencing the relationship between women and midwives, and also the interactions evident in interprofessional and intraprofessional teams. The skills of observing take time and patience to perfect; for example, most individuals tend to see only what they expect to see, and many others see only what they want to see. Obviously, this may be a more enjoyable visual impediment, but it is hardly clarity. The ability to see what actually exists and to accept this without an attempt to interpret or colour the picture is rare at the best of times. Not surprisingly, the most open-minded and self-aware midwife may end up jumping to conclusions. Spradley (1979) issues a wise dictum for contemporary midwives, in that it is the values and viewpoints of the person looking that largely determines what is seen.

The use of personal narratives

Another strategy to assist midwives in their quest for learning from experience through the process of reflection is the use of personal narratives, which Kirkham (1997) aptly refers to as 'story telling'. The use of stories helps to identify clear links between professional judgement and analysis. Critical incidents can also become integral to the process of personal narratives.

Support is a necessary accompaniment to the sharing of 'stories' and critical incidents. Support affirms the worth of colleagues, provides for collaborative and therapeutic relationships that can supply mutual benefits and rewards within the essential parameters of learning together, culminating in safe opportunities for critical reflection (Palmer 1997).

The interdisciplinary nature of midwifery practice often ensures that the sharing of experiences provide a lively exchange of views, feelings, values and beliefs. When there is support in midwifery practice the standpoint of others is respected. Midwives are empowered to recognize their difficulties, take responsibility for their actions, explore the central issues around critical incidents and personal narratives, and develop a strategy for change which will bolster self-reliance and fulfilment.

Equality in midwives' working relationships aids the understanding and tolerance of difference. Midwives may see the world in different ways, and approach some aspects of care

differently, but ultimately their basic humanity equips them to value others. Trust is therefore important when sharing 'stories' and critical incidents. No midwives will begin to expel their concerns until they feel sure that personal confidence will be kept and words uttered, respected. In reality this may require time, attention and positive regard for each other, to enable colleagues to explore their action, feelings and concerns in a collegiate climate of mutual trust where confidentiality and understanding are at the forefront. Midwives listening to colleagues may want to encourage objectivity in their exploration and reflection on practice. Bear in mind that when accompanying colleagues on their journey (be it happy or sad) this means that they retain control over events. It does not mean that you should take over the driving seat or the reins of control.

The central tenets of learning from 'stories' and critical incidents cannot be overemphasized. Midwives, perceived as the paragons of virtue—the linchpins to effective maternity care, are constantly confronted with many of these significant events when caring for women and their families. Such interactive encounters according to Graham (1995 p. 28) are: 'filled with much potential learning and development, yet often this learning goes unlearned and the development is not acknowledged'. It is time to break this impasse if midwives are to strive toward becoming reflective practitioners.

Graham (1995) identifies some useful markers to aid reflection. These are:

- being adaptable, flexible and responsive to change alongside the willingness to listen to the viewpoint of others
- being in control and taking an active part in personal self-development and practice
- being able to keep an open mind
- being responsible—this according to Graham (1995) increases professional autonomy and accountability
- being able to develop skills relating to critical thinking, for example fostering a questioning approach to care
- having a wholehearted approach in order to consider all sides of an argument; by so doing

the individual will resist the temptation to make assumptions and jump to conclusions based on value judgements (Schön 1983)
- being able to confront uncomfortable truths and consider the outcomes of actions in present and future practice.

ARTICULATING REFLECTIVE KNOWLEDGE

Reflection and reflective writing have a language of their own and therefore we need to develop a view of academic style which will accommodate this way of writing without compromising its authority. Often in articulating reflection it is more authentic to use the first person both in speech and in writing Sometimes, however, a traditional view of what constitutes an academic style precludes this. This means that we have to learn to write comfortably in the first person when appropriate, to draw on the interplay of all dimensions of professional knowledge. It is important to attempt to articulate intuitive and reflective knowledge as best we can, although the very nature of intuition defies articulation, and still enjoy academic credibility. Webb (1992) supports the use of the first person in academic writing and this has been the premise supporting its use in the writing of this chapter.

Summary

This chapter has explored the notion that there are many dimensions within the knowledge that informs midwifery practice. The conclusion drawn is that both rational and intuitive ways of knowing are valid. Reflection can help the professional to utilize the interplay between all dimensions of professional knowing, including intuition. It can help midwives prioritize what they do and how they can do it more effectively. Essentially, it empowers midwives to determine the 'best fit' (Egan 1994) from competing alternatives for action. Reflection can help practitioners to value what they do, identify flaws and apprehend their practice. Finally, it may also help with assessment, planning, implementation and evaluation/review of action plans/care plans, thus providing greater clarity, meaning and coherence in midwives day to day practice. Reflective writing demands that the first person is used to enable the authenticity of experiential meaning to emerge.

REFERENCES

Appleton J V 1993 An exploritory study of the health vistor's role in identifying and working with vulnerable families in relation to child protection. Master of Science thesis, King's College, London, University of London, London

Assagioli R 1974 Psychosynthesis. Viking Press, New York

Ayer A J 1956 The problem of knowledge. Pelican Books, UK

Belesky M F, Clichy B M, Goldberger N R, Tamile J M 1986 Women's ways of knowing. Basic Books, New York

Benner P 1984 From novice to expert—excellence and power in clinical nursing practice. Addison Wesley, London

Benner P, Tanner C 1987 How expert nurses use intuition. American Journal of Nursing January:23–31

Bolam v. Friern HMC[1957] 2 All ER 118.

Broudy H, Smith B, Burnett J 1964 Democracy and education in American secondary schools. Rand Mcnally, Chicago

Burnard P 1989 The 'sixth sense'. Nursing Times 85(50): 52–53

Carper B A 1978 Fundamental patterns of knowing in nursing. Advances in Nursing Science 1:13–23

Davis-Floyd, Davis E 1996 Intuition as authoritative knowledge in midwifery homebirth. Medical Anthropology Quarterly 10(2) June:237–294

DoH (Department of Health) 1992 Health Select Committee second report on the maternity service (Chair—Winterton). HMSO, London

DoH (Department of Health) 1993 Expert Maternity Group report: Changing childbirth (Chair—Lady Cumberlege). HMSO, London

Duff E 1997 Safe in our hands—report of the Royal College of Midwives annual conference 1997—Harrogate. Midwives 110(1314):164

Easen P, Wilcockson J 1996 Intuition and rational decision-making in professional thinking: a false dichotomy? Journal of Advanced Nursing 24:667–673

Egan G 1994 The skilled helper, 5th edn. Brooks/Cole, California

Eraut M 1985 Knowledge creation and knowledge use in professional contexts. Studies in Higher Education 10(2): 117–133

Flint C 1995 Communicating midwifery. Cromwell Press, Cheshire

Flint C, Poulengeris P 1987 The know your midwife report. Supported by S W Thames RHA and the Wellington Foundation

Freire P 1972 Pedagogy of the oppressed. Penguin, Harmondsworth

Gendlin E 1962 Experiencing and the creation of meaning. Collier MacMillan, Andover

Gendlin E 1981 Focusing, 2nd edn. Bantam Books, New York

Gendlin E 1993 Three assertions about the body. The Folio 12(1):21–33

Glen S, Clark A, Nichol M 1995 Reflecting on reflection: a personal encounter. Nurse Education Today 15:61–68

Graham I 1995 Reflective practice:using action learning mechanism. Nurse Education Today 15:28–32

Grey E, Pratt R 1992 Towards a discipline of nursing. Churchill Livingstone, New York

Heidegger M 1962 Being and time. Blackwell, Oxford

Jarvis P 1984 Professional education. Croom Helm, London

Jarvis P 1986 Reflective practice and nursing. Nurse Education Today 12:174–181

Jarvis P 1992 Reflective practice and nursing. Nurse Education Today 12:174–181

King L, Appleton J 1997 Intuition: a critical review of the research and rhetoric. Journal of Advanced Nursing 26:194–202

Kirkham M 1992 Labouring in the dark. In: Abbott P, Sapsford R(eds) Research into practice. OUP, Buckingham, pp 5–18

Kirkham M 1993 Communication in midwifery. In: Alexander J, Levy V, Roch S (eds) Midwifery practice: a research based approach. Macmillan, Basingstoke

Kirkham M 1994 Using research skills in midwifery practice. British Journal of Midwifery 2(8):390–392

Kirkham M 1997 Reflection in midwifery—professional narcissm or seeing with women. British Journal of Midwifery 5(5):259–262

Levin D 1985 The body's recollection of Being. Routlege Kegan Paul, London

McCormack B 1992 Intuition: concept analysis and application to curriculum development. I. Concept analysis. Journal of Clinical Nursing 1:339–344

McCormack B 1993 Intuition: concept analysis and application to curriculum development. II. Application to curriculum development. Journal of Clinical Nursing 2:11–17

Mezirow J 1990 A critical theory of adult learning. In: Tight M (ed.) Adult learning and education. Routledge, London. pp 124–138

Murphy K, Atkins S 1994 Reflection with a practice led curriculum. In: Palmer A, Burns S, Bulman C (eds) Reflective Practice in Nursing. The growth of the professional practitioner. Blackwell Science, Oxford, pp 10–17

Murphy-Black T, Falkner A (eds) 1990 Midwifery. Scutari, London

New English Dictionary (ed Baker E) 1932 Odhams, London

Orme L, Maggs C 1993 Decision making in clinical practice: how do expert nurses, midwives and health visitors make decisions? Nurse Education Today 13:270–276

Palmer A 1997 Learning to reflect. Nursing Times 1(2):3

Palmer A, Burns S, Bulman C (eds) 1994 Reflective practice in nursing. The growth of the professional practitioner. Blackwell Science, UK

Polanyi M 1966 The tacit dimension. Routledge Kegan Paul, London

Powell J 1989 The reflective practitioner in nursing. Journal of Advanced Nursing 14:824–832

Pyles S, Stern P 1983 Discovery of nursing gestalt in critical care nursing. The importance of the gray Gorilla syndrome. Image Journal of Nursing Scholarship 15(2):4–9

Rogers C 1967 On becoming a person. Constable, London

Rogers C 1983 Freedom to learn for the 80's. McMillan International, Columbus

Rose P, Parker D 1994 Nursing: an integration of art and science within the experience of the practitioner. Journal of Advanced Nursing 20(6):1004–1010

Ryle G 1949 The concept of mind. Penguin Books, London

Schön D 1983 The reflective practitioner: how professionals think in action. Temple Smith, London

Schön D 1987 Educating the reflective practitioner. Jossey Bass, London

Schön D 1991 The reflective practitioner. Avebury, Aldershot

Shraeder B, Fischer D 1987 Using intuitive knowledge in the neonatal intensive care nursery. Holistic Nursing Practice 1(3):45–51

Sleep J, Grant A 1987 West Berkshire perineal management trial: three year follow up. British Medical Journal 295:749–751

Sleep J, Grant A, Garcia J, Elbourne D, Spencer J, Chalmers I 1984 West Berkshire perineal management trial. British Medical Journal 289:587–590

Spradley J P 1979 The ethnographic interview. Holt Rinehart & Winston, New York

UKCC 1995 PREP and you—fact sheets 1–8. UKCC, London

Walsh M 1997 Accountability and intuition: justifying nursing practice. Nursing Standard 11(23):39–41

Webb C 1992 The use of the first person in academic writing. Journal of Advanced Nursing 17(6):747–752

Westcott M R 1968 Toward contemporary psychology of intuition. Holt, Rinehart & Winston, London

FURTHER READING

Agyris C, Schön D 1976 Theory in practice—increasing professional effectiveness. Jossey-Bass, London

Atkins S, Murphy K 1993 Reflection a review of the literature. Journal of Advanced Nursing 18:1188–1192

Atkins S, Murphy K 1994 Reflective practice. Nursing Standard 8(39):49–56

Baily J 1995 Reflective practice: implementing theory. Nursing Standard 9(46):29–31

Bellman L M 1996 Changing nursing practice through reflection on the Roper, Logan and Tierney model: the enhancement approach to action research. Journal of Advanced Nursing 24:129–138

Berger P, Luckman T 1971 The social construction of reality. Penguin, Harmondsworth

Boud D, Keogh R, Walker D (eds) 1995 Reflection: turning experience into learning. Kogan Page, London

Clarke M 1986 Action and reflection: practice and theory in nursing. Journal of Advanced Nursing 11(1):3–11

Cruikshank D 1996 The 'art' of reflection. Using drawing to uncover knowledge development in student nurses. Nurse Education Today 16:27–130

Denes-Raj V, Epstein S 1994 Conflict between intutive and rational processing: when people behave against their better judgement. Journal of Personality and Social Psychology 66(5):819–829

Dewey J 1933 How we think: a restatement of the relation of reflective thinking to the educative process. DC Heather Company, Boston, USA

Dewing J 1990 Reflective practice. Senior Nurse 10(l0):26–28

Easen P, Wilcockson J 1996 Intuition and rational decision-making in professional thinking: a false dichotomy? Journal of Advanced Nursing 24:667–673

English I 1993 Intuition as a function of the expert nurse: a critique of Benner's novice to expert model. Journal of Advanced Nursing 18:387–393

Farrington A 1993 Intuition and expert clinical practice in nursing. British Journal of Nursing 2(4):228–231

Gaskin I 1996 Intuition and the emergence of midwifery as authoritative knowledge. Medical Anthropology Quarterly 10(2):295–298

Gatley E 1992 From novice to expert: the use of intuitive knowledge as a basis for district nurse education. Nurse Education Today 12:81–87

Getliffe K A 1996 An examination of the use of reflection in the assessment of practice for undergraduate nursing students. International Journal of Nursing Studies 33(4):361–374

Greenwood J 1993 Reflective practice: a critique of the work of Agyris and Schön. Journal of Advanced Nursing 18:1183–1187

Holley M 1989 Writing to grow. Heinemann, New Hampshire

Honey P 1988 You are what you learn. Nursing Times 84(36):34–36

Johns C 1996 The benefits of a reflective model of nursing. Nursing Times 92(27):39–41

Jung CG 1959 The archetypes and the collective unconsciousness. Collected works of C G Jung, vol. 9, Part 1. Routledge Kegan Paul, London

Kenny C 1994 Nursing intuition: can it be researched? British Journal of Nursing 3(22): 1191–1195

Lawler J 1991 Behind the screens. Churchill Livingstone, New york

Lietaer, Rombauts J, Van Balen R (eds) 1990 Client-centred and experiential psychotherapy in the nineties. Leuven University Press, Belgium

Lister P 1989 Experiential learning and the benefits of journal work. Senior Nurse 9(6):20–21

Meerabeau L 1992 Tacit nursing knowledge: an untapped source or a methodological headache? Journal of Advanced Nursing 17:108–112

McCaugherty D 1993 Round the Benner? Nursing Standard 7(33):50–51

Miller V 1995 Characteristics of intuitive nurses. Western Journal of Nursing Research 17(3):305–316

Murray C 1994 Go back. Something's wrong. American Journal of Nursing 7(53):53

Newell R 1992 Anxiety, accuracy and reflection: the limits of professional development. Journal of Advanced Nursing 17:1326–1333

Paley J 1996 Intuition and expertise: comments on the Benner debate. Journal of Advanced Nursing 23:665–671

Paul R, Heaslip P 1995 Critical thinking and intuitive nursing practice. Journal of Advanced Nursing 22:40–47

Poole K 1995 Death of a patient 1: a personal reflection. British Journal of Nursing 4(4): 197–200

Richardson G 1995 Reflection on practice: enhancing student learning. Journal of Advanced Nursing 22:235–242

Robinson K, Vaughan B 1992 Knowledge for nursing practice. Butterworth Heinemann, Oxford

Schraeder B, Fischer D 1986 Using intuitive knowledge to make clinical decisions. Journal of Maternal—Child Nursing 11:161–162

Stuart C 1997 Reflective journals as a teaching/learning strategy—a literature review. British Journal of Midwifery 5(7):434–438

Temple A 1991 Reflection and the charge nurse. Nursing Standard 20(5):2632–2634

Teasdale K 1997 Becoming a reflective practitioner. Health Professional Digest 5(2):40–41

Wondrak R 1992 Intuitive actions. Nursing Times 88(33):41

3

Female genital mutilation: unveiled and deconstructed

Maureen D Raynor   Ransolina Morgan

CHAPTER CONTENTS

This chapter raises the fundamental question of how do we make sense of the cultural diversity of women's experiences of maternity care arising from the habits and dictum of socio-cultural influences. Differences in class, race, culture and ethnicity are key players in influencing the quality of health care women receive at the best of times; but what if women are survivors of female genital mutilation, what kind of prejudices and stereotypical attitudes will they encounter from health care professionals whose traditional custom and practices are at variance with their own? This chapter aims to unveil and confront some of the vexed issues surrounding female genital mutilation. The purpose of the chapter is to enable health care providers to examine their own attitudes, values and beliefs, which may make them at odds with women, who are survivors of genital mutilation. To this end the multi-complex but interrelated concepts of race, ethnicity and culture will be explored, and in the process hopes to provide a radical rethinking of these terms and their interactions.

INTRODUCTION

In Britain female genital mutilation affects women from minority ethnic groups, a practice which enters the core of marginalized communities who are often disenfranchised within the more dominant majority culture. The primary aim of this chapter, therefore, is to confront the challenges posed for midwives when caring for women with genital mutilation. The chapter begins by utilizing a sociological framework to focus on the multicomplex interrelations between race, ethnicity and culture. The intention here is to provide useful background information to enable the reader to examine critically the ways in which stereotypes and prejudices may oppress and silence women who are survivors of female genital mutilation. Indeed, the Royal College of Nursing (RCN 1996) asserts the importance of nursing and midwifery curricula exploring issues of culture and ethnicity, including prejudices and stereotypes created around the vexed issue of female genital mutilation, which many health care workers either remain ignorant of or absolve themselves from, as the practice may be seen as belonging to an 'other' culture.

Finally, in consideration of the dearth of research and information in the health care literature regarding this clandestine practice, the chapter also seeks to provide a concise explanation of its major dimensions. This will be brought to life by the use of case studies and a problem-solving approach to care planning. These activities should enable the reader to reflect on care more generally in order to identify effective strategies that they may need to implement in their own sphere of practice to ensure that the holistic needs of genitally mutilated women will be sensitively met.

It is assumed the reader has an understanding of:

- the anatomy of the normal external female genitalia
- the different types of episiotomies and their benefits and implications for maternal morbidity
- the psychosexual and physical functioning of the external female genitalia.

THE CHALLENGES OF HEALTH CARE WITHIN A MULTICULTURAL CONTEXT

Multiculturalism is a test to any health care professional's political correctness. This means that today's midwife must be culturally aware and sensitive to women whose cultural background is different. Yet, although multiculturalism as a concept highlights cultural differences and the individuality of women, illuminating cultural variance in a society where the presence of people from diverse cultures coexist with their multifaceted belief systems, behaviour, lifestyles and language, it often fails to account for the politics of race, ethnicity and culture.

The Changing childbirth report (DoH 1993) recognizes the cultural diversity of pregnant women, and has given midwives the opportunity to reappraise their practice, and the confidence to assert themselves as advocates of women in their care, in a way that many were beginning to think was no longer possible. For women to take control of their maternity care, their individuality has got to be respected and this should be reflected in service provision and delivery. The provision of good quality services will not have the desired effect unless they are complemented by sensitive delivery by individual midwives as this plays a big part in client satisfaction. Midwives need to appraise their capacity for providing truly individualized care as being accountable for their own practice demands that they should be able to: 'recognise and respect the uniqueness and dignity of each patient and client and respond to their need for care, irrespective of their ethnic origin, religious beliefs, personal attributes' (UKCC 1992: Clause 7). Maternity services have been criticized for not meeting the needs of minority groups (Audit Commission 1997, DoH 1992, Phoenix 1990). Stereotyping rather than correct information have informed care and needs assessment of these women resulting in a powerful and poisonous combination of frustration and ineffective care, creating and maintaining inequalities in health (Schott & Henley 1996).

BLOCKS TO EFFECTIVE CARE: CONFRONTING PREJUDICES AND STEREOTYPES

Prejudice—that is, preconceived views held by one person or group about another usually based on incorrect information—leads to discrimination. Prejudice has its roots in stereotyping and assumptions based on incorrect or partly correct information. In the absence of sound knowledge it is not uncommon to make assumptions based on the limited knowledge one possesses. It is often seen as acceptable to bridge gaps in knowledge by making assumptions, particularly when practitioners feel that they should have the knowledge (Schott & Henley 1996). The less we know, the more assumptions we make. Stereotypes often dwell on the negative aspects of the different culture, which sometimes become exaggerated. The obvious nature of black people's difference makes stereotyping more likely even though culturally they may be more comparable with the majority population than white minority ethnic groups whose difference is not always visibly obvious. Treating people as individuals will reveal the aspects of their culture that is relevant to them so that appropriate and responsive care can be planned and delivered in innovative, courageous and empowering ways. The message is clear: making assumptions prevents midwives from communicating effectively, obtaining accurate information, and may lead to care which is inappropriate—care which frustrates and may even result in non-compliance to care information and advice among service users (Schott & Henley 1996).

ETHNOCENTRICISM AND EUROCENTRICISM

The 'medical model' which has shaped health care service provision in Britain is based on a eurocentric and ethnocentric understanding of illness (Hopkins & Bahl 1993, McKenzie 1995). This has led to a highly standardized and inflexible structure within the NHS, with care focused to meet the needs of the dominant majority. At best the needs of women who are genitally mutilated are marked out as 'other', relegated to the ambiguous category of 'women with special needs'. Surely all women during pregnancy and childbirth have 'special needs' and want to have these needs met in a special way. Yet

paradoxically, the needs of women who have been genitally mutilated are often overlooked, seen as problems and considered as 'different'. Thus culminating in care which marks out artificial differences rather than similarities between this group of women and women from the majority culture. This is not in keeping with the philosophy of 'Changing childbirth' (DoH 1993) where the maternity service is meant to embrace the needs of women from a multifaith, multicultural and multiethnic society (Schott & Henley 1996).

Eurocentricism takes the perspective that the European culture is 'superior' to those of others, and adopts the view that minority cultures should assimilate its values and beliefs to be accepted in the majority culture. Conversely, ethnocentricism amounts to no more than 'cultural stereotyping' (Smaje 1995). This is where health care professionals may make value judgements and inappropriate assumptions about their clients' needs, either on the basis of the majority ethnic experience or on biased notions based on stereotypical images of clients' unique backgrounds. The concepts of race, ethnicity and culture are often used sparingly because of lack of understanding of their true meaning and partly because they are uncomfortable words which, for some, have negative connotations. But, in order to recognize, challenge and work against prejudices and stereotypes which may negate genitally mutilated women's experience of maternity care, midwives need to have knowledge and understanding of the overt and covert ways in which eurocentric and ethnocentric values and beliefs are effected.

RACE, ETHINICITY AND CULTURE
Race

The term 'race' is fraught with contradictions; it is often used to differentiate between people with different skin colour and bodily features placing them in positions of superiority and inferiority. Those belonging to the 'powerful' white-skinned 'race' relegate those with black skin to a position of inferiority. They deem the latter to be inferior in intelligence and civilization and incapable of self-care and therefore assign themselves as masters and caretakers of this inferior race. Although there is no biological or genetic justification to support this view, the visible physical characteristics are often used to create demarcation between what is perceived as 'different' races (Jones 1994). It seems sensible to argue, therefore, that all humans belong to one race, the human race, which disqualifies the superiority/inferiority assertion attached to skin colour. Thus, whilst sex is biologically determined, race is socially constructed and used to justify racism (Schott & Henley 1996).

The Race Relations Act of 1976 makes it illegal to discriminate against anyone on the grounds of colour, race or ethnicity, either directly or indirectly, in any aspect of life including provision and delivery of maternity services (CRE 1994). It was hoped that this would help to eliminate racial discrimination, but available evidence suggests that this has not been the case. Because of the insidious nature of indirect discrimination, and the difficulty involved in proving it, the Act has not made as much impact as it could have done. Women with genital mutilation may find that racism operates at both an individual and an institutional level. Providing effective care for these women means that midwives must be able to recognize direct and indirect racism, so that they can confront it and work against it.

Ethnicity

Ethnicity refers to a group with a common cultural identity. Therefore, a minority ethnic group represents a minority group within society or where the dominant group is perceived as 'different', it does not relate to black and white issues as all members of a given society belong to an ethnic group. Individuals talk about ethnic dress and ethnic food as strange and exotic in the same way as ethnic minority groups are perceived as 'strange' and other. Hopkins & Bahl (1993) claim that when carers concentrate on cultural differences and 'exotica' these merely excuse them to 'victim blame' the communities concerned when complaints about poor quality care is received. One's ethnicity is not always relevant in the same way in every context; it is relevant only in some situations and in the presence of certain people. Members of one ethnic group may identify with members of another ethnic group in certain aspects of life more than they identify with members of their own ethnic group. Class, age, gender and other social factors may affect ethnic identity; therefore it can be dangerous to generalize based on someone's perceived ethnicity. Minority ethnic groups are heavily concentrated in the lower social classes (Garcia, Kilpatrick & Richards 1990, Smaje 1995) and upward mobility has been difficult. This puts black women at a disadvantage at three levels—that is, race, gender and class (Schott & Henley 1996). Although the cause of the socioeconomic status of black people may be multifactorial, their ethnicity, which is historical, is a major contributory factor. Ethnicity is a useful sociological concept, which throws light on the complex issue of female genital mutilation.

Culture

Culture and ethnicity are sometimes treated synonymously, with culture seen as pertaining only to people from a different background. Yet culture is a way of life, including lifestyles, patterns of beliefs and values, customs and behaviour as well as family and other social arrangements. Culture may refer to the way of life of an entire society or to particular groups within a society with a shared ethnic identity (Smaje 1995). Culture would be better understood if it was not shaped and confined to differences between nations, but seen as differences between groups, for example families, classes, religious groups, occupational groups, social groups and so on.

Individuals in society are socialized into a particular culture from an early age in a subtle and insidious way, to the extent that values and beliefs unconsciously become the very core of one's existence, being perceived as normal and natural (Schott & Henley 1996). Culture, then, enables communities to function cohesively because of their shared norms and values. Culture is complex; while it shapes one's way of life and is part of one's existence, blurring of cultural boundaries may result from overlap. The dynamic nature of culture is due to the flexibility and permeability of these boundaries, which allows for reshaping of culture in the presence of certain influencing factors. Belonging to a particular culture does not neglect individuality so, while the cultural orientation of each client is important, the way that culture affects a woman's life is paramount. Her individual reaction to and interaction with the world at large will be determined by the uniqueness of her cultural background.

Culture is more than dress and diet; it involves strong beliefs and assumptions, which are reflected in individuals' thought processes and actions. It may be easier to change one's diet and one's dress than values and beliefs which are usually deeply entrenched, being shaped by a number of factors such as family background, religion and ethnicity. These microcultures account for the malleability of some beliefs, as in some cases family values may take precedence over ethnicity, or ethnicity over religious values, though in many cases all strands that make up culture are so intrinsically linked that separating them may be almost impossible. A woman whose culture is at odds with that of her midwife may find that these cultural differences are defined as 'special needs' requiring special provision and care. Marshall (1992) revealed that, while health professionals advocated cultural pluralism, they also expressed reservations in how these could be achieved. Neither practitioners nor clients can be expected to reject personal values and beliefs readily as they have been part of their socialization from an early age; however, as reflective practitioners, effort should be made to challenge possible negative feelings towards women with different cultural background. Lack of understanding or denial of the legitimacy of other cultures gives credence to the assimilationist perspective, which does not take account of the uniqueness of individuals and the value of culture. Integration of two cultures cannot occur unilaterally; the majority culture must be willing and able to accommodate the minority culture, but there is always the question of whether complete integration is ever possible. In relation to female genital mutilation the issue of culture is particularly problematic and will be explored in more depth later in the chapter.

THE SOCIAL MEANING OF FEMALE GENITAL MUTILATION

In the United Kingdom (UK) female genital mutilation (FGM) is an illegal practice enacted under the Prohibition of Female Circumcision Act 1985 (HMSO 1985). This Act deemed it an offence to excise, infibulate or otherwise mutilate the whole or any part of the labia majora or labia minora or clitoris of another person, or to aid, abet or procure this performance by another person of any of those acts on that other person's body (RCOG 1997). FGM is a global issue, which affects millions of women and female children occupying all corners of the globe. The World Health Organization (WHO 1996a) identifies the problem as a blatant abuse of human rights and a matter of public health. The recommendation is that strategies for the prevention and abolition of FGM should be included in existing political agenda, health service budgets and health education curricula alongside subject areas such as HIV/AIDS, safe motherhood and women's sexual health programmes. For contemporary midwives it is clear that FGM is an integral part of women's sexuality, their reproductive health and women's role in society. In the majority of cases mutilation is performed on young girls from as early as 1 day old and beyond. This means that 'these children and young people have no voice or knowledge to understand the implications of female genital mutilation' (RCN 1996 p. 4). Although for the young girl this must be the worst form of betrayal by her parents who have been the centre of her universe, who she is closest to and who she ultimately trusts more than anyone else, enforcing child protection laws should always be a last resort. The midwife needs to acknowledge that FGM is a recognized form of child abuse. This will necessitate collaborative networking with other health care workers such as health visitors and social workers to educate parents and deal with the issue in a sensitive and enlightening way.

Encountering a woman with genital mutilation may be a grim and sobering prospect, but is not as remote as some may think, especially with the increase in the number of refugee families from war-torn zones settling in Britain. The authors have been truly amazed by the number of student midwives who have shared critical incidents in relation to caring for women who have been genitally mutilated. They have all expressed concern and frustration about the sparsity of information in the more popular midwifery textbooks, in conjunction with the lack of clear guidelines on how to provide best care for these women. In order to conceptualize the 'special needs' of women who have been mutilated when discussing and planning their care, the midwife must have not only an understanding of the social meaning of this multicomplex phenomenon but also knowledge of the biophysical imperative and classification of FGM.

THE BIOPHYSICAL MEANING OF FEMALE GENITAL MUTILATION

A report by the World Health Organization (WHO 1996a p. 2) technical working group, condemns all forms of FGM and echoes unequivocally the calls for its eradication, defining the practice of FGM as: 'a range of procedures including excision of the prepuce (the fold of skin above the clitoris), the partial or total excision of the clitoris (clitoridectomy) and labia, and the stitching and narrowing of the genital orifice (infibulation)'.

In an effort to highlight the scale of the problem this definition has now been submitted by WHO for inclusion in the International classification of diseases, when it is next revised. 'Female genital mutilation' conveys the unflinching weight of the problem more than the more euphemistic, medicalized and misleading concept of 'circumcision'. It relates more transparently to the unwarranted removal of a healthy organ whether for customary or non-therapeutic

reasons (WHO 1997). Furthermore, the practice is on a far greater scale and entirely different from removal of the foreskin in the male infant. Nevertheless, it should be acknowledged that there are parallels to be drawn between the two practices, which some authors are quick to point out are equally abhorrent and questionable. Lightfoot-Klein (1997, personal communication) explains the similar attitudes and misconceptions towards removal of the infant male foreskin and the pressure that is being mounted, especially in North America, to challenge what is perceived to be an equally ritualized custom.

CLASSIFICATION OF FEMALE GENITAL MUTILATION

Attempts to categorize and classify FGM have been thwarted with difficulties owing to the variety of ways in which the act is performed, coupled with the ethnic diversity of groups who practise it. However, the nomenclature currently favoured by WHO (1996a p. 6) goes some way in achieving standardization for practice.

Type I

This is excision of the prepuce, with or without excision of part or all of the clitoris. A knowledge of the functions and anatomical structures of the external female genitalia is therefore crucial to the practice of every midwife. Figure 3.1 illustrates what the female genitalia may look like following removal of the clitoris—*clitoridectomy*, also referred to as *sunna circumcision* by some Muslim communities (Dorkenoo & Elworthy 1992).

Type II

This is excision of the prepuce and clitoris together with partial or total excision of the labia minora, known also as *nymphectomy* (Dorkenoo 1994). The author claimed that bleeding from the raw surfaces and from the clitoral artery is quite often arrested by a number of highly questionable remedies, from the insertion of catgut sutures to the application of homemade poultices such as

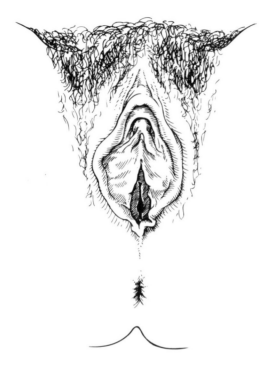

Figure 3.1 Diagram of clitoridectomy (type I) (the hatched area denotes the extent of the tissue removal; usually the clitoris and prepuce are removed).

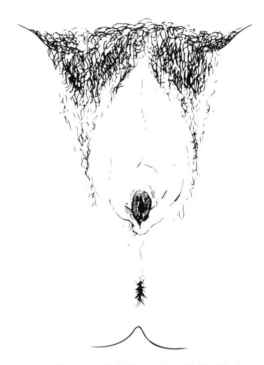

Figure 3.2 Diagram of infibulation (type III) (the blank space indicates the extent of the tissue removal; the labia minora and labia majora are removed along with the clitoris as depicted in the previous diagram; the woman is left with a tiny hole through which to menstruate, and an abundance of scar tissue which is unlikely to stretch during the birth process).

porridge and raw eggs. Not surprisingly, the very interventions employed to achieve haemostasis have major implications for the health of the young girl or woman. Young lives are further compromised by the operator, who is often a lay person from the local community with limited knowledge of anatomy, surgical techniques and aseptic procedures (WHO 1997). Utilization of little or no local anaesthetic when the excision is made means that the extent of the cut cannot be accurately controlled, as the acute pain and suffering experienced by the victim may cause her to move and writhe about in agony (Toubia 1994).

Type III

This is excision of part or all of the external genitalia and stitching/narrowing of the vaginal opening—known also as infibulation (Fig. 3.2). This is the most extreme form of mutilation which leaves only a small posterior opening for the passage of menstrual blood and urine, and is known commonly as *pharaonic circumcision* by communities from the Sudan, or *Sudanese circumcision* by the Egyptians (Dorkenoo 1994, WHO 1997).

Type IV

This is the unclassified category which WHO (1997) claims may involve mutilation such as:

- pricking, piercing or incision of the clitoris or labia, or both
- stretching of the clitoris or labia, or both, and cauterization by burning of the clitoris and surrounding tissues
- scraping of the vaginal orifice or cutting of the vagina
- the introduction of corrosive substances into the vagina to cause bleeding or other foreign matter such as herbs, intended as a means of tightening or narrowing the vagina.

WHO (1996a) acknowledges that some forms of FGM may not fall neatly into any of the given categories, thus pointing out that FGM encompasses any other procedures that fall under the umbrella of its definition previously outlined. However, whilst the definitions and classifications offered by WHO provide the midwife with useful factual information, they are often constructed as being oversimplistic, as the extent of the injuries may not be easily ascertained from the mere nomenclature. A degree of caution should therefore be exercised, warns Toubia (1994).

PREVALENCE OF FEMALE GENITAL MUTILATION

El Dareer (1992) and WHO (1996b) highlight the difficulties in trying to estimate with any degree of accuracy the true extent of the problem, which is thought to date back to the days of the Pharoahs. Others believe that 'the custom has been practised until quite recently in the UK and Europe as a 'remedy' against masturbation and to control the sexuality of women diagnosed as mentally ill' (RCN 1996 p. 4).

The practice, now rare and virtually extinct in many countries, is endemic in some African, Middle Eastern and Asian countries (Dorkenoo 1994; WHO 1997). Given the scale and nature of the problem, to date there has been no systematic means of enquiry or global surveys to reflect the true incidence of FGM, and some countries even fail to keep records. Consequently, WHO (1997) estimates that 100–132 million girls and women have been affected, with a further 2 million more being at risk annually; put into perspective this figure equates to 6000 a day, 4 a minute or 1 every 15 seconds. Types I and II are thought to account for 80% of the total number of cases, with type III (infibulation), the most severe form, accounting for the remaining 15–20% of all procedures.

HEALTH-RELATED CONSEQUENCES OF FEMALE GENITAL MUTILATION

As stated previously FGM is not only a health-related issue and major human rights problem

as it violates the integrity of women's psychosexual functioning, but it is also a recognized form of child abuse (Herdley & Dorkenoo 1992). Regardless of the type and degree of mutilation inflicted on the young female's genitalia, one thing is for sure: the insult caused is intractable and will leave indelible psychological imprints and scars. Hence the practice can never be justified as it has grave implications for women's physical and psychosexual health. This quells the argument of whether such practices should be conducted in the sterile and 'safe' environment of a hospital theatre in an effort to avoid backstreet operations. WHO (1997) warns about the dangers of medicalizing the practice, which would serve only to legitimize and perpetuate its continuance.

The resultant short and long term morbidity associated with FGM may take different forms but will ultimately depend on the extent of the injury caused. In some instances death may even be an unwanted, unexpected and unnecessary consequence (Toubia 1993). Problems may involve pain, dysmenorrhoea, haemorrhage, infection, urinary problems and psychosexual dysfunction on entering marriage, where sexual pleasure for the young bride is either gone completely or minimized (Toubia 1994, Walker 1992). Other complications may arise in trying to achieve a successful pregnancy, not to mention the problems which may arise during the process of childbirth. Table 3.1 summarizes some of the associated acute and chronic complications that may undermine the health of the affected female.

MEDICOLEGAL PERSPECTIVE

Detailed analysis of the legal and ethical debate surrounding FGM is outside the scope of this chapter. Nevertheless, it is important that midwives recognize that, even though FGM has been an illegal practice in the UK since 1985, implementing the law may pose a number of dilemmas, not least being the challenge of how to overcome the surreptitious ways in which the actual practice is performed.

Table 3.1 Summary of related health risks of FGM

Acute health-related problems	Chronic-health related problems
Pain	Dyspareunia/sexual dysfunction due to diminished sensitivity
Haemorrhage	Dysmenorrhoea
Shock	Recurrent urinary tract infections
Acute retention of urine	Pelvic infections (more common with infibulation) may extend to involve
Infection	Pelvic organs e.g. uterus and fallopian, tubes
Fracture or dislocation of bones such as the humerus, femur, humerus pelvic joints and clavicle, incurred during the excessive force and pressure employed by attendants to control the movements of the struggling girl at the time of the incision.	Infertility due to pelvic inflammatory disease/damage to reproductive organs
	Severe keloid scarring, which WHO (1997) reports may be so extensive that it could prevent penile penetration, with resultant long term psychosexual sequelae
	Abscess formation, possibly due to deep seated infection or an embedded suture
	Clitoral neuroma—leads to hypersensitivity and dyspareunia, caused mainly by the entrapment of the clitoral nerve by a suture or by the scar tissue surrounding the wound
	Fistulae formation—may involve bladder and vagina (vesicovaginal) or rectum (rectovaginal). May occur during the actual procedure, sexual intercourse or childbirth.
	The problem may be lifelong, severely compromising the health of the woman and could result in social ostracism

Source: Adapted from WHO (1996b; 1997).

FORWARD International (Foundation for Women's Health, Research and Development) the UK-based organization who are funded by the DoH, have worked arduously in educating professional groups as well as relevant immigrant communities on the dangers of FGM and its prevention. The organization continues to search for innovative and effective ways in which to stem the tide of tens of thousands of young females who may be at risk, either from illegal practices which are forced underground or more commonly the result of children being sent back to their parents' countries of origin for a 'holiday'; FGM is after all the custom in such communities.

This poses a real dilemma not only for the health care professionals but also for school teachers and social workers. The puzzle is, should they interfere in situations where traditional custom and traditional rituals collide with modernity and Western ideology, or should they refrain from meddling into what some may perceive as a practice firmly rooted in cultural mores? Dorkenoo (1994) argues that it is important to keep a clear focus on what is primarily a child protection and human rights issue, and placing FGM under the umbrella of 'culture' only disguises the enormity of the problem and shifts the focus, while excusing those with the most power and clout to effect change. She also cautions against the dangers of racism, constant interference from midwives, doctors and other professional groups allied to health, or those who generally care about the welfare of girls and women. But even though such confrontation may be misinterpreted and construed as meddlesome, divisive and downright racist, the issue of child protection is a real Achilles' heel as this cannot be perceived as a racist issue. Midwives and other members of the multidisciplinary team must therefore examine their own racist and stereotypical values and beliefs in order to differentiate between what is cultural affairs and what is blatant human rights abuse. Defining the problem as cultural is to respect and tolerate it. Likewise, forcibly removing parts of a young girl's or woman's genitalia is a part of no one's given culture.

Female genital mutilation can only be eliminated once there is a real understanding of the suffering of individuals and communities on a truly humanitarian basis that goes beyond culture and race, and embraces three salient points: the need to protect the child who cannot voice her opinion, the need to continue to heighten public awareness regarding the injustices of FGM and the need to recognize that efforts to maintain cultural integrity may silence women and young girls not to speak out about their experiences. Adamson (1992) conflates the debate by insisting that personal and institutional racism must be opposed to be able to offer care that is sensitive, empathetic and respectful of the cultural diversity reflected within current health care provision. In justifying her claims the author reiterates that FGM is not only a human rights issue but it is also an equal opportunities issue. Midwives practising in the UK who are from the majority culture should, therefore, appreciate that sexism is no less an oppressive and sinister force than is racism.

For many midwives it may seem essentially contradictory and even absurd that women who are perhaps one of the most vulnerable groups in any society are the main perpetrators of FGM. These women are often refugees and may command a limited grasp of English; midwives should also recognize that some of these women are parents who are poor, and who may even be isolated from their communities (Adamson 1992). It is important to note, however, that the practice also cuts across the social divide, and is not unknown among the more affluent and well-educated sectors of some communities. Adamson (1992) stresses that, to be effective in caring, midwives will require a lot of courage, self-awareness and a clear vision to listen and learn and constantly readjust their cultural perspectives, a practice which minority groups in general are very accustomed to.

The truth is, the law introduced in the UK in 1985 to outlaw the practice of FGM is difficult to enforce. This raises a couple of poignant questions: first, why does the tradition of FGM continue to be seen by some communities as such a valued and ritualized practice? Secondly, why do mothers who themselves are often survivors of FGM, who are fully aware of the physical and mental scars, who go on to bear the pain of childbirth, and who are at the forefront regarding the nurturance and protection of their young subject their daughters to the operation? The answers to these questions will unfold by examining the main reasons for the continued practice of FGM.

REASONS FOR THE CONTINUED PRACTICE OF FEMALE GENITAL MUTILATION

WHO (1997) and pressure groups such as FORWARD international acknowledge that the roots of FGM cannot be confined to any one specific ethnic group as its origins remain obscure. None the less the reasons for its use are multifactorial and deeply embedded in ideological and historical influences of the given societies in which the practice has emerged. FGM throws light on the social meanings surrounding traditional customs, values and beliefs, power and powerlessness and their contribution to health inequalities, and the general compliance of women to the dictates of their community custom and traditional values (WHO 1996b). WHO identifies a number of reasons for the continuance of FGM, which may be categorized as follows:

- psychosexual
- sociological
- hygienic and aesthetic
- traditional myths and beliefs
- religious.

Psychosexual reasons

Marriageable status of the young woman appears to be an overriding factor in some societies. Reducing the sensitivity of the female genitalia attenuates any sexual desire that may result in her losing her virginity before marriage. This may affect the bride price, and the honour of the family as well as the young woman's suitability to enter matrimony, to be seen as unfit to marry carries a stigma in some communities, and is a curse to be avoided at all cost. FGM is also a means of controlling female sexuality not only outside marriage but inside marriage as well, thus serving to increase male sexual pleasure (Dorkenoo 1994, Toubia 1994). From a social and legal perspective, then, it can be seen how this internal struggle becomes a real thorn in the side for some families. The obvious concern for these families is not whether or not the excision is necessary, but is more a question of which law to break. Do they ignore the UK legislation or do they ignore the unwritten law that exists in their communities, where their daughters will be at risk of being treated as a social outcast as their purity is in doubt, culminating in shame and disgrace for the whole family? Understandably, with lack of greater insight into the wider ramifications of mutilation, many parents choose to send their daughters back 'home' thus freeing them from the constraints of the law, which is ineffective in such situations. Given that the law only deals in certainties, it remains highly questionable whether it is at all feasible or even advisable to prosecute perpetrators retrospectively under the 1989 Children Act (HMSO 1989), when the

net effects on the parent–child relationship are considered.

Sociological reasons

Ceremonial rites of passage are a necessary ritual in all societies and punctuate all of the life cycle from birth to death. FGM in some communities is one way in which a girl makes her transition from childhood into womanhood, a practice which identifies with the heritage of the girl's parents' traditions and customs, and assists in the maintenance of social cohesion and integration of the young woman in society (Toubia 1994, WHO 1996b).

Hygiene and aesthetic reasons

Because female sexuality is seen by some as being dangerous, rampant, unpredictable and deviant, the external genitalia are feared, deemed unclean and unsightly, and as such should consequently be removed to promote hygiene and aesthetic appeal (Toubia 1994).

Traditional myths and beliefs

Bearing in mind the influences of the so-called 'old wives tales' on childbearing women in the UK, it should not be difficult for midwives to conceptualize how traditional myths and beliefs may influence the practice of FGM, since it is mistakenly thought to enhance a woman's fertility without any consideration of the accompanying physical and psychosexual sequelae (WHO 1996b).

Religious reasons

These are frequently identified as a valid reason for FGM, especially from those families practising under the auspices of the Islamic faith. However, WHO (1996a) has dismissed this notion, emphasizing that, although FGM is deeply embedded in some ethnic communities' traditional belief system, the entire issue of FGM is not the domain of any one religious denomination. Because the practice predates Islam, the charge that it is a religious requirement of Islam is refutable and based on conjecture, as the Koran makes no allowance for the practice. This has led WHO (1996a p. 3) to conclude that FGM is a multifaith issue:

including Muslims, Christians (Catholics, Protestants and Copt), animists and also non-believers in the countries concerned … it is important to note that neither the Bible nor the Koran prescribe to the practice, although it is frequently carried out in some Muslim communities in the genuine belief that it forms part of Islam.

CARING FOR THE INFIBULATED WOMAN—IMPLICATIONS FOR MIDWIFERY PRACTICE

When a woman who has been infibulated becomes pregnant a number of issues will need to be considered. The following scenarios (Case studies 3.1 and 3.2) and accompanying reflective activities will illuminate some of the key points that the midwife will need to address. On review of the studies, complete Activities 3.1 and 3.2.

Case study 3.1

Antepartum period

Iman is a 24-year-old Muslim woman who originates from North Africa, but has been living in the UK since winning a scholarship to study law at a prominent university in England. She is married to Riaz, a 32-year-old paediatrician, who was born and brought up in the UK. The couple are expecting their first child.

After the death of her grandmother, who was Iman's main guardian and who she thought all along was her mother, Iman's upbringing was transferred to her aunt who lived in a small community, where community elders still believed in the ritual practice of female genital mutilation as marking a young woman's rite of passage into womanhood. Indeed, Iman was subjected to the procedure of infibulation following the loss of her 'mother' when she was 15 years old.

At 12 weeks' gestation the named midwife meets the couple for the first time whilst visiting them at home to conduct the antenatal 'booking interview'. The midwife took a detailed history reflective of Iman's relevant medical, obstetrical, psychological and surgical background. However, Iman failed to disclose to the midwife her surgical history (i.e. the fact that she suffered the worst

Case study 3.1 Continued

form of genital mutilation as a teenage girl—infibulation), as she felt uncomfortable in talking about such a painful and personal matter. Equally the midwife failed to pick up on the cues when the question was posed … 'tell me, have you had any surgical procedures in the past?' Iman paused, failed to maintain eye contact with the midwife as she felt torn between her family's traditional values and those of her British counterparts, she felt the midwife would not understand and therefore remained silent; praying that she would be able to maintain her composure as the tears began to well up inside her and pricked at the corners of her eyes.

The midwife who had several other visits to make, continued with her paper exercise and continued to ask a series of closed questions to elicit the information which she deemed was important, in order to complete the process as quickly as possible.

Activity 3.1

1. Critically analyse the possible determinants and antecedent factors which may create tension in this mother–midwife relationship.
2. Assuming that Iman felt safe to disclose details relating to the genital mutilation she experienced, outline a plan of care during the antenatal period that may meet the holistic needs of this family.
3. Identify the counselling skills which may enable the midwife to be effective when caring for Iman.
4. What professional or voluntary support agencies could this family contact for support, information and counselling?

Discussion of Case study 3.1

Deinfibulation should be discussed during the antenatal period to prevent and arrest some of the possible complications which may develop during labour, such as obstructed labour, haemorrhage, and severe trauma coupled with the risk of fistulae formation (RCN 1996). Networking with specialist centres who can offer expert advice in dealing with women who have been infibulated, such as Northwick Park Hospital in London, is strongly recommended by Dorkenoo (1994). The RCN (1996) emphasizes the benefits to be gained by working collaboratively with multidisciplinary and interdisciplinary agencies in order to create clear guidelines for dealing with individual cases of FGM.

Ideally every effort should be made to realize continuity of care with carer where trust and mutual respect can be more easily cultivated. A birth plan, reflective of Iman's wishes should be devised between herself and her carer(s), with the midwife clearly documenting the assessment, planning, implementation and continued evaluation of the effectiveness of such care to aid effective communication and to ensure continuity of care. The midwife should also recognize the need for healthy partnerships when working with families, colleagues, advocacy agencies and other voluntary organizations (Aston 1997, RCN 1996).

Case study 3.2

Intrapartum and early postpartum periods

Iman was admitted at 37 weeks' gestation to her local maternity unit in spontaneous labour accompanied by Riaz. On admission to the labour suite the named midwife noticed how distressed and frightened Iman was with each uterine contraction, and quickly explained the admission procedure to the couple. Iman's birth plan was then explored to try and elicit what coping strategies she had in mind for dealing with pain. It was at this time that the midwife noticed two entries on the birth plan were written in bold and underlined in red ink—'I do not consent to any vaginal examinations and I do not want any male doctors to attend me in labour'.

After she had completed reading Iman's birth plan the midwife thought she would explain the significance of vaginal examinations to the couple as a means of assessing progress in labour. Iman had also indicated her wish to have an epidural (the importance of performing a vaginal assessment before the administration of pharmacological means of analgesia during labour was strongly impressed upon the midwife during her education and training). Riaz then explained that his wife's genitalia had been infibulated and feared the pain and discomfort that she would incur as a result of the routine digital assessments. Iman then started to sob, informing the midwife in between sobs how helpless and terrified she was at the prospect of a vaginal birth.

The midwife had never encountered anyone with female genital mutilation in her practice, knew very little about the varying types and health consequences of this procedure and felt completely at a loss for words.

Following a 10 hour labour Iman, assisted by the aid of an episiotomy, gave birth to a live female infant weighing 2.7 kilograms at birth.

Activity 3.2

1. Outline the action that the midwife should take on disclosure of the information by the couple highlighted in the above scenario.
2. Identify the physical, psychological, sociocultural and counselling needs of Iman and Riaz during the labour process.
3. Discuss the responsibilities of the midwife and the entire interdisciplinary team in providing effective care for this couple.
4. Describe the potential problems which may arise during this labour and devise a plan of action which may prevent or alleviate them.
5. What type of episiotomy should have been performed in Iman's case?
6. Discuss the professional and medicolegal implications that the midwife should consider before the episiotomy is repaired?
7. What factors should be taken in consideration when planning care for this family during the post-delivery period?

Discussion of Case study 3.2

Midwives should be conversant with the needs of women who are mutilated to be able to convey empathy and sensitivity. This means that the woman's right to choices and her right to dignity and privacy during labour must be respected. It is part of the professional responsibility and moral duty of the midwife to protect the woman from harm and to act as her advocate. In Iman's case, she must not be made to feel that she is a 'freak' when she is at her most vulnerable; neither should intimate examinations and labour room procedures be turned into a circus and a 'peep show' (Adamson 1992). The RCN (1996) instruct midwives to avoid destructive forces that may impact on the midwife–mother relationship such as being 'judgmental and punitive'.

Midwives, like obstetricians who are at the cutting edge of maternity care, have a duty to know the facts about the medico-legal implications of FGM. The RCN and The Royal College of Obstetricians and Gynaecologists (RCOG) have both been proactive in this arena, issuing guidelines for their members. More recently the Royal College of Midwives (RCM) have issued guidelines (1998) to their members regarding their professional and medicolegal responsibilities when caring for genitally mutilated women.

The ubiquitous four Cs of current reports influencing maternity care within the UK (DoH 1992, 1993) should underpin the care the woman receives (i.e. choice, control, continuity and communication). Every opportunity should be provided to encourage the woman to discuss her needs and to play an active part in the decision-making process, which should be communicated and respected. Confidentiality and other ethical considerations, such as informed consent to any intervention, should also be uppermost in the midwife's mind. An advocacy service should be readily accessible to reduce the potential for conflict and to overcome communication barriers. It is paramount though that any links made, or assistance, is not provided by an organization with a vested interest in the continuance of the practice of FGM (Adamson 1992).

It is prudent to anticipate problems during labour, such as: difficulties with vaginal examinations as the discomfort and intrusion encountered by the woman by this invasive procedure may increase her perception of pain, fear, stress and anxiety, thus negating her experience of childbirth (Aston 1997). Dorkenoo (1994) attests that the use of an epidural analgesia during labour may be inappropriate as it may lead to a woman's feelings of powerlessness and loss of control over her body; the sensation of touch could trigger 'flashbacks' to when she was mutilated. Respecting the heterogeneity of women is therefore crucial to care provided in labour as it is dangerous to make assumptions about the needs and wishes of individual women without first offering them an opportunity to communicate their wishes. Since vaginal examinations can pose a number of difficulties and may prove particularly traumatic for the infibulated woman, the midwife should be able to adapt to the demands of the situation. Skills in looking for more subtle signs of the imminent second stage of labour should be honed, for example anal gaping, progressive change in maternal behaviour and expressive noises in response to the expulsive nature of uterine contractions, may serve to alert the midwife to progress in labour. However, because such observations are subjective and difficult to quantify, coupled with the anticipated

problems of severe perineal trauma, vesicovaginal fistula or rectovaginal fistula and their associated haemorrhage, it should come as no surprise to know that the incidence of an operative delivery for infibulated women may treble. This decision will also be influenced by the obstetrician's inexperience at managing such cases (Aston 1997, Dorkenoo 1994, Toubia 1994).

Dorkenoo (1994) also warns that other invasive interventions which necessitate access to the woman's genitalia, such as artificial rupture of the membranes, application of fetal scalp electrodes, bladder catheterization and doctors attempting to perform fetal blood sampling, may be extremely difficult if not nigh impossible to achieve. It is important that the midwife remembers that, regardless of the dictates of the maternity unit's protocols, the woman's consent must be sought before any procedure is undertaken.

The skills of the non-directive approach to counselling need to be developed and honed so that the dynamics of the mother–midwife relationship are positively effective, and are maintained through the core conditions of counselling (i.e. genuineness, acceptance and empathy). These may be conveyed by being non-judgmental in one's approach and actively listening and attending to the woman's and family's concerns (Dorkenoo 1994). The woman and her partner will need appropriate information and psychosexual counselling regarding the advantages of deinfibulation and the dangers of reinfibulation, preferably during the antenatal period. To reinfibulate the perineum following vaginal delivery is to be in breach of the 1985 Prohibition of Female Circumcision Act, and is, therefore, illegal. With this in mind RCOG (1997) issued a policy statement to its members which stressed the guidelines to be followed regarding repair of the genitalia following childbirth, which should be in accordance with the law:

repair of the vulva of a woman who has been delivered of a baby vaginally following a previous infibulation surgery can be performed for purposes connected with that labour or birth, but it is illegal to repair the labia intentionally in such a way that intercourse is difficult or impossible.

CONCLUSIONS

The chapter has unveiled and deconstructed some of the vexed issues pertaining to female genital mutilation, arguing that the practice is unacceptable for many reasons, not least being the ways in which the rights of children are ignored and women's bodies violated. Not only does it silence and suppress female sexuality but it also amounts to no more than a flagrant disregard for the rights and dignity of women. Midwives who are at the cutting edge to influence change have a duty to offer care that 'counteracts rather than violates women's bodies' (Kitzinger 1992 p. 219). Against this background the chapter has examined the complexities of female genital mutilation and how these impact upon a woman's childbearing experience. Thus bringing to the fore the vulnerability of these women and their families within our wider multicultural and multiethnic society. Emphasis has been placed on the need for research, education and continuing professional development among midwives coupled with the need to reflect on attitudes, values and beliefs in order to recognize how racism, stereotypes and prejudices operate at an individual and institutional level and the ways in which they interact to prevent effective care.

Providing effective care for women with genital mutilation, therefore, places a great onus upon the midwife's self-awareness and interpersonal abilities to be sensitive and non-judgmental when caring. Fundamentally the microcosms of our multicultural and multiethnic society affect us all as culture is integrally related to every aspect of caring. Our knowledge, beliefs, values and attitudes are not realities which exist and continue independently of each human existence, but are produced and continued as a result of our unique human action and interaction. Critical enquiry of ourselves and being able to explore the concept of personhood (i.e. who we are and the ways in which we become a product of our socialization) will enable us as midwives to understand the more multicomplex issue of some minority ethnic groups wanting to adhere to their communities' traditional values and beliefs.

Finally, since women are not a homogeneous group, not all women share similar positions in life, have similar experiences and enjoy similar lifestyles, so the needs of individual women who are genitally mutilated will be different. We must therefore continue to search for innovative, empowering and courageous ways to care for these families.

Box 3.1 Practice check

- Are you suitably informed to care for women sensitively who are survivors of genital mutilation?
- How will you ensure confidentiality, privacy and dignity when caring for genitally mutilated women and their families?
- What guidelines and protocols are readily accessible which empower you to plan care sensitively for genitally mutilated women?
- Do you know the contact number and address of one support group, advocacy agency or other organization that may be of assistance when caring for a genitally mutilated woman?
- Are you able to recognize how prejudice, stereotypes and racism may operate at an individual and institutional level in order to work against racist attitudes or care which discriminates against women in your care?

Summary

Female genital mutilation has serious health consequences for a woman's psychosexual and physical well-being. Female genital mutilation impacts upon midwifery care because it is closely linked to a woman's sexuality, her reproductive health and a woman's role in society. Female genital mutilation violates the integrity of women's rights and is also a form of child abuse.

Health promotion and education will be more appropriate when the midwife collaborates with women's health services, pressure groups and advocacy agencies.

Anticipate problems with vaginal examinations to assess progress in labour. Guidelines should be available regarding deinfibulation and repair of the perineum following childbirth.

Counselling skills will increase personal effectiveness at listening and attending.

ACKNOWLEDGEMENTS

The authors would like to thank Vanessa Davies and Rachel Sykes, two former student midwives (now practising midwives) for sharing their critical incidents which related to the care of a genitally mutilated woman. Their powerful narratives were humbling and empowering, acting as the catalyst for much of this chapter.

APPENDIX: USEFUL CONTACT ORGANIZATIONS AND ADVOCACY GROUPS

The groups and organizations from around the globe that are actively involved in the human rights of women and minority groups are too numerous to mention; therefore, the list identified is not intended to be exhaustive.

Equality Now, PO Box 20646, Columbus Circle Station, New York 10023, USA
This is a grassroots organization, run by female lawyers. It is an international network which gathers and scrutinizes data on the human, political, economic and social rights of girls and women.

FORWARD International (Foundation for Women's Health Research and Development), 40 Eastbourne Terrace, London, W2 3QR
Tel: 0171 7252606; fax: 0171 7252796;
email: forward@dircon.co.uk
This is a government-funded organization with extensive experience in the subject of FGM. FORWARD also publishes excellent resources e.g. videos, books, postcards, leaflets and posters, which are useful teaching aids for health care professionals working in a variety of settings. Training is also provided in relation to policy, intervention strategies and support.

Minority Rights Group, 379 Brixton Road, London, SW9 7DE
This is a small organization which publishes books and other useful literature on issues related to women's health issues and other information related to minority groups.

The Royal College of Nursing, 20 Cavendish Square, London, W1M 0AB
Tel: 0171 8720840
The RCN has produced an excellent guide on FGM for use by midwives, nurses, health visitors and others.

WIN (Women's International Network) NEWS, Fran Hosken (editor), 187 Grant Street, Lexington, MA 02173, USA
WIN News contributes a regular column on FGM as well as distributing the 'Childbirth Picture Book' free to African groups on request.

World Health Organization, Division of Family Health, CH-1211 Geneva 27, Switzerland
The World Health Organization have published a number of reports, booklets and training kits relating to female genital mutilation, many of which can be ordered free of charge.

REFERENCES

Adamson F 1992 Female genital mutilation: a guide for professionals. FORWARD International, London
Audit Commission 1997 Executive briefing: first class delivery—improving maternity services in England and Wales. Audit Commission, London
Aston G 1997 Sexuality during and after pregnancy. In: Andrews G (ed.) Women's sexual health. Baillière Tindall, London, pp 124–125
Commission for Racial Equality 1994 Race relations code of practice in maternity services. CRE, London
DoH (Department of Health) 1992 House of Commons Health Committee second report—Maternity services, session 1991–1992, vol. 1. HMSO, London
DoH (Department of Health) 1993 Report of the Expert Maternity Group: Changing childbirth, parts 1 and 2. HMSO, London
Dorkenoo E, Elworthy S 1992 Female genital mutilation: proposals for change. Minority Rights, London
Dorkenoo E 1994 Cutting the rose—female genital mutilation: the practice and its prevention. Minority Rights, London
El Dareer A 1992 Women, why do you weep? Zed Books, London
Garcia J, Kilpatrick R, Richards M (eds) 1990 The politics of maternity care. Oxford University Press, Oxford
Herdley R, Dorkenoo E 1992 Child protection and female genital mutilation. FORWARD International, London
HMSO 1985 Prohibition of Female Circumcision Act. HMSO, London
HMSO 1989 Children Act. HMSO, London

Hopkins A, Bahl V (eds) 1993 Access to health care for people from black and ethnic minorities. Royal College of Physicians, London, pp 78–79
Jones L 1994 The social context of health and health work. Macmillan, London
Kitzinger J V 1992 Counteracting, not re-enacting, the violation of women's bodies: the challenge of perinatal care givers. Birth 9(4):219
Marshall H 1992 Talking about good maternity care in a multicultural context. In: Nicolson P, Ussher J (eds) The psychology of women's health and healthcare. Macmillan, London, pp 200–224
McKenzie K J 1995 Racial discrimination in medicine. British Medical Journal 310:478–479
Phoenix A 1990 Black women and the maternity services. In: Garcia J, Kilpatrick R, Richards M (eds) The politics of maternity care. Clarendon Press, Oxford, pp 274–299
RCM (Royal College of Midwives) 1998 Female genital mutilation and the role of the midwife. RCM Midwives Journal 1(7):218–219
RCN (Royal College of Nursing) 1996 Female genital mutilation. RCN, London
RCOG (Royal College of Obstetricians and Gynaecologists) 1997 Female circumcision: female genital mutilation. RCOG, London
Schott J, Henley A 1996 Culture, religion and childbearing in a multicultural society. Butterworth Heinemann, London
Smaje C 1995 Health, race and ethnicity. Kings Fund Institute, London

Toubia N 1993 Female genital mutilation: a call for global action. INK, New York

Toubia N 1994 Female circumcision as a public health issue. New England Journal of Medicine 331(11):712–716

UKCC (United Kingdom Central Council) 1992 Code of professional conduct for nurses, midwives and health visitors. UKCC, London

Walker A 1992 Possessing the secret of joy. Harcourt and Brace, New York

WHO (World Health Organization) 1996a Female genital mutilation: report of a WHO Technical Working Group, General 12–19 July 1995. WHO, Geneva

WHO (World Health Organization) 1996b Female genital mutilation: the practice—a briefing kit. WHO/FRH/WHD/96.26. WHO, Geneva

WHO (World Health Organization) 1997 Female genital mutilation: a joint WHO/UNICEF/UNFPA statement. WHO, Geneva

FURTHER READING

Hindley J, Montagu S 1997 Midwifery care and female genital mutilation. In: Kargar I, Hunt S C (eds) Challenges in Midwifery Care. London, MacMillan, pp 63–75
A very useful chapter which examines the medicolegal, physical, sociocultural, and psychosexual implications of female genital mutilation alongside the professional and counselling issues that should be considered by midwives and other health care professionals when providing care for women who are survivors of genital mutilation.

Kassindja F, Miller-Bashir L 1998 Do they hear you when you cry? Bantam Press, London

This book details a moving and powerful account of a young woman who was able to flee to the West to escape the threat of genital mutilation following her forced arranged marriage to a man old enough to be her father. This personal narrative opens a window of opportunity and provides a good example of how traditional practices may collide with modernity.

McConville B 1998 A blood tradition. Nursing Times 94(3):34–37
The article reports on a visit to Mali, West Africa and urges readers to support the international efforts towards the eradication of female genital mutilation.

4

'Cultural conceptions': lesbian parenting and midwifery practice

Nicki Hastie

The aim of this chapter is to challenge the invisibility often experienced by lesbians as users of health services by emphasizing the need to suspend stereotypical attitudes and heterosexist assumptions. Some health issues identified are key concerns for lesbians and will be discussed in order to demonstrate to midwives, and other professionals allied to health, how important it is to display sensitivity around sexuality and identity, regardless of whether a woman chooses to disclose her sexuality. The decision to have children, the experience of pregnancy, childbirth and maternity care, how a woman experiences body image and her experience of personal and family relationships raise issues for lesbians which do not always fit comfortably within conventional medical or midwifery practice. A further positive aim of the chapter is to demonstrate how lesbian experience and culture need not remain hidden to health professionals if health services address the significance of current lesbian-focused research.

It is assumed that the reader has some underpinning knowledge of the following:

- opposing theories and ideologies of female sexuality
- the relationship between gender and sexuality
- sociocultural influences on sexuality.

A CULTURAL HEALTH SERVICE

Health care for the most part takes place not in clinical settings but in cultural settings. Health practitioners, both as professionals and as individuals, function every day in an institutionalized framework which reinforces the cultural dimensions of health, illness and health care. One of the clearest examples of this is our system of health care in the UK: the NHS. Having celebrated its 50th anniversary in 1998, the NHS has undergone many changes and challenges since it was set up. This is because the workings of the NHS are dependent on the economic and social policies of the day, and any ensuing government legislation which impacts on the nation's health and strategies for health care provides a benchmark by which to measure wider sociocultural attitudes, beliefs and assumptions, including who is deemed eligible for particular treatments.[1]

Concern over the cost of treatments and how to choose which service users are given access to certain therapies or surgery will be familiar themes to health professionals. They are uncomfortable truths that the health service has found hard to admit and to come to terms with, but truths which are none the less guiding the future of health care. This changing medical agenda can only be fully understood through a sociological framework which places anxieties regarding health care provision and responses to gaps in that provision within the context of the values of contemporary society and changes in social attitudes. Sociocultural issues are everywhere in health care practice, and recognition by practitioners of cultural aspects and influences on health can help to improve the quality and equality of health care delivered to all users of health care services.

Cultural anxieties, fears and beliefs and difficulties with access to health care are key factors

impacting on the health of lesbians. This chapter begins by providing a wider cultural context to the prejudice lesbians face in society before moving on to look at examples of good practice in a midwifery context. This background information is provided on the understanding that health practitioners cannot fully respect the individual needs of lesbians in their care if they have never considered issues relating to sexual orientation and sexual identity. Many of the issues raised will be relevant to all health care professionals; others have particular significance for midwifery practice and for the practice of those who have a clear role to play in pre-conception, antenatal, labour and postnatal care.

The mixture of lesbian (and gay male) sexuality and parenting can instil horror and disgust even in individuals who would otherwise say they 'accept' same-sex relationships. Prejudice, false assumptions and stereotyping have created an image of 'the lesbian' as 'unfit mother', whether she be a biological or non-biological parent figure. More and more lesbians are choosing parenthood and our late-1990s society continues to struggle with deep-seated anxieties and confused morals around the upbringing of children. In 1998, the RCM considered whether to introduce guidance notes for working with lesbian clients, based on members' suggestions and needs (Kaufman 1998, Kaufman, personal communication, 1998). The philosophy of good midwifery practice may be to respect the rights of all women to equal treatment, but midwives also need to consider the cultural oppressions which impinge on women's lives so that they can avoid perpetuating prejudice and stereotypes. It is possible that midwives may themselves feel the pressure of cultural disapproval for supporting lesbian clients, and this chapter aims to provide examples of good practice and pointers to resources which can assist midwives in providing an equality of health care.

SILENCES AND STEREOTYPES

I have always been struck by the depth of people's anxieties about saying the word 'lesbian'. The censorship and self-censorship which operate around this

---

[1] I am thinking here, for example, of The health of the nation (DoH 1992), which sets out priorities for health promotion and research. Such a document begins to govern education in state schools, and reflects, for example, on what society deems appropriate to teach children about sex education. Also, debate over the Human Fertilization and Embryology Act (HMSO 1990) continues to demonstrate social opinion and concern about parenthood and who may take part in parenthood.

cultural category prohibit speaking it aloud, especially in public places.... Any visibility, any open expression of affection, any desire for recognition is perceived as excessive: two lesbians are a crowd; seeking acknowledgement of one's relationship is pushy. The central message continues to be that it's safer, and nicer, to remain silent and keep it hidden.

(Stacey 1997 p. 66)

Supposedly progressive people ... who oppose oppression on every other level, balk at acknowledging the societally sanctioned abuse of lesbians and gay men as a serious problem. Their tacit attitude is 'Homophobia, why bring it up?'   (Smith 1993 p. 100)

'Why mention lesbians?' has often been the attitude of practitioners in mainstream health care as well as society in general. But this lack of attention represents more than casual disinterest; it amounts to wilful abuse and neglect. Lesbians are scarcely visible in health research, in health education programmes, as health providers or as health service users. Lesbians are invisible amongst the category of women and often ignored in studies which do address sexual orientation issues, but focus on the lifestyles and needs of gay men. Lesbians are silenced by sexism, heterosexism and homophobia: silenced through societal embarrassment, fear, ignorance and direct hostility and prejudice. This also means that lesbians are forced to silence themselves in order to seek protection from negative reactions.

Homophobia and heterosexism are the result of oppressive social structures which teach that there are cultural 'norms' of sexuality and seek to enforce such 'norms' through legislation which discriminates against lesbians and gay men.[2] Such legislation gives social sanction to the oppression of lesbians and masks the fact

that sexual 'norms' and sexual identities are socially and culturally constructed (Caplan 1987, Kitzinger 1987, Weeks 1985). Lesbians do not have the same access to health care as heterosexual women because of homophobia and heterosexism.

Homophobia is more than the fear of same-sex closeness and sexuality which might be implied by the term 'phobia'. Homophobia is often expressed as a complete hatred and intolerance of lesbians and gay men, and although irrational is accepted by and acceptable to society. *Heterosexism* is the assumption that heterosexuality is the norm, that other people are heterosexual and that heterosexuality is the only acceptable expression of sexuality.

While many of the health issues which affect lesbians are those which affect all women, invisibility adversely affects experiences of health care for lesbians. O'Hanlan (1995) adapts the definition of women's health issues as employed by the Office of Research on Women's Health, to state that: 'lesbian health issues are those issues to which lesbians are "more susceptible, may have greater prevalence, or may be unique in developing, or be affected by differently" than heterosexual women'. Key issues which negatively impact on the health of lesbians and the provision of health care to lesbians are wide ranging, as reflected in Box 4.1.

The realities of lesbian experience are hidden from the mainstream heterosexist society and so stereotypes are rife among health practitioners. Stereotypes held by nurses in training include the belief that lesbians seduce heterosexual women, lesbians want to be men and can be recognized by a masculine appearance, lesbians are

---

[2] For example, section 28 of the Local Government Act 1988 (HMSO 1988) states:

1. A local authority shall not:
   (a) intentionally promote homosexuality or publish material with the intention of promoting homosexuality;
   (b) promote the teaching in any maintained school of the acceptability of homosexuality as a pretended family relationship.
2. Nothing in subsection (1) above shall be taken to prohibit the doing of anything for the purpose of treating or preventing the spread of disease.

Wilton (1995 p. 192) points out that 'Subsection (2) was, of course, added in order to protect those charged with educating people about HIV/AIDS and, as such, reinforces in British law the unhelpful and offensive link between homosexuality and disease.'

There is no protection for lesbians and gay men in British employment law, nor protection as partners and parents. Stonewall, the political lobby group campaigning for legislative change to end the discrimination of lesbians and gay men, have launched the Equality 2000 campaign to highlight the fact that lesbians and gay men are denied basic human rights (Mason & Watson 1997).

Box 4.1 **Key points for practice; negative issues impacting on the health of lesbians**

- prejudice and discrimination (which is exacerbated by state legislation)
- assumptions of heterosexuality—asking a woman if she is sexually active and then offering her contraception is a standard process in primary health practice
- anticipation of or previous experience of negative reactions from health providers—24% of lesbians surveyed by Reagan (1981) delayed seeking health care because of concerns that they would receive negative responses from health professionals
- inadequate care through lack of knowledge of lesbian culture and community networks
- disregard for partners of the same sex, including exclusion of a female partner during examinations and counselling (Kenney & Tash 1993) and refusal to acknowledge a same-sex partner as the next of kin. Compounding the reaction of health care staff is the isolation many lesbians experience within their biological families. Families can deny lesbian partnerships and exclude the female partner even when it is the patient's wish that her partner acts as primary carer (Swissler 1997)
- concerns over confidentiality—25% of lesbians would not come out to health care providers if sexual orientation would be recorded on health records (Zeidenstein 1990).

a bad influence on children and lesbians are a common source of HIV/AIDS and other sexually transmitted diseases (Eliason, Donelan & Randall 1993). In an earlier study, Good (1976) found that 25 out of 72 gynaecologists who claimed they had treated a lesbian stated that they could tell a patient was a lesbian through clinical observation and judgement. One wonders what they can have been looking for! Mental health professionals are also biased in their contact with lesbian clients (Murphy 1992) and some mental health professionals continue to blatantly oppress their lesbian clients by promoting the stereotype that a lesbian sexual orientation is *caused* by previous sexual abuse and trauma, or even suggest mental health problems are directly attributable to lesbian sexuality (Golding 1997). Given this lack of awareness it is not surprising that Stevens & Hall (1988) document ostracism, invasive personal questions, shock, embarrassment, unfriendliness, pity, condescension and fear as typical responses lesbians have received from health care providers.

All of these factors should concern health providers because oppression and invisibility damage health. The reply from those in the caring professions to the question 'Homophobia: why bring it up?' should be that homophobia is itself a health hazard (O'Hanlan et al 1997).

Health professionals can make a positive difference to support the health of lesbian health service users if they are sensitive to the experience of lesbians. It is important that health care providers know how to access research on lesbian health and that heterosexual practitioners become more familiar with lesbian cultures and communities.

Two comprehensive reviews of literature available on lesbian health were by Stevens (1993), who looked at research from 1970 to 1990, and O'Hanlan (1995), who updated the picture to 1995. Between them they have built a long list of references. Many studies, however, have been small and unfunded, conducted by lesbian health activists in local communities. This in no way invalidates these studies because they provide valuable information to be followed up in further research, but it does mean that they will have gone unrecognized by a medical profession which prioritizes writing in clinically oriented peer-reviewed journals. Both overviews of research have a North American focus, but the US and British cultures share similar experiences of oppression and findings in American studies are beginning to be replicated in British journals and reports (Morrissey 1996). Another important source is the volume edited by Stern (1993), published as a result of the success of a special issue of the journal Health Care Women International on lesbian health. Most of the available research focuses on the experiences of white, middle class lesbians. Reflecting the even greater marginalization and invisibility of black lesbians in society, there are few studies which adequately explore cultural experiences of race and sexuality (Cochran & Mays 1988).

While preparation for motherhood is a pressured and vulnerable time for all women, the many inaccuracies which circulate about lesbians due to silencing and stereotyping make it necessary to consider separately the additional needs and experiences of lesbians who choose motherhood.

LESBIAN PARENTHOOD

Parenthood is an area where many assumptions are made about 'family life' and the 'heterosexual norm'. Politicians and the popular media continue to act as if the traditional family still exists, ignoring shifts in societal attitudes and beliefs which, in the 1990s perhaps more than ever, show the family (and parenthood) to be a constantly changing social and cultural construct (Mason 1994, Sandell 1994). There are many ways in which lesbians may be mothers or have a parenting role. A lesbian may have children from a previous heterosexual relationship. She may co-parent a female partner's child(ren). She might adopt or foster. Other lesbians are choosing to become parents and may do so as single women, within lesbian partnerships, or by creating a wider 'family structure' around them which could include lesbian friends, gay male friends, the biological father, and others who have no direct biological connection to the child. Some women choose donor insemination, either by finding a donor themselves and self-inseminating, or arranging insemination through a clinic; others may have sex with a man in order to become pregnant.

The decision to have children is a key one for all women and no practitioner concerned with women's health can afford to ignore the lesbian perspective. Consider the issues in Activity 4.1.

Activity 4.1

Make a list of the dilemmas and decisions for lesbians around parenthood which you think most clearly differ from heterosexual women's experiences.

Kenney & Tash (1993) identify three key areas which may pose challenges for the lesbian woman:

- how to conceive
- how and where to find a lesbian-sensitive health care provider

- how to handle personal, family and lesbian social relationships.

Lesbians may wish to minimize their contact with health care staff because of concerns over negative responses and instead choose non-traditional health services (Harvey, Carr & Bernheine 1989), or they may delay seeking professional care until absolutely necessary. Cultural and social issues specific to the lesbian experience include whether to choose a known or unknown sperm donor, how to balance a co-parenting relationship with a lesbian partner when only one partner is legally recognized as a parent, whether or not to involve the biological father after birth, and overcoming societal assumptions that children live in a heterosexual household.

Lesbians can face hostility from other lesbians or feel isolated from some parts of the lesbian community which is still itself struggling with lesbian parenthood. While lesbians have often been at the forefront of campaigns for improved facilities for women with children, it is only relatively recently that lesbian mothers have become users of these services in any great number. Lesbian-only social venues and events have not traditionally felt the need to make provision for child care and lesbian communities are still adapting to what is sometimes referred to as a 'baby boom'. This can cause difficulties for a new mother who fears ostracism and prejudice from the wider heterosexual society and needs to seek support from a community which understands and reflects her lesbian identity.

Midwives need to be able to direct lesbian clients to lesbian parenting support groups (most major cities now have at least one) and to relevant client care information just as they would for heterosexual women. There is a growing range of literature by and for lesbians which addresses health issues. By accessing these resources, and being encouraged to do so through the inclusion of such items on reading lists in professional education and training, midwives can improve their own understanding of the cultural issues outlined above. It is here that the pertinent issues are likely to be discussed honestly from the inside and to reflect sociocultural influences rather than the practice and experience of maternity care developed in more traditional settings.

Lisa Saffron's (l998) *Challenging conceptions* is a useful practical guide for UK lesbians planning a child by self-insemination. Lesbians are otherwise faced with preparing-for-parenthood books assuming the mother's heterosexuality or books on donor insemination which assume the partner's infertility. Reading relevant stories from other women at this time of change can be empowering:

I needed to read the accounts by women who had done it, to hear what they really thought about it all. I didn't know many women who had DI [donor insemination] babies. Talk of a 'lesbian baby boom' might make sense in the United States, but the numbers in Britain still aren't that great.   (Rodgerson 1994 p. 54)

Cheri Pies' (1985) *Considering parenthood: a workbook for lesbians* is another book which assists lesbians to plan parenthood and to consider the whole balance of personal, social and family relationships. Pies focuses in depth on lifestyle changes and cultural aspects of parenthood which heterosexual couples may never consider in the process of becoming parents, given that heterosexual culture assumes a right to parenthood.

RESPONDING SENSITIVELY TO LESBIANS IN MIDWIFERY PRACTICE

The previous section introduces some of the broader cultural issues associated with lesbian parenthood which can assist midwives in understanding the needs of their lesbian clients. But how women will react and interact with their health care providers from planning conception through to birth is always going to be personal and individual, and many lesbians will make a deliberate choice not to disclose their sexuality. It is not the woman's responsibility to disclose her sexuality in order to receive an equality of health care which is able to incorporate and comprehend her lifestyle and behaviours. There is no way of knowing which women in the general practitioner (GP) surgery waiting area or in the antenatal class are heterosexual and which

are not. Practitioners don't need to ascertain a client's sexuality in order to support her effectively and sensitively; but they do need to ensure they are not assuming heterosexuality. Many midwives will already have supported lesbian mothers, perhaps unknowingly, and have provided excellent care if they have been open and non-judgmental.

Case study 4.1 is included to help apply issues more directly to practice. After reading the scenario, try answering the questions in Activity 4.2.

Case study 4.1

Background
Julie* is white and working class and has lived as a lesbian since her late teens. She was aged 35 at the birth of her first and only child. Julie self-inseminated using a known donor and chose a home birth. Julie conceived within a stable lesbian relationship and her partner provided support and encouragement, but it was not a co-parenting decision. Her partner was not present during inseminations and did not accompany her to consultations. Julie's partner worked at the hospital where Julie saw her consultant and may have been 'outed' as a lesbian had she attended consultations. Julie did not disclose her sexuality at any time to any of the health professionals involved in caring for her throughout the pregnancy and birth. She felt it was not safe for her to say she was a lesbian. Health professionals also did not know that she had self-inseminated. She presented as a single woman.

Planning pregnancy
The pregnancy was carefully planned. Julie did 6 months' research and planning before the first self-insemination. This included putting together her own birth plan, which was a comprehensive plan combining a medical and herbal perspective. Julie had knowledge of and training in herbalism. This process was assisted by Julie making contact with the local home birth group. All other women in this group were white, heterosexual and middle class; they did not know Julie's sexuality. The sperm donor was younger than Julie and she had known him for most of his life. His involvement after the birth would be to see the child but not take on a parenting role. Julie self-inseminated for 7 months, three to six times each month before the first conception. She miscarried at 10 weeks. Julie did not seek medical advice at this stage and instead used herbal treatments. She conceived again after 5 more months of self-insemination, using herbs to promote fertility, a therapy she also found useful throughout the pregnancy.

*Julie is a pseudonym.

Case study 4.1 Continued

Contact with health professionals throughout pregnancy

Julie approached her GP only after the time that the usual tests would be offered. She wished to avoid as many 'invasive' tests as possible. The GP was unhappy and unwilling for Julie to have a home birth because of her age. He told Julie he wanted 'a live baby and a live mother'. The GP referred Julie to midwives and made an appointment for her with a consultant. The consultant, a woman, spoke more positively with Julie about her plans and took her birth plan seriously. The consultant also had concerns about a home birth for a first child. Midwives attached to Julie's local GP practice were supportive but wanted her to have a series of ultrasound scans. Julie agreed and had one early and one late scan. Julie kept all of her antenatal appointments at hospital and with the midwives. She was anaemic and this was monitored through blood tests, folic acid, careful diet and her own use of herbs. There was no pressure on Julie from any health professionals to name the father. Midwives were concerned about the support Julie would have during and after the birth, but remained non-judgmental.

Birth

Midwives were very supportive at the home birth and reassured by the support from other women Julie had chosen to attend the birth—her partner, Julie's mother and a lesbian friend. The midwives continued to be non-judgmental and supportive in the visits they made to Julie's home after the birth when it must have been obvious that Julie was in a lesbian relationship. Julie believes the midwives empowered her. By responding positively to her birth plan they made her feel safe, in control and comfortable. The GP attended on the day of birth and carried out the usual checks.

Postnatal support

Midwives visited regularly for a while, as did a health visitor. Following her refusal to have her baby vaccinated, the GP wrote to Julie to say he was removing her from his list. Julie wrote a detailed letter in response but received no reply.

Discussion on Case study 4.1

The three issues identified by Kenney & Tash (1993)—how to conceive, the need to give careful thought to interactions with health providers and how to balance personal, social and family relationships—are central to the way Julie's experience is described in Case study 4.1. Another woman's story would, of course, have slightly different elements emphasized, but a

Activity 4.2

Look again at Case study 4.1 and answer the following questions:

1. Discuss the ways in which Julie was able to retain power and control over her pregnancy/birth experience.
2. Critically analyse the factors which may have influenced Julie's decision to have her baby at home.
3. Although Julie's birth expectations were fulfilled, reflect again on the scenario and try to identify the factors which may easily have led to a negative birth experience for Julie.

key aspect of parenthood for all lesbians is planning to conceive. This is not only to do with the fact that lesbians are unlikely to be engaged in, or want to engage in, sexual relationships with men and so need to plan insemination, but because oppression contributes the additional pressure of having already to plan at the preconception stage clear relationship structures with other significant adults for when the child is born. Given the lack of legal structures to support lesbian parenting and society's anxiety at lesbians bringing up children, co-parenting options with the biological father to be or a supportive lesbian partner will require careful negotiation, not to mention how to cope with the varied reactions of extended family members. Some lesbian couples decide not to become parents because they fear their own parents' reactions (Kenney & Tash 1993).

Achieving conception if you are a lesbian requires a great deal of forethought and planning. Rodgerson (1994 p. 54) comments: 'The hostility faced by lesbians and gay men who want to be parents is ironic considering how well planned and desperately wanted most of our children are'. Julie undertook detailed research in order to put together a comprehensive birth plan which could include her own knowledge and belief in complementary therapies as well as examples from conventional medical practice. It was important that health professionals respect her birth plan and take it seriously so that she could retain power and choice throughout her pregnancy. A key point is that lesbians are aware that they are already 'outsiders' and therefore disadvantaged within mainstream health care settings, even before they disclose their sexuality.

Julie chose not to disclose her sexuality at any time throughout the pregnancy. Whether or not a woman has experienced negative responses during previous contact with health professionals, and however confident and self-assured she may be in planning and managing her pregnancy, the daily experience of living as a lesbian in a culture where heterosexism and homophobia dominate means that she will often choose to stay silent about her sexuality to protect herself and others close to her from abuse. It is significant that Julie did not seek medical advice after her miscarriage. Avoiding contact with and intervention by health care practitioners and delaying asking for medical advice are consistent findings in numerous research studies on lesbian experiences of health care (e.g. Smith, Johnson & Guenther 1985, Stevens & Hall 1988, Zeidenstein 1990).

This should be of real concern for practitioners and can cause damaging conflicts. A home birth may feel the only option for a lesbian who desires a birth with more intimacy and privacy, and one where she can choose a variety of people to attend the birth without needing to explain their relationship to herself or the child. If she is an 'older' mother she may be advised to have greater medical attention and intervention. This could cause extreme distress for the woman in leaving her at greater risk of receiving prejudicial treatment and disapproval. The explicit support of the midwife is needed in helping the woman to feel relaxed and in control of her birth. Careful use of non-heterosexist language on the midwife's behalf can help to reassure a lesbian client that her professional carer is 'not just another blinkered heterosexual' (Wilton 1996 pp. 129–130) and help to promote open communication so that a lesbian woman can disclose what she wants, including, perhaps, explaining her fears in their specific context.

A woman can be given entirely inappropriate information if communication is not as open and clear as it could be. As Wilton (p. 129) states, 'Even simple questions like "When did you last have sex?" or "What form of contraception do you use?" will not result in appropriate or useful information if "sex" means different sets of activities to the woman and her midwife'. Practitioners cannot properly advise a woman on relationship changes and sexuality after surgery or the life- (and body-) changing experience of childbirth if they do not allow for the possibility that she may not be having sex with a male partner.

Wilton (p. 129) suggests a question such as 'I haven't met your partner yet; does he or she work full-time?' can demonstrate that you are not assuming a client's heterosexuality. This is a useful example, but practitioners may find the repeated use of 'he or she' clumsy in conversation after a while, and if they only see a pregnant mother irregularly they will need to find some way of recording the information they gain from the individual so they can develop their future practice accordingly. Confidentiality of client disclosures is another issue which requires careful attention as the word 'lesbian' on a woman's health records can have serious consequences for her future treatment. For instance, a lesbian who finds she could be infertile may regret a previous disclosure if her status as a lesbian denies her the chance to have her infertility comprehensively and clinically investigated.

An example of positive practice identified during research for this chapter is of a woman GP who was considered by lesbians in her local community to be a 'lesbian-friendly GP'. If a woman disclosed her sexuality, she would encode this information for her own use on the client records. This meant that in all future sessions with the client she could avoid irrelevant questions which could be seen to assume heterosexuality. Lesbians attending the practice felt supported and would talk more honestly about their health as lesbians. By word of mouth, this GP became known as a lesbian-sensitive health care provider, and more lesbians joined her caseload. In turn, through the growing number of lesbians using her practice, the GP gained increased experience and confidence in working with lesbians as an effective lesbian-sensitive health care provider.

Publications

Health practitioners can take steps to adjust heterosexist language structures and improve their familiarity with lesbian culture by reading non-medical material written from a lesbian perspective. The lesbian press (books, newspapers, magazines, journals) and lesbian community support networks are a crucial resource for lesbians and a valuable link for health care providers wanting to improve their care for lesbian health service users. The anxiety involved in contacting mainstream health services means that lesbians turn to their familiar and trusted networks to check facts and to collect advice. Lesbian health workers already familiar with lesbian cultural resources play a key role in circulating research and good practice among lesbian communities. Lesbians should not lose out because of lack of information dissemination to lesbian cultural venues and networks.

Articles on lesbian health have appeared in professional journals across all health specialities. Other key journals for up to date information and research include the Journal of Homosexuality, Journal of Lesbian and Gay Social Services, and Journal of the Gay and Lesbian Medical Association, the world's first peer-reviewed multidisciplinary journal dedicated to lesbian, gay, bisexual and transgendered health. This new journal was launched in April 1997. Professionals themselves need a 'safe space' in which to have work accepted and published, and the editors believe this journal will increase the body of literature available for use in medical school curricula (Gay and Lesbian Medical Association 1997).

Networks

Lesbian health promotion networks have begun to develop in the UK, and the national health promotion group LesBeWell, which produces a bimonthly newsletter Dykenosis, for women who have sex with women, has been particularly

successful. A growth in sexual health projects and programmes in response to HIV/AIDS has also begun to recognize lesbians as a cultural group in need of specialist health services. These services aim to cross the divide between lesbian culture and mainstream health care by providing specialist clinics staffed by health practitioners who are also lesbian. The Bernhard Clinic was established in 1992 within the Department of GenitoUrinary Medicine at Charing Cross Hospital to provide specialist sexual health care to women who have sex with women. The immediate response to the Bernhard Clinic confirmed there was a need for more clinics (Conway & Humphries 1994), and a second lesbian sexual health clinic followed, the Audre Lorde Clinic at the Royal London Hospital. The clinics promote regular breast and gynaecological screening for all lesbians and remove the worry for lesbians that good health promotion and education support provided in their own communities could be compromised by mixed messages received in mainstream health settings. Of the women who have had smears at the two London clinics, 18% have shown abnormalities (Gill 1996).

The quality of health care can also be improved if health providers have a secure environment in which they too can come out as lesbian and gay. Cultural identification is a key concept in building self-esteem for all minority groups. Marginalized communities gain strength from visibility and this can have an important impact on an individual's ability to negotiate access to and receive appropriate health advice. A Canadian family physician practised for many years without identifying a single gay client. When he came out, 15 of his clients also revealed that they were gay (Robb 1996).

Networks of lesbian (and gay) health workers are already in existence within well-established professional associations. The RCN has a Lesbian and Gay Nursing Issues Working Party (Platzer 1993) and the Gay and Lesbian Medical Association in the USA provides a forum for medical students and physicians. These networks, as well as lesbian health promotion networks such as LesBeWell, can be useful contacts for health professionals seeking information and guidance on how to support lesbian health service users. These networks also act to make lesbian and gay issues visible at all levels of medical practice.

Examples of good practice can also be extracted from the voluntary sector and information made available to workers in mainstream health services. Practitioners should be aware that there are self-help groups and community support networks which specifically meet the health needs of lesbians. As well as self-insemination and parenting groups for lesbians, other networks allow for a lesbian-specific focus on experiences of disease and illness. For instance, Cancerlink has a Lesbian Network for lesbians and partners affected by cancer, and Breast Cancer Care is recognizing the importance of diverse cultural experience and expanding its peer support network by actively recruiting lesbian volunteers.

Research

Lesbians remain invisible if research does not recognize the needs of lesbians as a separate population. Research on lesbian health is a sensitive issue and regular review and evaluation of research is necessary to assess gaps in the literature available and to consider good practice issues when conducting research with marginalized groups. Some methodological questions are posed in Platzer & James (1997). Current and future research projects include sponsored research such as that proposed by the US National Gay and Lesbian Health Foundation, which aims 'to develop a national research agenda that could impact national policy' (DeAngelis 1994), and ad hoc research carried out by lesbian academics or activists. Both are needed. Lesbian researchers recently advertising for survey respondents in lesbian community newspapers include McIntosh (1997), investigating experiences of disclosure of sexuality to health professionals among lesbians in the Aberdeen area, and Fish (personal communication, 1997) who is aiming to conduct the biggest ever lesbian health survey in the UK. Fish (1997)

is researching lesbians' experiences and perceptions of breast and cervical screening and how lesbians view their risk of these cancers, especially in relation to heterosexual women.

Lesbian health is more than sexual health

In the same way that mainstream women's health programmes and government health targets have been crticized for their lack of sociocultural awareness, for their over-emphasis on women's reproductive potential and for reducing women's health concerns to a collection of diseased female bodily parts (Hastie, Porch & Brown 1995), it is important to move beyond the view that lesbian health is centred on *sexual* behaviours. Should specialist lesbian health clinics be based within departments of genitourinary medicine, thus continuing a focus on sexual health and sexual behaviours, or should they take a wider focus to embrace all aspects of lesbian culture? Lesbians surveyed by Trippet & Bain (1993) cited the failure of traditional health care to provide holistic care as one reason for not seeking contact with health services. While lesbian sexual health clinics can offer greater potential for holistic care for lesbians by promoting an environment which is encouraging and affirming of lesbian experience rather than embarrassed or intolerant, such clinics may continue to isolate women who identify as lesbian but are not necessarily 'sexual' with women. Lesbian culture emphasizes that 'lesbian' is a sociocultural identity as well as a sexual identity. It is also a self-defined identity and many women remain invisible within the category of lesbians because they do not conform to stereotypical and assumed patterns of behaviour which are imposed both inside and outside of lesbian communities.

Lesbian communities should be invited to set the agenda on where and how lesbian-positive health services should be developed. Separate, specialist clinics may not always be the preferred option as they can reinforce the isolation and otherness of already marginalized groups. Respondents in Mind's survey of lesbian, gay and bisexual mental health service users stressed the responsibility of the NHS in ensuring that *all* of its services are accessible and relevant to *all* groups within the communities it serves (Golding 1997).

CONCLUSIONS

The key to the development and dissemination of good practice is the integration of sexuality and sexual orientation issues within all areas of medical and health professionals' education and training. Assumptions need to be challenged constantly, both in education and training and during all interactions with women. Culturally sensitive health care acknowledges the adverse effects on health of marginalization and oppression and places health in a wider social context where what is meant by 'health' is constantly in need of redefinition. A culturally sensitive health service needs to be a constantly evolving service and cannot operate successfully if health care providers, on having their awareness raised, again lapse into complacency and stereotyping. Increased visibility of lesbians as a specific *group* in health care should also support a focus on the needs of women as *individuals*, thus reflecting the philosophy of a woman-centred approach to care as embraced in Changing Childbirth (DoH 1993). Pregnant women cannot always be neatly classified and assigned to one or another cultural category. Lesbians may or may not identify themselves as lesbians publicly, but whether or not a woman's sexuality is known by her health care provider she should receive a quality of care which recognizes options other than heterosexuality. Individuals live very varied lifestyles, may belong to many communities and prioritize different cultural experiences and identities at different times.

Supportive responses to the needs of lesbians as health service users and providers of care must cut across all health services and departments and all ages, and must not become hidden as a subcategory within areas of medicine, midwifery and nursing which already specialize in women's health. The new lesbian mother will one day be the parent of a child in the paediatric ward (Perrin & Kulkin 1996). This same woman will also demand her rights to be positively supported as a lesbian within maternity care, health care of the elderly services and other professions allied to health (Connolly 1996).

At the time of writing, the RCM has not yet selected the themes which will be taken forward for development into policy guidance documents, although 'lesbian mothers' has been one of this year's suggested themes. Midwives and their lesbian clients should be encouraged to write to the RCM to document their experiences and practice-related questions. Some questions for midwives which may benefit from the policy support of the RCM are included within the practice check detailed in Box 4.2.

Box 4.2 Practice check

- During your professional training have the needs of lesbian clients been discussed and to what response?
- Do you know of a midwifery colleague or a colleague in a related field who has come out as lesbian or gay within a professional context?
- If you are a lesbian midwife, are you able to contribute your understanding of lesbian health resources and networks for the benefit of other practitioners? What would have to happen to make this possible and safe?
- How can an integrated package of care be introduced which is culturally sensitive and appropriate for a lesbian client across the range of health providers a pregnant woman will need to consult?
- Would you feel confident to challenge the homophobia and heterosexism of colleagues in the rest of the care team?

Summary

Lesbians do not have the same access to health care as heterosexual women because of heterosexism and homophobia. Oppression and invisibility damages health—homophobia is itself a health hazard. Lesbians may tend to avoid contact with and intervention by health care practitioners and delay asking for medical advice for fear of negative reactions.

Prejudice, false assumptions and stereotyping have created an image of the lesbian as 'unfit mother', whether a biological or non-biological parent. Family and parenthood are constantly changing social and cultural constructs—there are many ways in which lesbians may be mothers or have a parenting role.

Summary (*Continued*)

Lesbians may not feel safe to disclose their sexuality even in an apparently supportive environment—health care professionals can be supportive by not assuming heterosexuality. The explicit support of the midwife is needed to help the woman feel relaxed and in control of her birth, including careful use of non-heterosexist language.

Confidentiality should be maintained on patient records—use of the word 'lesbian' on records may be prejudicial to a woman's future health care, although it should not be.

Health care providers need to access research on lesbian health and become more familiar with lesbian cultures and communities. Health care providers can access information from a range of lesbian health networks which have begun to develop in the UK.

Health research should recognize the needs of lesbians as a separate population.

The quality of health care can be improved if health care providers have a secure environment in which they too can come out as lesbian or gay. Lesbian communities should be invited to set the agenda on where and how lesbian-positive health services should be developed.

APPENDIX: USEFUL CONTACTS

Stonewall, 16 Clerkenwell Close, London EC1R0AA
Tel: 0171 336 8860
A campaign organization working for lesbian and gay equality.

LesBeWell, PO Box 4048, Moseley, Birmingham B13 8DP
A national lesbian health promotion group.

London Lesbian and Gay Switchboard,
(24 hours a day)
Tel: 0171 837 7324
Provides information and advice on all issues relating to lesbians, gay men and bisexuals; can refer callers to organizations and groups in their local area.

London Lesbian Line
Tel: 0171 251 6911
Provides information and advice for lesbians; can refer callers to lesbian lines throughout the UK and Ireland.

A useful website address at:
http://glma.org/publications/jglme/j.htm

REFERENCES

Caplan P (ed) 1987 The cultural construction of sexuality. Tavistock, London

Cochran S D, Mays V M 1988 Disclosure of sexual preference to physicians by black lesbian and bisexual women. Western Journal of Medicine 149(5):616–619

Connolly L 1996 Long-term care and hospice: the special needs of older gay men and lesbians. Journal of Gay and Lesbian Social Services 5(1):77–91

Conway M, Humphries E 1994 Bernhard clinic meeting need in lesbian sexual health care. Nursing Times 10–16 August:40–41

DeAngelis T 1994 First data released on lesbian health [WWW] http://www.scn.org/fp/l/lgbt/neighborhoods/wellness/lesmenthelth.txt (23 August 1997). Originally published in Monitor July 1994:53

DoH (Department of Health) 1992 The health of the nation: a strategy for health in England. HMSO, London

DoH (Department of Health) 1993 Changing Childbirth: report of the Expert Maternity Group, vol 1 and 2. HMSO, London

Eliason M, Donelan C, Randall C 1993 Lesbian stereotypes. In: Sterny P N (ed) Lesbian health: what are the issues? Taylor & Francis, London, pp 41–54

Fish J 1997 Letter. Diva (letter), December:5

Gay and Lesbian Medical Association 1997 Journal of the Gay and Lesbian Medical Association [WWW] http://www.glma.org/journalvision.html:(23 August 1997)

Gill E 1996 Three cheers for smears. Diva, October: 54–55

Golding J 1997 Without prejudice: Mind lesbian, gay and bisexual mental health awareness research. Mind, London

Good R S 1976 The gynecologist and the lesbian. Clinical Obstetrics and Gynecology 19:473–482

Harvey S M, Carr C, Bernheine, S 1989 Lesbian mothers: health care experiences. Journal of Nurse Midwifery 34(3):115–119

Hastie N, Porch, S, Brown, L 1995 Doing it ourselves: promoting women's health as feminist action. In: Griffin G (ed) Feminist activism in the 1990s. Taylor & Francis, London, pp 13–27

HMSO 1988 Local Government Act. HMSO, London

HMSO 1990 Human Fertilization and Embryology Act. HMSO, London

Kaufman T 1998 Diva (letter), February:4

Kenney J W, Tash D T 1993 Lesbian childbearing couples: dilemmas and decisions. In: Stern P N (ed) Lesbian health: what are the issues? Taylor & Francis, London, pp 119–129

Kitzinger C 1987 The social construction of lesbianism. Sage, London

McIntosh J 1997 Request for participants in Pink Paper 25 July:29

Mason A 1994 The scientific baby and the social family: the possibilities of lesbian and gay parenting. In: Healey E, Mason A (eds) Stonewall 25: the making of the lesbian and gay community in Britain. Virago, London, pp 137–149

Mason A, Watson M 1997 Equality 2000. Stonewall, London

Morrissey M 1996 Attitudes of practitioners to lesbian, gay and bisexual clients. British Journal of Nursing 12–25 September:980–982

Murphy B C 1992 Educating mental health professionals about gay and lesbian issues. Journal of Homosexuality 22(3–4):229–246

O'Hanlan K A 1995 Lesbian health and homophobia: perspectives for the treating obstetrician/gynecologist. [WWW] http://www.ohanlan.com/lhr.htm (15 November 1997) Also published in Current Problems in Obstetrics, Gynecology and Fertility 18:94–133

O'Hanlan K A, Lock J, Robertson P, Cabaj R P, Schatz B, Nemrow P 1997 Homophobia as a health hazard: Report of the Gay and Lesbian Medical Association [WWW] http://www.ohanlan.com/phobiaiihzd.htm (15 November 1997)

Perrin E C, Kulkin H 1996 Pediatric care for children whose parents are gay or lesbian. Pediatrics 97(5):629–635

Pies C 1985 Considering parenthood: a workbook for lesbians. Spinsters Ink, San Francisco

Platzer, H 1993 Ethics: nursing care of gay and lesbian patients. Nursing Standard 13–19 January:34–37

Platzer, H, James T 1997 Methodological issues in conducting sensitive research on lesbian and gay men's experience of nursing care. Journal of Advanced Nursing 25(3):626–633

Reagan P (1981) The interaction of health professionals and their lesbian clients. Patient Counselling and Health Education 3(1):21–25

Robb N 1996 Medical school seeks to overcome 'invisibility' of gay patients, gay issues in curriculum. Canadian Medical Association Journal 15 September:765–770

Rodgerson G 1994 Review of Challenging conceptions: planning a family by self-insemination by Saffron L. Diva, June:54

Saffron L 1998 Challenging conceptions: planning a family by self-insemination, 2nd edn. Saffron, London

Sandell J 1994 The cultural necessity of queer families. Bad Subjects 12:March 1994 [WWW] http://english-www.hss.cmu.edu/bs/12/sandell.html (15 November 1997)

Smith B 1993 Homophobia: why bring it up? In: Abelove H, Barale M A, Halperin, D M (eds) The Lesbian and Gay Studies Reader. Routledge, London, pp 99–102

Smith E M, Johnson S R, Guenther S M 1985 Health care attitudes and experiences during gynecologic care among lesbians and bisexuals. American Journal of Public Health 75:1085–1087

Stacey J 1997 Teratologies: A cultural study of cancer. Routledge, London

Stern P N (ed) 1993 Lesbian health: what are the issues? Taylor & Francis, London

Stevens P E 1993 Lesbian health care research: a review of the literature from 1970 to 1990. In: Stern P N (ed) Lesbian health: what are the issues? Taylor & Francis, London, pp 1–30

Stevens P, Hall J 1988 Stigma, health beliefs, and experiences with health care in lesbian women. Image: Journal of Nursing Scholarship 20:69–73

Swissler M A 1997 Breast cancer—out of the closet. Curve, March:35

Trippet S E, Bain J 1993 Reasons American lesbians fail to seek traditional health care. In: Stern P N (ed) Lesbian health: what are the issues? Taylor & Francis, London, pp 55–63

Weeks J 1985 Sexuality and its discontents. Meanings, myths and modern sexualities. Routledge & Kegan Paul, London

Wilton T 1995 Lesbian studies: setting an agenda. Routledge, London

Wilton T 1996 Caring for the lesbian client: homophobia and midwifery. British Journal of Midwifery 4(3):126–131

Zeidenstein L 1990 Gynecological and childbearing needs of lesbians. Journal of Nurse Midwifery 35(1):10–18

5

Ethical dilemmas in midwifery practice

Janet L Charity   Beverley A Ord

CHAPTER CONTENTS

This chapter has the following aims:

- to develop midwives' intuitive knowledge of ethics
- to explore the language of ethics
- to apply ethical decision-making frameworks to dilemmas in midwifery practice
- to reflect upon ethical dilemmas in relation to reproductive technology

INTRODUCTION

This chapter explores ethical dilemmas which may confront midwives in their clinical practice. Definitions of ethics and morals are provided and a description of an ethical dilemma is given. Approaches to, and frameworks for, ethical decision making are offered; the frameworks selected will then be applied to real-life scenarios.

The contents of this chapter are intended for midwives and students who wish to develop their intuitive knowledge of ethics. Intuition is interpreted by Thompson & Melia (1988) as 'an integrative ability of the imagination to take the confusing variety of data and phenomena in a situation and make some kind of sense out of them' (p. 20). As intuition is an important starting point for midwives, a more simplistic version considers that midwives act in accordance with previous experiences and or because it 'feels right', without necessarily any formal learning in the area of ethics. This version is endorsed by Douglas (1991) who considers that, in the past, there have been assumptions that ethically 'correct' decisions can be made without such formal input. Kohner (1996) asserts that practitioners need to develop an awareness and understanding of ethics as it is argued that formal input in relation to ethics will contribute positively towards a midwife's accountability (see Ch. 6).

Primary sources of authors who have written in depth on the subject of ethics have been utilized throughout this chapter and it is not the intention of the current authors to supersede these in any way. The purpose of this work is to bring together the development of a knowledge of ethics, incorporating the initial stance of intuition, and ultimately explore an ethical decision-making framework which midwives can make use of in order to inform their autonomous decisions.

The latter part of this chapter is focused upon an overview of the ethical challenges for midwives in relation to women who have undergone assisted conception. This overview seeks to provide the midwife with an understanding of the dilemmas, which both the woman and the midwife may be confronted with, from their first interaction in the context of the provision of maternity services.

There are many contemporary issues relating to a midwife's practice which make a knowledge of ethics essential rather than just an option. The outcomes of programmes of education leading to admission to Part 10 of the register state that student midwives have to achieve 'an understanding of the ethical issues relating to midwifery practice and the responsibilities which these impose on the midwife's professional practice' (UKCC 1998 p. 13). The numerous developments, which also incorporate ethical issues and thus have impact on midwifery practice, include the review of the maternity services (DoH 1993). This review portrays the ethical principle of autonomy as the main focus of the recommendations contained within it. Choice and control are two essential ethical issues that are embodied within the principle of autonomy. The NHS Patient's Charter in relation to maternity services implicitly refers to the principle of autonomy also, by stating the rights of women in relation to the care they can expect (DoH 1996a). Risk management within the NHS is also considered to be an important activity and is concerned with, amongst other aspects, the reduction of loss of life (DoH 1996b). Risk management is clearly related to the Code of professional conduct (UKCC 1992); The Code affirms that midwives must safeguard and promote the well-being of women. The final development to be considered is in relation to reproductive technology, which is governed by the Human Fertilisation and Embryology Act 1990 (Morgan & Lee 1991). The rights of women and avoidance of the causation of potential harm are embraced by the Human Fertilisation and Embryology Authorities's Code of practice (1995), which provides guidelines for all practitioners involved. The aforementioned developments must be considered in conjunction with the fact that women receive more information and are much more articulate than ever before (Richards 1997).

It is evident, therefore, that the preceding developments demand a knowledge of ethics. Fryer (1995 p. 341) further qualifies how useful such a knowledge may be as follows:

- ethical enquiry and debate are essential to the professional practice of midwifery
- an understanding of ethics within a programme of education provides an opportunity to explore the wider implications of autonomy in practice for both midwives and women in childbirth
- codes of practice and conduct should be used to facilitate ethical reasoning rather than to provide some moral judgement of behaviour
- midwives need to combine an understanding of the ethical principles underlying professional codes of practice and conduct, with a greater appreciation of ethical and legal boundaries, if they are to contribute effectively to any ethical debate.

In addition to the benefits highlighted by Fryer, a knowledge of ethics can positively assist midwives with the avoidance of prejudice in the workplace (see Chs 3 and 4), and may also assist supervisors of midwives, as their role embraces supporting midwives with ethical dilemmas (see Ch. 10).

Midwives have always been confronted with ethical issues and dilemmas. However, what may be less familiar to midwives is the language of ethics and it is critical that familiarity with the language is gained to contribute effectively towards any ethical debate. As part of a professional group, midwives encounter situations and dilemmas of a moral kind which exceed the experience of lay people and therefore Hussey (1996) argues that a heightened sensitivity and improved ability to reason and decide ethically can only benefit the midwifery profession further.

THE MEANING OF ETHICS, MORALS AND ETHICAL DILEMMA

It is necessary to understand what the word 'ethics' means. Purtilo (1993 p. 6) defines it as 'a systematic reflection on and analysis of morality'. This is, in fact, what midwives are constantly undertaking within their every day professional practice. A further definition is offered by Jones (1994 p. 15), as she considers that ethics is 'the application of processes and theories of moral philosophy to a "real situation". It is concerned with the basic principles and concepts that guide human beings in thought and action, and which underline their values'.

Reflection and morality are embodied within both of these definitions. All midwives are readily familiar with the concept of reflection, but there is a need to consider what morality is. Thompson & Melia (1988 p. 2) define morals as 'the standards of behaviour actually held or followed by individuals and groups' compared with ethics, which they define as 'the science or study of morals'. Both terms 'ethics' and 'morals' can and still are used interchangeably and this is the stance taken within this chapter.

Tschudin (1986 p. 118) describes the features of a dilemma as follows: 'A problem can be solved, but a dilemma cannot be solved; there is only a choice between two equally difficult, or bad, alternatives'. From this description it is evident that, when midwives are faced with often-complex dilemmas, an ethical decision-making framework would provide a supportive function.

The next part of this chapter now focuses upon an overarching approach to ethics, which provides the background to ethical decision-making frameworks.

Approaches to ethics

Ethics is viewed by Beauchamp & Childress (1989) as a generic term for several ways of examining moral life; therefore approaches to ethics require demarcation. Use is made of one of the two approaches discussed within these authors' work, specifically normative ethics. Within this approach, ethical theories are used in an attempt to determine which actions are right and which are wrong and these may be applied to dilemmas which occur within midwifery practice. This approach, when combined with methods of analysis, is known as 'applied normative ethics'. The second approach is termed 'non-normative ethics', which includes descriptive and metaethics. These are concerned with factual investigation and analysis of the language and concepts of ethics respectively, and will not be focused upon further within this chapter.

Frameworks for moral reasoning

As stated previously, the approach 'applied normative ethics' makes use of ethical theories and methods of analysis. In conjunction with this approach, the concept of a framework for moral reasoning requires exploration, as it ultimately serves to guide the midwife in decision making and the right thing to do. The Code of professional conduct (UKCC 1992) is considered to be a framework for moral reasoning. It was formulated with regard to the broad ethical principles embraced by the profession (Hussey 1996) and provides the standard expected for professional behaviour (ENB 1997). Hussey identifies the following functions that might be fulfilled by the Code:

1. *Guidance*—codes serve to aid, guide and facilitate the professionals in their work.

2. *Regulation*—codes prescribe some of the 'role norms' of the professional group: the moral

responsibilities, standards of correct behaviour and values necessitated by the peculiar demands and licences of the profession.

3. *Discipline*—code of conduct allows transgressions to be identified and justifies penalties, thus becoming an instrument of the authority of a governing body, where such exists.

4. *Protection*—to the extent that codes of conduct perform functions 1, 2 and 3 (above), they also perform the function of protecting the public in general and those who become patients in particular.

5. *Information*—to the extent that a code is known outside a professional group, it tells clients, colleagues, employers and society what standards to expect, so promoting confidence and trust.

6. *Proclamation*—the very existence of a code proclaims that the group aspires to the status of a profession, with moral respectability and autonomy.

7. *Negotiation*—the code can serve as a tool in negotiations and disputes with professional colleagues, employers, governments, etc., by explaining or justifying a stance or course of action.

However, the Code of professional conduct is not without its critics. Clarke (1996) claims that it contains ambiguous statements, which at first glance could appear to be deceptively simple, but which, in reality, are difficult to interpret. Furthermore, Hussey (1996) emphasizes that sometimes the ethical principles within the Code are implicit rather than explicit. In addition, the clauses within the Code are often quoted to and by midwives, yet an actual forum for discussion of the 16 clauses contained within it could be limited and may be perceived as being used in a punitive way only. These criticisms provide the justification for an explicit ethical framework to support and justify courses of action taken by a midwife when confronted with an ethical dilemma.

One framework for moral reasoning is outlined within the work of Beauchamp & Childress (1989), who describe four levels within a framework. Edwards (1996) elaborates upon

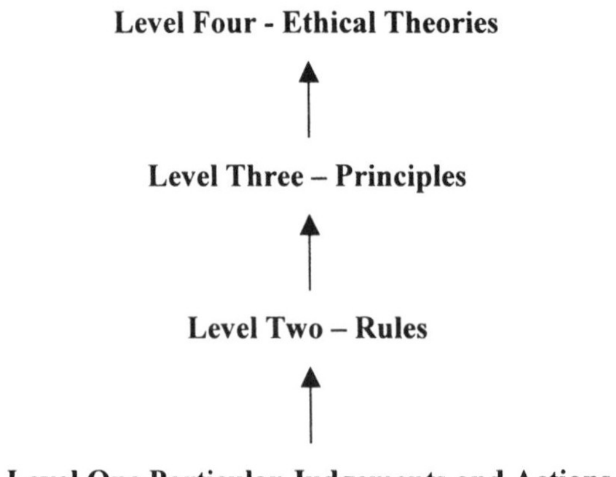

Level Four - Ethical Theories

↑

Level Three – Principles

↑

Level Two – Rules

↑

Level One Particular Judgements and Actions

Figure 5.1   Four level approach (From Beauchamp & Childress 1986 p. 6).

this frame-work and provides examples of application. This four level approach makes use of the approach to ethics previously referred to, namely normative applied ethics. This four level approach is outlined in Figure 5.1. Further description of these levels will now be provided and then applied to a midwifery case.

Level one—judgements and actions. When midwives are confronted with an ethical dilemma, they make a particular judgement and decide upon a course of action. This makes use of their intuition, and usually midwives reflect on their own experiences or that of a colleague's.

Level two—rules. The rules defined within this framework are the rules of veracity (truth telling), of privacy, of confidentiality, and of fidelity (promise keeping). Midwives are familiar with these rules as they are embodied within the Code of professional conduct (UKCC 1992) and Guidelines for professional practice (UKCC 1996), which assists in the interpretation of the Code.

Level three—principles. There are four main ethical principles which are usually applied within health care and midwifery practice specifically. These are:

1. *Autonomy*—concerned with self-governance, liberty rights and individual choice.

2. *Beneficence*—concerned with promoting the welfare of clients. Also, doing your best for others.
3. *Non-maleficence*—concerned with the non-infliction of harm on others. 'Primum non nocere' – above all, do no harm.
4. *Justice*—concerned with fairness. Equal distribution of benefits and burdens (Beauchamp & Childress 1989, Richards 1997).

Level four—ethical theories. There are two popular Western ethical theories, namely *utilitarian* theory and *deontological theory*. These theories are summarized and differentiated below:

1. *Utilitarian theory*—this theory is also referred to as 'teleological theory' (from the Greek '*telos*', meaning end or purpose). It is concerned with the consequences of an action and maximizing the amount of happiness for the greatest number (Thompson & Melia 1988). Raphael (1981 p. 41) declares that utilitarianism has a 'beautiful simplicity' and that the nineteenth-century utilitarians' Jeremy Bentham and others, particularly John Stuart Mills, held that 'the standard of morally right action is the increase of happiness (or the decrease of unhappiness) as much as possible for as many people as possible. Criticism of this particular ethical theory is concerned with defining the word 'happiness' and also the fact that, for some individuals, some unhappiness may be inflicted.

Examples of the application of utilitarian theory are evident in many aspects of midwifery practice, an example of which is antenatal screening tests. By offering all women screening tests to detect fetal anomalies, the consequences are that women will be prepared for the birth of a handicapped child or choose to have the pregnancy terminated. Proud (1995) reiterates that another argument in favour of such routine screening is for monitoring the 'at risk' fetus and thereby improving perinatal outcome. Conversely, unhappiness may be evoked for some women as anxiety is associated with the choice to have or not have such a test. In addition, it may be difficult to calculate the long term consequences of antenatal screening tests as the short term actions are usually focused upon.

Utilitarianism is sometimes referred to as 'consequentialism'. Seedhouse (1989) clearly differentiates between these, and considers that consequentialism is the more global ethical theory and, within this theory, the rightness or wrongness of an act should be judged only on the ground of whether its consequences produce more benefits than disadvantages. Utilitarianism is a major subset of this global category and hence 'the greatest good of the greatest number' is derived. Seedhouse (1989 p. 109) emphasizes the artificiality of distinguishing between utilitarianism and consequentialism so they could be used interchangeably, on a parallel with the terms ethics and morals.

2. *Deontological theory*—Deontology is derived from the Greek work '*deon*', meaning duty. Kantian deontology was formulated by an 18 century German metaphysician, Immanuel Kant. He formulated his theory in terms of the right thing to do *without regard to the consequences*. Kant's theory reflects that to act morally is concerned with acting out of respect for duty. Within this theory, moral rules are applied to everyone. The main example cited is that one should never lie, regardless of the situation or the circumstances (Henry 1996). Kant believed that rational beings were bound by what he called the 'supreme moral law' (Gillon 1992) and this supreme moral law could be expressed in several ways:

- the agent should 'act only on that maxim through which you can at the same time will that it should become a universal law'
- 'no person should be treated merely as a means, but always as an end' (Gillon 1992 p. 16).

The first point emphasizes that an action can be moral only it can be applied to everyone as a universal law. The second point concerns Kant's regard for human beings as he believed them to be autonomous and rational moral agents and should be respected as such (Edwards 1996). The application of this theory is evident within the Code of professional conduct (UKCC 1992) previously referred to. The clause relating to confidentiality states: 'Protect all confidential information concerning patients and clients obtained in the course of professional practice' (Clause 10). However, the UKCC encompasses utilitarian theory as it recognizes that the consequences of upholding confidentiality in some instances might not be appropriate. Child protection issues, for example, raise the need to disclose in the best interests of the child. The Code, therefore, provides guidance in this instance regarding when disclosure should be made.

A comparison of both theories, utilitarianism and Kantian deontology, is within an exemplar by Henry (1996). She cites the example of routine patterns of antenatal care and, in relation to introducing a team approach to care, underpins this team approach with utilitarian theory (concerned with consequences and maximizing happiness for the majority). The assertion with the team approach would be that women have continuity of carer, greater choice and more control in the decision-making process. However, women receiving traditional care may not enjoy the benefits as previously detailed in relation to 'the team approach' group. From a utilitarian perspective, the consequences of a team approach would benefit the majority, yet in the process of introducing change some women could be denied the benefits of this type of care and inequality could occur.

Henry (1996) then contrasts this approach by utilizing deontological theory. Within this theory, achieving a 'good' end (continuity of carer, greater choice, more control), will never justify the means, as in the former theory. Therefore, the introduction of a change that is considered to provide a better outcome would be offered equally, to all women, regardless of consequences. The consequences of this course of action could well mean poor preparation of change and poor outcomes. It will be obvious to the reader that this would not be desirable as the consequences of this nature could have far-reaching effects on the provision of midwifery care. Gillon (1992) also criticizes this theory for its excessive formalism.

Now that the four levels within this approach have been reviewed, Case study 5.1 is used for the application of these levels.

 Case study 5.1

Within a busy delivery suite, a woman who is in labour has identified to her named midwife that incorrect information has been recorded within her previous records. The error is related to histology results following a spontaneous abortion. The histology results contained details that inferred maternal blame, and the woman was very upset and angry. She asks the midwife to correct the error immediately; her psychological well-being is clearly affected. The midwife is also caring for another woman who is in active labour.

Level one—judgements. Midwife A may judge that the incorrect information will not affect the woman's physical care. It would not be a priority to deal with the records at this particular point as a consequence of dealing with it would take up valuable time, possibly to the detriment of the other women in the midwife's care. Midwife B may judge that the error highlighted by the woman is so important to her psychological well-being that she seeks to address the situation immediately, as demanded by the woman. Moral judgements have been made in both instances, based on the midwife's intuitive stance.

Level two—rules. It could be reasoned that in relation to midwife A's decision, the rule that has particular relevance in terms of supporting decision making is that of veracity (truth telling). The midwife will have been honest during the discussion with the woman and will have expressed the need to maintain the safety of both women receiving care. The rule of veracity, therefore, supports the judgement made at level one.

With reference to the decision made by midwife B, it is asserted that the rule supporting the decision-making process is also that of truth telling, in addition to that of fidelity (promise keeping). The midwife has acknowledged that an error has been made (veracity) and makes a promise (fidelity) in order to remedy the psychological distress the woman is experiencing.

The rules of confidentiality and privacy are not considered to have particular relevance in relation to this scenario.

Level three—principles. Both midwives could claim that their decisions are supported by the principles of beneficence and non-maleficence (see p. 81). Midwife A believes that she would be promoting the welfare of both clients, and seeks to avoid harm by not neglecting the physical care of both women. These principles also support midwife B's action, as the welfare of the woman involved is paramount and no further psychological harm is inflicted.

The principle of justice also supports midwife A's decision, as this midwife considers that there is a duty of care to both women. The principle of autonomy would be a priority to midwife B, as this midwife considers the woman's right to have her records corrected to be of paramount importance.

Level four—theories. Utilitarian theory has informed midwife A's decision not to take immediate action in relation to the woman's records. Maximizing happiness for the majority has been achieved through this decision. The majority in this instance may be viewed as the woman, the other woman in the midwife's care and midwifery colleagues who would have been required to provide care to the other woman if this decision was reversed. The consequences were considered by this midwife and the woman's physical care was considered to be the immediate priority. However, by utilizing this theory, the midwife's decision may have considerable impact on the woman's psychological well-being.

Kantian deontology has informed midwife B's decision to take immediate action. This theory upholds the moral rule of promise keeping without regard to the consequences. This promise must be upheld and supports the theoretical stance that, in formulating a rule, it should become a universal law—that is, be applied to everyone. By following a deontological stance, however, the midwife could be compromising the care of the other woman. This analysis is also supported by Henry (1996) who highlights that this theory cannot be adhered to in absolute terms in all circumstances.

Through the application of both ethical theories to the scenario portrayed, it is evident that the decision making could be problematic and may not always provide satisfactory answers to the dilemma posed. Midwives need to make use of both theories, whereby decision making is informed by the formulation of rules, and consider also the consequences of the action to be taken.

When using this four level approach, the use of intuition (level one) is a significant starting point in terms of decision making. Levels two and three (rules and principles) challenge further the midwife's original decision. With the application of level four (ethical theories), it may not be possible to make a decision based on one theory alone. A further area of concern regarding this four level approach which affects midwives is the lack of explicit reference to the Code of professional conduct (UKCC 1992). Despite its critics, the Code needs to be referred to when considering dilemmas.

SEEDHOUSE'S ETHICAL GRID

Seedhouse (1989) created a framework for ethical decision making with health professionals in mind (see Fig. 5.2) and considers that this framework is a precis of the elements necessary for thorough moral reasoning. The grid is depicted in four coloured layers; blue, red, green and black (depicted in Fig. 5.2 by different shading), which will be referred to as the inner layer, second layer, third layer and outer layer respectively (Marsh 1996). Seedhouse & Lovell (1992) describe each layer as follows:

- *the inner layer*—(equates to the blue layer) the principles behind health work
- *the second layer*—(equates to the red layer) the duties he believes he has
- *the third layer*—(equates to the green layer) the general nature of the outcome to be achieved
- *the outer layer*—(equates to the black layer) the pertinent practical features

Each layer contains a number of boxes (see Fig. 5.2) for consideration during the decision-making process. The midwife may make use of some or all of the boxes within one or all of the layers. Seedhouse (1989) emphasizes that the

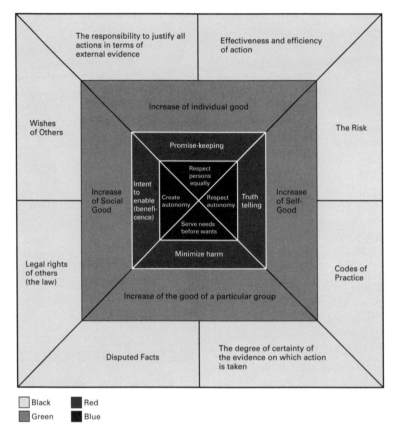

Figure 5.2 The ethical grid (From Seedhouse 1989 p. 141 Ethics, the heart of health care, Copyright John Wiley & Sons Ltd. Reproduced with permission.)

preferred manner of use depends upon the practitioner, which gives midwives the opportunity to exercise their autonomy. Seedhouse gives the following recommendations in relation to the use of the grid, which midwives may find useful.

• Consider the issue intuitively, without reference to the grid. Try to understand the extent of the ramifications of possible action. Clarify the issue by key aspects. Attempt to list basic pros and cons of the various options for action. Arrive at an initial intuitive position.

• Consider the grid. Consider the first layer, which is felt to be the most significant. This will often be the (inner) blue layer since this layer contains the rationale of work for health, and no genuine health work intervention can ignore every box of the (inner) blue layer.

• Consider all other levels of the grid, selecting—after appropriate weighing and balancing—those boxes which appear to offer the most appropriate solution (that is, those which seem most likely to produce the highest degree of morality).

• Arrange the boxes 'over' the dilemma, (that is, apply them to the mental picture of the proposed intervention). In this way, a course of action will have been decided, and the means to justify it in moral terms will be available (Seedhouse 1989 p. 142).

As stated previously when exploring the four level approach, two midwives may arrive at different decisions following analysis of an ethical dilemma. The use of Seedhouse's grid enables midwives to gain further support for their decisions in terms of the highest degree of morality. Whenever a dilemma occurs, the midwife may refer to the grid—this could be immediately when confronted with a situation, or after the event, in order to reflect upon the incident.

Application to midwifery

Seedhouse (1989) affirms that the grid comes to life only when applied to real situations. A number of Case studies will now be presented. The grid will be applied to Case studies 5.2 and 5.3, demonstrating how two midwives may arrive at different decisions. The remaining Case studies 5.4 and 5.5 will afford midwives with the opportunity for discussion with colleagues or as an exercise in reflective learning which may meet the requirements for post-registration education and practice (PREP). The dilemma will be analysed in accordance with the authors' perception.

Case study 5.2: Termination of pregnancy

At first sight, within Case scenario 5.2, there does not appear to be a need for the use of an ethical decision-making framework. The midwife could claim the right to exercise a conscientious objection (UKCC 1992). It has been highlighted, however, that there is no statutory definition of conscientious objection and this may cause difficulty for some midwives (RCM 1996).

 Case study 5.2

Ann is pregnant for the first time. The pregnancy was planned and Ann had been attempting to conceive for the past 18 months. Both Ann and her partner were very excited about the pregnancy. Routine ultrasound at 18 weeks' gestation revealed the condition gastroschisis. Advice was given to the couple regarding the fact that the abdominal defect may be operable but that a number of operations would be required and it was difficult to predict the long term consequences.

Ann requested a termination of pregnancy and is now on the labour suite.

The midwife is confronted with the dilemma of providing care for Ann, as the midwife does not agree with the reason for Ann's termination of pregnancy.

The dilemma that is asserted within this scenario is that the midwife can either provide care for this woman or not provide care for this woman. Two sets of reasoning are offered, utilizing a step-by-step approach within the grid.

Midwife A—the midwife who provides care for Ann. This is the initial intuitive stance taken. The midwife feels that a duty of care is owed. The midwife does not personally agree to the reason for this termination, yet does not feel strongly enough to raise a conscientious objection and respects the woman's decision.

- *The inner layer.* Midwife A 'respects autonomy'. Autonomy is a major part of the core rationale of the International code of ethics for midwives (see Appendix, p. 92). The midwife acknowledges that there is also the 'creation of autonomy' through the Abortion Act 1967 as amended within the Human Fertilisation and Embryology Act 1990 (Morgan & Lee 1991). This Act provides Ann with the option to terminate the pregnancy. The box 'serve needs before wants' is also fulfilled by the midwife supporting Ann, as her psychological needs are paramount.
- *The second layer.* The box 'intent to enable (beneficence)' is the ultimate goal for this midwife by providing Ann with support during the termination of pregnancy. Beneficence may be considered in conjunction with 'minimize harm', although the midwife recognizes that Ann may still experience unintentional harm from a bio/psycho/social/perspective. 'Promise keeping' has already been fulfilled by the two registered medical practitioners who were satisfied that the requirements of the Abortion Act were met. The midwife would be seen, therefore, to be working within a collaborative and co-operative manner with these health care professionals (UKCC 1992) by supporting such a promise.
- *The third layer.* The importance of this layer is reflected within the theory regarding consequentialism (see p. 81). This midwife has considered the consequences of the decision and considers that the provision of care would be 'the most beneficial outcome for the patient', which in this instance is Ann. It could also be

considered that the care given would also be 'the most beneficial outcome for a particular group' if the group in this instance is defined as other women who need to undergo termination of pregnancy. 'Increase of social good' could also be claimed in these circumstances, as antenatal screening for fetal anomalies is now an expectation of society and the midwife is supporting the woman's choice to terminate the pregnancy when the legal criteria are met.

• *The outer layer.* This outer layer of the grid is of great significance to midwives and provides the boundaries in which to work. Consideration of these external factors may have the greatest influence on a midwife's decision. Midwife A considers that 'the law' facilitates the decision made by Ann within the Abortion Act. 'Codes of practice' also make clear the stance which can be taken; specifically the Code of professional conduct Clause 7 'recognise and respect the uniqueness and dignity of each patient and client, and respond to their need for care, irrespective of their health problems or any other factor' (UKCC 1992). There are also guidelines by the document 'Termination of pregnancy for fetal abnormality' (RCOG 1996) This document assists in the interpretation of the law pertaining to abortion and specifies criteria for good practice, specifically 'women should be cared for by expert sympathetic staff' (p. 2).

Midwife B—the midwife who does not wish to provide care to Ann. This is the midwife's intuitive stance. The midwife feels very strongly about the issue of termination and is aware of the right to exercise a conscientious objection.

• *The inner layer.* Midwife B's decision is also supported by the boxes 'respect autonomy' and 'create autonomy'. A woman's autonomy is a central tenet and there would have to be significant justification to override it. Ann's ability to choose to have a termination and her freedom of choice is not affected in any way by midwife B's decision.

• *The second layer.* The box 'truth telling' has particular relevance in relation to this midwife's decision. The principle of veracity (truth telling) is an important principle of human conduct

(Seedhouse 1989). This midwife will be fulfilling Clause 8 of the Code of professional conduct: 'report to an appropriate person or authority, at the earliest possible time, any conscientious objection which may be relevant to your professional practice.' The RCM (1996) suggests that, because the onus is on the midwife to prove conscientious objection, it should be considered good practice to raise objection before a situation arises where a midwife may have to participate in the care of a woman during termination of pregnancy. This would then support the box 'intent to enable (beneficence)' as the midwife's manager can then arrange the off-duty to ensure that, as far as possible, there would be staff who do not object to care for women undergoing termination of pregnancy. 'Promise keeping' for this midwife would relate to keeping promises to self with regard to moral thinking and therefore uphold self-respect without compromising strongly held beliefs.

• *The third layer.* 'Increase of individual good', 'increase of good of a particular group' and 'increase of self-good' are supported by midwife B's decision. The elements within the first two boxes would be supported, as by not providing care the midwife seeks to safeguard the woman's best interests (UKCC 1992). Increase of 'self-good' is interlinked with the box 'promise keeping' in the second layer previously elaborated upon.

• *The outer layer.* External considerations also have relevance to midwife B's decision. Again, 'the law' supports this midwife's right to exercise a conscientious objection, as does the box 'Codes of practice', specifically the Code of professional conduct (UKCC 1992). This midwife may also refer to the RCM (1996) document, which elaborates upon conscientious objection and thus makes use of the box 'the responsibility to justify all actions in terms of external evidence.' The box 'effectiveness and efficiency of action' would also have been taken into consideration by this midwife, as the midwife should have informed the relevant manager at the earliest opportunity about the conscientious objection held. The box 'the risk' has particular relevance to midwife B's decision, as it may need to be reversed. The Abortion Act emphasizes the duty of care that exists in an emergency situation. This means that the midwife has to participate regardless of conscientious objection.

It can be seen from the analysis of the decision making relating to two midwives that each midwife is able to support their stance taken, which in turn supports a moral course of action. Not all of the boxes within each layer have been made use of—only those considered to have particular relevance were selected.

Case study 5.3: Evidence-based practice

As only a minority of midwives voice their conscientious objection (RCM 1996), and midwives may encounter this scenario only occasionally, exploration of a different scenario (5.3) is undertaken. An ethical analysis is again offered, utilizing Seedhouse's ethical grid.

 Case study 5.3

A team of community-based midwives always strive to base their practice on evidence-based findings. Several women have commented to team members that one of the midwives working within the team gives advice that conflicts with the advice already given to them by other team midwives. This particular midwife has worked within the team for a considerable number of years. The midwife is popular with both the other team members and the women receiving care. Examples provided by the women in relation to the conflicting advice concern the use of 'soothers' and cord care.

The dilemma confronting this team is whether or not they should inform this midwife about the comments made.

Team A. Team A choose to inform the midwife of their concerns. This is the intuitive decision of the majority of the team. The midwives acknowledge that they have a duty of care to the women receiving their care (UKCC 1996).

• *The inner layer.* The team's intuitive stance is supported by the box 'respect persons equally', with specific reference to the Code of

professional conduct (UKCC 1992). The moral elements within this box are embraced within the Code; Clause 6 emphasizes the need for midwives to collaborate and cooperate with colleagues within their team, and Clause 14 calls upon midwives to assist their colleagues in developing professional competence in the context of their own knowledge. 'Serve needs before wants' applies as the team will be fulfilling the needs of their client group by ultimately providing consistency of advice.

• *The second layer.* By informing the midwife of the women's views, the box 'intent to enable (beneficence)' enables women to receive evidence-based care. This is directly supported by the box 'minimize harm' as providing care that is evidence based seeks to avoid the causation of harm. 'Truth telling' is an important box to apply, as the team do not want to deceive their colleague and this further endorses the respect afforded to the midwife. 'Promise keeping' is linked implicitly to the Code, specifically Clause 1 (promote and safeguarding interests) and Clause 2 (no action or omission being detrimental to women). By informing the midwife of their concerns, the promises contained within these clauses will be fulfilled.

• *The third layer.* The team could justify that the box 'societal good' supports their decision, as they ultimately seek to protect the public (UKCC 1992). For the midwife involved, 'individual good' is the team's concern, as this practitioner's awareness of deficits in relation to knowledge will hopefully be changed for the better (UKCC 1992 Clause 3). The outcome would also benefit all clients within the midwife's care as they would have consistency and continuity of advice, thereby supporting the box 'increase of the good of a particular group'.

• *The outer layer.* This layer provides boundaries in which the team can work. 'The degree of certainty of the evidence on which action is taken' would influence team A's decision and the majority of the team must have that evidence in respect of the advice provided by their colleague to clients. This box would be inextricably linked to 'disputed facts' as the team needs to explore all of the facts either prior to the midwife being informed or with the midwife to clarify issues. 'The risk' of informing this midwife will have been considered by the team, in terms of future working relationships, and will have been placed in the context of the greater benefits to the women overall.

Team B. Team B intuitively choose not to inform their colleague of the issues raised by their clients.

• *The inner layer.* The box 'respect autonomy' is applied by the team, in order to support their initial intuitive stance. The team consider that this midwife is exercising the right to practise autonomously.

• *The second layer.* 'Minimize harm' also supports the team's decision and may be considered in several ways. The team do not consider that any real harm is being inflicted upon women receiving care and therefore this is not in conflict with Clauses 1 and 2 of the Code (UKCC 1992). In addition, the dynamics of the team will not be disrupted, which would contravene Clause 6 of the Code, which is concerned with working in a collaborative and cooperative manner with colleagues. Such disruption could impinge on the care of women. This outcome also gains support from the box 'intent to enable (beneficence)' as harmonious relationships would be maintained within the team.

• *The third layer.* 'Increase of the good of a particular group' is supported within team B's decision. The particular group in this instance is the team itself as the ICM (1993) states that 'midwives should support and sustain each other, nurturing each others' self-worth' (p. 4).

• *The outer layer.* Team B took into consideration the box 'the degree of certainty of evidence on which action is taken' and did not consider that there is sufficient evidence from the women upon which to act. This is considered in conjunction with 'disputed facts,' which also informed their decision. 'Wishes of others' were also taken into account—that is, all members of the team. 'The risk' is an important issue for the team before finally confirming the initial intuitive stance and they ultimately perceived that

there was no risk to the women. This was also considered within the red layer in the box 'minimize harm'.

From the analysis offered in relation to the decisions of two teams, it may be evident that one team's decision has more moral value than the other. This does not necessarily mean that one is 'right' and that the other is 'wrong'. Moreover, this analysis serves to provide midwives with a tool for further discussion and critical debate and to facilitate accountability in terms of their ethical decision-making ability.

Case studies 5.4 and 5.5 provide further opportunities for discussion and reflection:

 Case study 5.4

It is Susan's second pregnancy. Although Susan's first pregnancy was uncomplicated, she is anxious about this pregnancy. At 18 weeks' gestation, Susan received an ultrasound scan, which subsequently revealed that the fetus had dilated renal pelves. The only information imparted to Susan was that she was to be rescanned at 24 weeks' gestation. The GP was informed of the results but decided not to inform Susan of the results on the grounds that 'it would only make her anxious'. Susan subsequently asks her midwife the reason for the repeat scan at 24 weeks' gestation.

The dilemma confronting this midwife is whether the decision made by the GP should be overridden or whether to abide by his decision and not tell Susan about the dilated renal pelves owing to Susan's anxiety.

 Case study 5.5

Jane is 20 years old and married to Simon. She is a Jehovah's Witness. Jane is admitted to the delivery suite with severe pre-eclampsia and is subsequently delivered of a live child. She suffers a massive postpartum haemorrhage and her vital signs indicate hypovolaemic shock. Jane is also sedated as part of the management of her raised blood pressure. Jane's condition is rapidly becoming life threatening. The midwife has been asked to commence a blood transfusion. Simon refuses to allow Jane to have a blood transfusion based on religious grounds.

The dilemma confronting this midwife is whether to commence the blood transfusion or comply with the husband's wishes.

CHALLENGES FOR MIDWIVES IN RELATION TO REPRODUCTIVE TECHNOLOGY

The Human Fertilisation and Embryology Act 1990 (HMSO 1990) is of great practical importance to the increasing number of women wishing to take advantage of infertility treatments in order to have a child (Douglas 1991). The importance of midwives having knowledge of assisted conception techniques is emphasized by Malone (1995). She emphasizes that such a knowledge positively contributes towards the midwife's awareness of the subsequent psychological and physical stresses on the couple.

This raises the question 'what are the psychological adjustments that have to be made by these couples?' Sidebotham (1997) reveals that there is very little information available to either parents or the midwife regarding adjustment to pregnancy, owing to the relative newness of this field of science. Contained within Sidebotham's informative work, guidelines are outlined for midwives in order that they may provide this essential support during pregnancy and it also provides information regarding life with a new baby and the potential development of the child.

The following case studies serve to illustrate the issues regarding infertility problems of some women, which have resulted in pregnancy. The case studies will highlight the dilemmas which confront women and also the competing dilemmas for the midwives involved in the provision of care. An increased awareness of these dilemmas concurs with the view held by Malone (1995), who considers that midwives are best placed by maintaining a smooth transition from the fertility clinic to the antenatal clinic. It is contended, therefore, that insight into dilemmas facing couples who have successfully received fertility treatment will positively enable such a transition.

Delineating the couple's dilemmas serves to evoke discussion amongst midwives. The ethical position advocated by the authors to confront the competing dilemmas for midwives is expressed through the use of Seedhouse's grid. Where several dilemmas are given, the initial dilemma only will be analysed, supported by the utilisation of the four layers and boxes previously described. The analysis, in conjunction with a rationale, is provided afresh within a tabular format for ease of reference.

Case study 5.6: Donor sperm

Read Case study 5.6 and then consider the potential dilemmas.

 Case study 5.6

An Asian couple live very closely to their immediate and extended family. After much thought and consideration, they have agreed to the use of donor sperm to achieve a pregnancy. Donor sperm is contradictory to their religious beliefs yet the couple's desire to have a child has overridden their cultural constraints.

The couple's dilemmas

- Will the midwife enquire regarding the donor sperm as complete secrecy must be maintained? The family would not accept their decision to use donor sperm.
- Will their cultural and religious demands on their emotions cause them perhaps to have doubts during their pregnancy?
- Will the potential father fully accept the child?

Competing dilemmas for the midwife

The couple divulge during the booking interview details about the use of donor sperm and the concerns that they have.

- How can the midwife ensure that confidentiality is maintained?
- Should the midwife pass on her concerns regarding the potential for maternal anxiety to her colleagues?
- Should the midwife initiate action early regarding concerns for paternal attachment?

Table 5.1 provides a guide to the ethical position in this situation.

Table 5.1 Use of Seedhouse's ethical grid in relation to the issue regarding donor sperm

Intuitive stance	Layer	Box	Rationale
Maintain confidentiality	Inner	Respect autonomy	Embodied within Changing childbirth (DoH 1993)
	Second	Intent to enable (Beneficence)	Promotes confidence for further interactions
	Third	Increase of individual good	Women expect to have confidential disclosures respected
	Outer	Codes of practice	Maintain confidentiality— Code of professional conduct (UKCC 1992), making disclosures only with consent

Case study 5.7: Down's syndrome

Now read Case study 5.7, which involves assisted conception for a mature couple.

Case study 5.7

A couple have been happily married for 18 years. They have been undergoing assisted conception treatment for 15 years. Pregnancy has finally been confirmed. The woman is 39 years of age and her partner is 56 years of age. They are financially secure and have a supportive family. An amniocentesis has revealed Down's syndrome.

The couple's dilemmas

- Should they terminate this very precious pregnancy with the knowledge that the woman may not become pregnant again?
- Is it 'better' to have a baby with a handicap than no baby at all?
- Would the husband be able to care for the child in later years should they decide to continue with the pregnancy?
- Will they be able to cope with a handicapped child?

Competing dilemma for the midwife

- The couple ask the midwife for advice in relation to termination of the pregnancy.

Refer to Table 5.2 for a presentation of the ethical position in this case study.

Case study 5.8: Surrogacy

Finally read Case study 5.8 and reflect on the dilemmas in the case of surrogacy.

Case study 5.8

A couple, both in their mid thirties, are unable to have children. The woman's sister offered to have a child for the couple. The surrogate mother used her own eggs through a stimulated in vitro fertilization cycle. These were fertilized with the sperm from the adoptive male parent. Embryos were subsequently transferred and the surrogate mother became pregnant with twins.

The couple's dilemmas

- The commissioning couple wish to be present at the birth. The birth mother wants her own partner to be present instead.
- The birth mother wishes to give birth in accordance with her own choices and the adoptive parents are keen for the quickest, safest delivery for both babies.

Competing dilemma for the midwife

- The commissioning couple wish the midwife to involve them in the 'arrival' of the twins and yet the relationship between them and the birth mother is clearly strained.

Again Seedhouse's grid (Table 5.3) provides a guide to the ethical position.

Table 5.2 Use of Seedhouse's ethical grid in relation to the issue regarding Down's syndrome

Intuitive stance	Layer	Box	Rationale
Midwife must be unbiased	Inner	Serve needs	The couple have the right to choice despite the feelings of the midwife
	Second	Intent to enable (Beneficence)	Choices should be presented to the couple
	Third	Increase of individual good	The couple will be empowered through choice
	Outer	The risk	The long term consequences will not be able to be calculated

Table 5.3 Use of Seedhouse's ethical grid in relation to the issue regarding surrogacy

Intuitive stance	Layer	Box	Rationale
Support the birth mother	Inner	Serve needs before wants	Although the commissioning couple wish to be involved, the needs of the birth mother are paramount
	Second	Promise keeping	Implicit with the Code of professional conduct—Clauses 1 and 2
	Third	Increase of individual good	Priorities lie with the birth mother and are the immediate responsibility of the midwife
	Outer	The law	The midwife's legal duty of care lies with the interests of the birth mother and child

Summary

Ethical dilemmas are not new to midwives. Contemporary developments in midwifery practice highlight the need for midwives to develop further their intuitive knowledge base. The language of ethics is outlined and an approach to ethics is suggested, namely applied normative ethics. Two frameworks for decision making are discussed, namely the Code of professional conduct and the four level approach. Advantages and limitations to both frameworks are acknowledged within the discussion.

Seedhouse (1989) considers that the ethical grid is a precis of all the necessary elements for thorough moral reasoning; the use of this grid develops further the framework previously explored. The layers of the grid have been applied working from the inner layer to the outer layer. The boxes which offered the most appropriate 'solution' have been selected in the context of the case studies analysed. (Seedhouse does, however, indicate that there is flexibility with the use of the four layers and respective boxes.)

Midwives are influential in relation to the psychological adjustments that have to be made by women who become pregnant following assisted conception techniques. Case studies have been employed to feature the dilemmas which face some couples. The competing dilemmas this may create for the midwife are explored, making use of the ethical grid (Seedhouse 1989) within a table in order to facilitate ease of reference.

APPENDIX: INTERNATIONAL CODE OF ETHICS FOR MIDWIVES

I. Midwifery relationships

a. Midwives respect a woman's informed right of choice and promote the woman's acceptance of responsibility for the outcomes of her choices.
b. Midwives work with women, supporting their right to participate actively in decisions about their care, and empowering women to speak for themselves on issues affecting the health of women and their families in their culture and society.
c. Midwives, together with women, work with policy and funding agencies to define women's needs for health services and to ensure that resources are fairly allocated considering priorities and availability.
d. Midwives support and sustain each other in their professional roles, and actively nurture their own and others' sense of self-worth.
e. Midwives work with other health professionals, consulting and referring as necessary when the woman's need for care exceeds the competencies of the midwife.
f. Midwives recognize the human interdependence within their field of practice and actively seek to resolve inherent conflicts.

II. Practice of midwifery

a. Midwives provide care for women and childbearing families with respect for cultural diversity while also working to eliminate harmful practices within those same cultures.
b. Midwives encourage realistic expectations of childbirth by women within their own society, with the minimum expectation that no women should be harmed by conception or childbearing.
c. Midwives use their professional knowledge to ensure safe birthing practices in all environments and cultures.
d. Midwives respond to the psychological, physical, emotional and spiritual needs of women seeking health care, whatever their circumstances.

e. Midwives act as effective role models in health promotion for women throughout their life cycle, for families and for other health professionals.
f. Midwives actively seek personal, intellectual and professional growth throughout their midwifery career, integrating this growth into their practice.

III. The professional responsibilities of midwives

a. Midwives hold in confidence client information in order to protect the right to privacy, and use judgement in sharing this information.
b. Midwives are responsible for their decisions and actions, and are accountable for the related outcomes in their care of women.
c. Midwives may refuse to participate in activities for which they hold deep moral opposition; however, the emphasis on individual conscience should not deprive women of essential health services.
d. Midwives participate in the development and implementation of health policies that promote the health of all women and childbearing families.

IV. Advancement of midwifery knowledge and practice

a. Midwives ensure that the advancement of midwifery knowledge is based on activities that protect the rights of women as persons.
b. Midwives develop and share midwifery knowledge through a variety of processes, such as peer review and research.
c. Midwives participate in the formal education of midwifery students and midwives.

(ICM 1993)

REFERENCES

Beauchamp T L, Childress J F 1989 Principles of biomedical ethics. Oxford University Press, Oxford
Clarke R 1996 In: Frith L (ed) Ethics and midwifery: issues in contemporary practice. Butterworth Heinneman, Oxford, pp 205–220
DoH (Department of Health) 1993 Changing childbirth part 1, Report of the Expert Maternity Group. DoH, London
DoH (Department of Health) 1996b Risk management in the NHS. DoH, London
DoH (Department of Health) 1996a NHS The patient's charter: maternity services. DoH, London
Douglas G 1991 The Human Fertilisation and Embryology Act 1990. Family Law March:110–116
Edwards S D 1996 Nursing ethics: a principle-based approach. Macmillan, Basingstoke

ENB (English National Board) for Midwifery and Health Visiting 1997 Preparation of supervisors of midwives: managing professional conduct Module 4.
Fryer N 1995 How useful is a knowledge of ethics? British Journal of Midwifery 3(6):341–346
Gillon R 1992 Philosophical medical. John Wiley, Chichester
Henry C 1996 In: Siddiqui, Kendrick K (eds) Popular ethical theories: their use and function in midwifery. British Journal of Midwifery October 4(10):519–521
HMSO 1967 Abortion Act. HMSO, London
HMSO 1990 Human Fertilisation and Embryology Act. HMSO, London
Human Fertilisation & Embryology Authority 1995 Code of Practice. HFEA, London

Hussey T 1996 Nursing ethics and codes of professional conduct. Nursing Ethics 3(3):250–252

ICM (International Confederation of Midwives) 1993 International code of ethics for midwives. ICM, London

Jones S 1994 Ethics in midwifery. Mosby-Year Book Europe, London

Kohner N 1996 The moral maze of practice: a stimulus for reflection and discussion. Kings Fund, London

Marsh B J 1996 The right to choice and the value of ethics. British Journal of Midwifery 2(4):82–86

Malone C 1995 Managing multiple births. Modern Midwife September:12–16

Morgan D, Lee RG 1991 Blackstones guides to the: Human Fertilisation & Embryology Act 1990 (Abortion & Embryo Research, the new law). Blackstones,

Proud J 1995 Ethics and obstetric ultrasound. British Journal of Midwifery 2(2):79–82

Purtilo R 1993 Ethical dimensions in the health professions. W B Saunders, Philadelphia

Raphael D D 1981 Moral Philosophy. Oxford University Press

RCM (Royal College of Midwives) 1996 Proceedings of the Ethics Committee 1993–1996. RCM, London

RCOG (Royal College of Obstricians and Gynaecologists) 1996 Termination of pregnancy for fetal abnormality in England, Wales and Scotland. RCOG, London

Richards J 1997 To choose about choice: the responsibility of the midwife. British Journal of Midwifery 5(3):163–168

Seedhouse D 1989 Ethics, the heart of health care. John Wiley & Sons, Chichester

Seedhouse D, Lovell L 1992 Practical Medical Ethics. John Wiley, Chichester

Sidebotham M 1997 In: Karger, Hunt S (eds) Challenges in midwifery care. Macmillan, London

Thompson I E, Melia K M 1998 Nursing ethics. Churchill Livingstone, New York

Tschudin V 1986 Ethics in nursing: the caring relationship. Heinemann Nursing, London

UKCC 1992 Code of professional conduct. UKCC, London

UKCC 1996 Guidelines for professional practice. UKCC, London

UKCC 1998 Midwives rules and code of practice. UKCC, London

FURTHER READING

RCM (Royal College of Midwives) 1997 Surrogacy. Defining Motherhood Position Paper No 18 August. RCM, London

Provides legal aspects and definitions in relation to surrogacy. Guidelines provided in relation to the midwives' role during the antenatal, intrapartum and postnatal periods. Requirements for birth registration stated.

6 Responsibilities and accountability

Carol Newton   Chris Johnson   Colleen Drury

The aim of this chapter is to examine the accountability and responsibility of midwives with particular emphasis on the legislation which governs their practice.

HISTORY OF STATUTORY ACCOUNTABILITY FOR MIDWIVES

The aim of United Kingdom legislation relating to midwifery practice has always been to protect the public. Long-standing efforts to achieve this aim by regulating and controlling midwives finally culminated in the Midwives Act of 1902 (HMSO 1902) (1915 for Scotland). This Act has not fundamentally altered for almost a hundred years despite major changes in the delivery of service and free movement of people within the European Union.

Midwives Acts

The first Act of 1902 'to secure better training and supervision for midwives' sanctioned the setting up of the Central Midwives Board (Cross 1996 p. 5) which was to be independent of the General Medical Council (GMC) and directly responsible to the Privy Council. The Central Midwives Board was given very wide powers under the Act. See Box 6.1.

The title of midwife was now protected but this original legislation gave the medical profession a lot of influence over midwives and their practice. This was reflected in the membership of the Central Midwives Board where midwives were in the minority.

Midwives rules

The Central Midwives Board formulated rules for the practice and training of midwives with the first set being issued in 1903. One of the earliest examples of medicalization of childbirth can clearly be seen in the 1919 version of Midwives rules in which is set out requirements for summoning medical aid, which the midwife was required to do in all cases of illness of the patient or child or any abnormality occurring during pregnancy, labour or lying-in period. Midwives were also required to make various notifications to the local supervising authority (LSA) for reasons identified in Box 6.2.

The 1902 Act was intended to be an enabling Act; however Clarke (1995) portrays this Act as preserving the midwife in name who, in return for the benefits of education and registration, had to surrender to medicine's control of midwifery and accept a reduced sphere of competence and practice. Professional regulation in the

form of supervision of the practising midwife had now come into being. Midwives Acts since 1902 have introduced only minor amendments or have been consolidating Acts. The major change between 1902 and 1979 was the introduction of a salaried midwifery service which made local authorities responsible for the provision of maternity services, and midwives became employees. The Midwives Act 1951 (HMSO 1951) consolidated the previous Midwives Act and amendments into one. There was no major change in the statutory position of the midwife and the same statutory framework remained unchanged until the Nurses, Midwives and Health Visitors Act 1979 (HMSO 1979).

Nurses, Midwives and Health Visitors Act 1979

The midwifery profession is still governed by a statutory framework which highlights the recognition and importance society places upon the status of such professionals. The statutory framework that was established with the Midwives Act 1902 determined the sphere of midwifery practice, which was reflected in the Nurses, Midwives and Health Visitors Act 1979. The 1979 Act enabled the establishment of the United Kingdom Central Council for Nursing, Midwifery and Health Visiting (UKCC) to regulate these professions by establishing and improving standards of nursing, midwifery and health visiting in order to serve and protect the public.

THE UNITED KINGDOM CENTRAL COUNCIL FOR NURSING, MIDWIFERY AND HEALTH VISITING

The key tasks of the UKCC are identified in Box 6.3. In 1989, the UKCC and National Boards were reviewed which culminated in a new Nurses, Midwives and Health Visitors Act 1992 (HMSO 1992). The aim of this new Act was to strengthen the UKCC's position as the regulatory body for practitioners. This effectively enabled each of the three professions to become self-regulating by election of members to Council

Box 6.3   **Key Tasks of the UKCC (UKCC 1997)**

- To maintain a register of qualified nurses, midwives and health visitors
- To set standards for nursing, midwifery and health-visiting education, practice and conduct
- To provide advice for nurses, midwives and health visitors on professional standards
- To consider allegations of misconduct or unfitness to practise due to ill health.

and that professional conduct function to be centralized at Council level. The national boards became smaller executive bodies responsible for accreditation of institutions and validation of courses in accordance with the UKCC's requirements regarding standard, kind and content. It was now the responsibility of the statutory midwifery committee of the UKCC to make rules regarding standards to be observed in relation to supervision of midwives, with the national boards issuing advice and guidance consistent with these.

The statutory framework comprises therefore the primary legislation, namely the Nurses, Midwives and Health Visitors Acts 1979, 1992 and 1997. This primary legislation is implemented via the secondary legislation or statutory instruments of which the Midwives rules form part. The Midwives rules (UKCC 1998) implement the statutory framework within which midwives practise. The UKCC is also responsible for standards of practice and exists to ensure practitioners are accountable to the public for their actions.

ACCOUNTABILITY

Midwives have historically been answerable to their professional body since the Act of 1902 which implicitly made midwives accountable through a series of Midwives rules and Codes of practice, and more recently, the Scope of professional practice (UKCC 1992a). However, the word accountability was only first documented in the first editions of the Code of professional conduct in 1984. Discussion on the subject of accountability has come to the forefront following the publication of this Code, the concept of which has been the cornerstone in the regulations of midwifery and the way in which the profession progressed (Kitson 1993). Midwifery's concern with accountability stems from two sources, the consumer and the profession.

The consumer

The consumer was highlighted in the Second report on the maternity services (House of Commons 1992). The committee representing women's views acknowledged their desire for the provision of continuity of care and carer throughout pregnancy and childbirth, and the majority of the committee regard midwives as the group best placed and equipped to provide this (para. 49). It also raised the issue that most women want a wider choice of place of delivery than the existing concentration in obstetric hospitals allows.

Women also want more say in the type of care they receive at all stages—care which should always make them feel in control of their own bodies (paras. 50–55). Consumers want more reliable information about the advantages and disadvantages of specific procedures and freedom to give or refuse consent and thus feel as partners in the process. This was further elaborated upon in the report of the Expert Maternity Group, entitled Changing Childbirth (DoH 1993), stating that 'The woman must be the focus of maternity care. She should be able to feel that she is in control of what is happening to her and be able to make decisions about her care, based on her needs, having discussed matters fully with the professionals involved' (DoH 1993 p. 9). This statement highlights the relationship between a woman and the health care professional involved in her care during childbearing. The statutory framework which the midwife works within must allow the flexibility to meet these needs whilst defining clearly the sphere of responsibility and accountability.

The Changing Childbirth Group acknowledged that women want a maternity service that offers safety, continuity of care and carer; this inspires confidence, responds to individual's needs and enables them to feel in control. It should allow women an informed choice of options. The consensus was that even when professionals believe that the mother's choice may increase the risk of harm to herself or her baby they do not have the right to impose their views. In extending control to the woman it enables real decision making. This does not mean responsibility is abdicated. It is necessary to inform women of the possible dangers some choices may entail. If a woman exercises her right to informed choice it is appropriate for her to take responsibility for her actions.

The professional

Secondly it is necessary to consider the midwife as a practitioner who is legally and professionally bound by the Midwives rules and code of practice (UKCC 1998a). This states that the midwife is accountable for her practice and that the needs of the mother and her baby must be the primary focus ensuring that the mother is enabled to make decisions about her care based on her needs. The result of such recommendations has significant implications for maintaining and improving professional knowledge and competence (UKCC 1992b). In addition to the pre-registration education and training of midwives, practising midwives need to adapt to new roles and acquire a broader range of skills, as allowed for by the Midwives rules and code of practice (UKCC 1998a pp. 27–29). In order to examine the various dimensions of the role of the midwife, the concept of accountability needs to be analysed.

A model of accountability

Bergman (1981) cites Murray and Zetner's definition of accountability as: 'being responsible for one's acts and being able to explain, define or measure in some way the results of decision making' (p. 54). Tshudin (1989) also highlights accountability as arising out of responsibility by stating that one is responsible for professional actions and therefore accountable for them. In examining the Midwives rules and code

of practice (UKCC 1998a) it is the word 'responsibility' which occurs more frequently than the word 'accountability'. In Bergman's model of the preconditions leading to accountability, responsibility is the second of three preconditions (Fig. 6.1), the first being ability.

Ability: knowledge, skills and values

Accountability includes the midwife being able to explain and justify any decision making and demonstrating the reasons for any decisions made (UKCC 1996, 1998b). Practice therefore requires a sound knowledge base upon which to make decisions based on professional judgement. Bergman identifies this prerequisite as ability based upon knowledge skills and values in order to decide on a specific issue. This knowledge should be research based and up to date, which has implications for continuing education (see Ch. 12) as a basis for accountability in practice and is expected by the Code of professional conduct (UKCC 1992b), Midwives rules

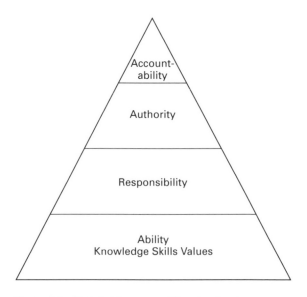

Figure 6.1 Model of the preconditions leading to accountability (From Bergman 1981, reproduced by kind permission from the International Council of Nurses 1998).

and code of practice (UKCC 1998a) and Scope of professional practice (UKCC 1992a). Rule 33 of Midwives rules lists the expected outcomes of programmes of education providing the knowledge base enabling admission to part 10 of the UKCC register. This list is an explicit statement of the sphere of accountability by which the midwife is professionally and legally bound. It is suggested therefore that a practising midwife cannot choose to exercise accountability for only some of the stated list. It may be argued that a midwife may specialize but must undergo professional updating in order to offer the full range of midwifery skills if this is required. Despite the code of practice giving clear guidelines to practitioners regarding their responsibility for maintaining and updating skills, as well as the acquisition of new skills, a study by Reid (1994) demonstrated that 2% of midwives were unwilling to support women requesting a home confinement and 1% were unwilling to support women requesting water, acupuncture or hypnosis as methods of pain relief. Rule 33 also states the student should use 'relevant literature and research to inform the practice of midwifery' (UKCC 1998a, p. 13). There is a tension here in that practising midwives are expected to be competent to provide intrapartum care but they might have had no opportunities to develop skills in less common methods of pain relief. Added to this the research evidence is sometimes conflicting. This reinforces the concept of professions striving to develop knowledge for the benefit of clients. Practice that is based in 'custom and practice' is no longer acceptable; evidence must now inform practice.

The UKCC Code of professional conduct (UKCC 1992b) does not cover specific circumstances in which decisions are made but presents principles which must be applied to practice. Therefore, whatever judgements are made, the midwife must be able to justify the actions taken. The decisions made by the midwife must be research based (Kitson 1993), a view supported by Fraser (1995) and McKay (1997). Entry to the register is only the beginning of a lifelong commitment to professional development and maintenance of competence enabling the midwife to practise with confidence and the required knowledge and skills for day to day practice.

Responsibility

Bergman's hierarchical model makes it clear that ascending to the next stage needs not only the personal acceptance of responsibility but also knowledge of the requirements of legislation and understanding that the midwife is responsible for her own actions. This model, which relates to nursing as opposed to midwifery, does not address the safeguard of statutory supervision for midwives through which a midwife can gain support from the supervisor of midwives whilst still accepting responsibility for her own practice (UKCC 1998a).

Batey & Lewis (1982) discuss responsibility as denoting a charge or activity, that one is willing to fulfil. A midwife, in accepting the charge or activity or the task, equally accepts the responsibility for carrying out that particular action. Therefore responsibility may be viewed as the care and consideration for the outcome of one's actions and legal liability, hence accountability. Thus highlighted by these authors is the interrelatedness of responsibility within the definition of accountability. Soothill, Mackay & Webb (1995) point out that the terms of 'accountability' and 'responsibility' are often used as if they were interchangeable and synonymous. However, there is a distinct difference even though there are inextricable links. Pearson & Vaughan (1986) support his point but acknowledge that there is a clear difference between them. Kendrick (1995) highlights the confusion which surrounds the concept of accountability and responsibility, stating that using the terms synonymously or interchangeably leads to lack of clarity. According to Mander (1995) accountability cannot exist without responsibility having been granted and accepted. The acceptance of responsibility is dependent upon the education and thus the ability and experience of the midwife. A midwife may not be held accountable or have accountability imposed for an action unless she is given and accepts the responsibility.

Responsibility is granted to the midwife by virtue of her job description, supported by the activities of a midwife (UKCC 1998a) and the Midwives rules, particularly Rule 40 (UKCC 1998a). The concept of responsibility goes beyond that of duty and relates to what a professional both does and says. The term responsibility can also be found in the Code of professional conduct (UKCC 1992b). Responsibility may be described as having two components, responsibilities assigned by members of the profession and responsibilities assigned to the profession by external sources such as a NHS trust protocol or policy. Trust policies might constrain midwifery practice; therefore incongruence occurs between assumed and the assigned responsibilities (Batey & Lewis 1982, Clarke 1995). To act responsibly the midwife must use the professional rules and codes and exercise clinical judgement. However, there may be conflict when the midwife is acting under constraints of trust protocols with which she is expected to comply. Bradshaw & Bradshaw (1997) argue that, although the midwife's central duty is to care for the client, it is more likely to be secondary to the control exerted by organizational constraints and regulations. In fact Dimond (1994) calls for the protection of midwives who may be under pressure from managers to work outside their sphere of practice as their range of duties enlarge.

The definition of a midwife and activities of a midwife are explicit, indicating the boundaries of practice (UKCC 1998a). Robinson, Golden & Bradley (1983) identified a substantial proportion of midwives who practised in situations where they were not required to exercise fully the degree of responsibility for which the midwife is trained. This was particularly evident with regard to antenatal care provision. A more recent study by Pope et al (1997) highlights that the midwife's practice base will effectively determine the responsibility undertaken, for example, hospital or community based. Reid (1993) found that 85% of midwives felt confident to offer total care to women with uncomplicated pregnancies although they did not feel their current role allowed them to do so. It was also considered by

68% of midwives that their present practice did not reflect the full role of the midwife.

Midwives rules identify the midwife as provider of care to 'normal' women but also to act in an emergency or where a deviation from normal is recognized. It must be absolutely clear where ultimate responsibility lies for the care and safety of mother and baby, in all situations and in all locations. For example 'As a registered nurse, midwife or health visitor, you are personally accountable for your practice and, in the exercise of your professional accountability, must acknowledge any limitations in your knowledge and competence and decline any duties or responsibilities unless able to perform them in a safe and skilled manner' (UKCC 1992b, para. 4). The midwife's primary responsibility is to the mother and baby; this does not mean that the midwife controls but rather practises in partnership with the woman and her family. The midwife is responsible for providing skilled care, up to date research-based knowledge and information as well as psychological support to the woman and her family. The woman in return has a responsibility within the partnership of reporting on her condition and in decision making regarding her wishes and needs.

Authority

Authority is the last of Bergman's preconditions for exercising accountability and may be defined as the right to make decisions and then implement them. The UKCC provides midwives with the authority to undertake the duties they are trained for. Midwives can facilitate women assuming authority by providing information and encouraging women to make their own decisions.

Lewis & Batey (1982) discuss the importance of authority accompanying responsibility and consider it to have three sources:

1. *Authority of situation*—this arises from, for example, an emergency situation whereby the authority to do what is necessary is accorded to those present even when under normal circumstances that authority need not exist. This is

supported by the UKCC's decision to amend rule 40 (UKCC 1998a), which now states that

1. 'A practising midwife is responsible for providing midwifery care to a mother and baby during the antenatal, intranatal and postnatal periods.
2. Except in an emergency, a practising midwife shall not provide any midwifery case, or undertake any treatment which she has not, either before or after registration as a midwife, been trained to give or which is outside her current sphere of practice.
3. In an emergency, or where a deviation from the norm which is outside her current sphere of practice becomes apparent ... a practising midwife shall call ... such other qualified health professional who may reasonably be expected to have the requisite skills and experience to assist her.'

2. *Authority of expert knowledge*—granted in recognition of a midwife's qualification and registration and uniqueness of role. Society expects midwives to have skill and knowledge to provide midwifery care and highlights the need for sound knowledge base to inform practice. Hunt (1984) states midwives should be allowed to use research findings innovatively if this means challenging established practices and procedures. Clarke & Renfrew (1992) argue practice is influenced by a number of factors including skills, experience and research.

3. *Authority of position*—this considers the right to act linked to a formal position such as a midwife having a right to carry out the duties of a midwife because she is registered and employed or self-employed. Copp (1988) states that power in the form of authority must be given for the professional to be accountable.

Bureaucratic organizations like the NHS often insist on lines of accountability or chains of command, with adherence to policies and little flexibility for the individual practitioner. Managers assume the ultimate responsibility and authority as they are supported by trust policies and guidelines which may impinge on the midwife's sphere of practice within the organization.

Hunt (1984) argues that those with authority to effect change may not want to, whilst would-be innovators do not have the necessary authority. According to Hutton (1994) women want midwives to have more power and authority. It could be argued that increasing authority would result in increased responsibility even when deviations from normal arise. This may be supported by protocols but restricted by the rules (UKCC 1998). Clearly there are tensions in what the Midwives rules and codes expect and what employers require of their employees.

This critical incongruence between the expectations of midwives and those of others in the health care system can contribute to negative consequences in the organizational work environment of midwives and in turn affect the provision of maternity care (Batey & Lewis 1982). The midwife must have the authority needed to carry out actions in such a way as to accept accountability by virtue of the right expertise and power to make decisions about the course of action in any given situation (Batey & Lewis 1982, Johns 1989, Jones 1996). The point of registration provides midwives with the legal right to practise as a responsible midwife with a defined sphere of practice (UKCC 1998). However, this may be problematic and fraught with difficulties if the paternalism of obstetricians and GPs, which has beset midwifery practice during the decades of medicalization, continues and causes midwives to become deskilled and disempowered.

Accountability

If professionals claim to be professional care givers, then they become accountable to their client group, to other members of their professions, to their employer and finally to themselves. All are inextricably linked and cannot be considered in isolation. The public have a right to expect and demand a high quality maternity service. Changing Childbirth (DoH 1993) sought to redress the medicalization of care and enable the midwife to take the lead role where appropriate. This stance has been encouraged by consumer groups supporting the view of the midwife utilizing her full skills. In order to do this, a midwife must be aware of best evidence and professionally competent in order to pass on information and discuss options for care knowledgeably. Women want freedom of choice and midwives who have become deskilled must regain their full role and accept responsibility for it. As practice develops the rules and codes provide guidance on a midwife's role and responsibilities as they develop. This clarity is essential for defining the responsibilities of the profession and the individual midwife but there will inevitably be some incongruence as to the responsibility with changing environments. McKay (1997) suggests that if midwives want autonomy then they must assume greater responsibility and accept their accountability. Any adjustment to practice should, however, be firmly based on Midwives rules, codes guidelines and the Scope of professional practice (UKCC 1992a,b, 1996, 1997, 1998a,b).

Schott (1993) suggests that many midwives have lost their confidence in the birth process and in their own abilities as experts in normal pregnancy and birth. Some may need to develop new skills and to increase their flexibility and confidence as independent practitioners and also members of maternity service teams. Roles and responsibilities need careful examination in the light of change. Tensions have been highlighted between professionals, especially in relation to the 'lead professional' since the publication of Changing Childbirth (DoH 1993).

According to Hartley (1997) the Midwives rules (then UKCC 1993) prevent the midwife remaining the 'lead professional' should there be a deviation from normal. In contrast the Midwives code of practice (UKCC 1998a) acknowledges that the midwife may be required to develop new skills and as such these may become 'an integral part of the role of the midwife'.

It is well established that an uncomplicated pregnancy and normal labour may be managed by a midwife, who remains responsible for all the midwifery care given until she transfers that responsibility to a doctor if a complication arises, but even then she must assist in a competent manner and is still responsible for her own actions.

Each professional in this situation retains clinical accountability for their own practice (UKCC 1998a). No one else can answer for you and it is no defence to say you were acting on someone else's instructions. As a practitioner a midwife is accountable for both commission and omission (Bergman 1981, UKCC 1992b). Although protocols can clarify respective roles and responsibilities of both medical and midwifery staff, the accountability of the midwife is separate from but complementary to the accountability of the doctor, though the roles are interrelated. Midwives can work beyond the recognized role without statutory limitation as long as they have been trained to do so and there is a local agreement or protocol; examples include intravenous cannulation, augmentation of labour and acupuncture.

Therefore the constraint is to be trained in new skills and theoretical knowledge, the midwife having freedom to accept responsibility and hence accountability. Entwhistle (1993) urges midwives to consider the motives for widening their sphere of practice, recommending that research must show that the development is for the benefit of mothers and babies and not for financial reasons or to cross professional boundaries. Midwives today are assuming a wider role and an increased responsibility for the overall care of women. New patterns of care include, for example:

- midwifery-managed delivery units
- team midwifery
- case load management
- midwifery group practices
- midwifery-managed services.

The wider role of the midwife has enabled a decrease in the number of hours worked by junior doctors, whilst achieving continuity of care by undertaking such procedures as perineal suturing and intravenous cannulation. However, Ramsay (1997) cites an instance where midwives who encompass this wider sphere with no increase in staffing levels may be in breach of the Code of professional conduct (UKCC 1992b).

Continuity of care and carer has been highlighted in many government reports as an important issue for women. In addition women want more choice, continuity and control in their care and the birth of their babies. Team midwifery has been seen as a way of providing women with continuity of care, but many units have since abandoned this (Wraight et al 1993).

Activity 6.1

Drug administration

A doctor prescribes an antibiotic, by intravenous injection, for a postnatal mother. The ward is busy and the midwife is responsible for the care of six mothers one of whom has undergone a lower segment caesarean section 3 days ago and is now pyrexial. The midwife has not achieved competency in giving drugs via the intravenous route though the trust has a protocol which allows practitioners to develop competency in this skill.

Question
What action should the midwife take in recognition of fulfilling her accountability?
Try to give your own response to this question before reading the response given below.

Response
If she administers the drug she will be in breach of the Rules and Codes. If she does not administer the drug she needs to ensure another competent practitioner does so to avoid an omission of care.

She should acknowledge her limitations, if the midwife acts outside her sphere of competency she may be negligent as it is the midwife who is responsible for her actions. The doctor who delegated the task still retains some responsibility and the practitioner carrying out the task is accountable to the practitioner delegating. This is termed 'indirect accountability'.

When considering accountability the emphasis is often on doing or commissioning. It is however equally important to acknowledge that accountability includes omission or not doing. (UKCC 1992b)

Activity 6.2

GPs and antenatal care

A GP provides antenatal care personally to his clients. He does not allow the midwife to participate in providing antenatal care for these women. The midwife is aware that the GP implements a medical model and only supplies the physical component of care and examination. There is no discussion instigated by the GP regarding choices, infant feeding or education needs.

Question
Identify the key issues which relate to the midwife's responsibility and accountability in the situation.
Answer this question yourself before reading the response below.

Response
The midwife has a duty to provide antenatal care (Rule 33). The defined activities of a midwife suggest that not to provide care would be a breach of duty of care and therefore failing in her responsibility and accountability. The mother may have legal recourse in terms of lack of midwifery care if health promotion advice is not received and the mother, baby, or both, suffer as a direct consequence.

the woman's care if this meets her needs more effectively. The scenarios in Activities 6.1 and 6.2 should help to explain the midwife's responsibility and accountability in two different situations.

LEGAL DIMENSIONS OF ACCOUNTABILITY AND RESPONSIBILITY

The law has a number of functions in relation to midwives' accountability and responsibility. It structures the relationship between women and the midwife, and between employer and employee. It also sets limits to acceptable practice on behalf of society. Midwives are in a unique position in relation to the law, with a very well-defined sphere of practice. The profession can therefore use the law in a positive way to practise to full potential and to reinforce professional standards rather than undermine them. The sphere of practice of midwives has been clearly defined, which in practice gives the midwife clinical responsibility and independence

Page (1995) considers group practices as a progression of team midwifery aimed to provide continuity of care. One to one midwifery practice is, it is argued, an even better way of providing continuity of carer for women (McCourt & Page 1996). If the midwife is to provide this type of care effectively she must be aware of her responsibilities and sphere of practice. Page (1995) reaffirms that women have equal rights in the relationship which develops between themselves and the midwife. In providing continuity of carer the midwife practises with more responsibility. Dimond (1994) states midwives are legally accountable to their clients, society, employer and the UKCC and, whilst the midwife might be the woman's lead carer, it is also the midwife's responsibility to involve others in not shared in the same way by nurses. However, implementation of The scope of professional practice (1992a) and the review of the Nurses, Midwives and Health Visitors Act (1997) may address this in the future. For example, the title of 'nurse' may well be protected in law as 'midwife' has been, although the definition of the role of a nurse is likely to be more difficult than that of a midwife owing to the huge diversity of clients and patients and practice areas in nursing.

The definition in statute of the midwife's sphere of practice may be defined as the accountability for normal childbirth, and responsibility is demonstrated when a midwife exercises that accountability. Staying within the law and remaining accountable as well as responsible does not always guarantee a career free from involvement with litigation, and not all midwives give thought to this unique blend of legislation, professional accountability and responsibility until things go wrong, compensation is being sought, or they are involved in a disciplinary investigation.

In recent years there has been a steep rise in the volume of obstetric litigation, often for cerebral palsy, which affects around 1 in 400 babies. Obstetric and midwifery litigation claims are currently estimated to be about 5000 new claims against the NHS each year and are the most expensive as well as some of the most frequent. These cases are usually heard in High Court and the sums claimed may be up to £4.8 million. It is estimated that, despite the increase in claims, only 10–20% of cerebral palsy is actually caused by birth asphyxia (Colditz & Henderson-Smart 1990). The other 80–90% are multifactorial and may have been apparent regardless of the mode of delivery. It stands to reason that if this is the case then these claims could be reduced by implementing some risk management strategies that demonstrate reasonable care was, in fact, given during the birth (see Ch. 9). Within the profession there are fears that the risk of litigation could result in defensive practice. Instead what must be demonstrated is that practising midwives act in the capacity of reasonably skilled professionals, and would be judged accordingly. The test is the 'Bolam' standard, that is to say, the midwife would be judged as such by a

responsible body *of reasonably skilled midwives* (*Bolam v. Friern Hospital Management Committee* [1957]). The Bolam standard was approved in *Whitehouse v. Jordan* [1981] 1 All ER 267, in which an obstetrician was found to be not liable for damage caused to a baby during a difficult, failed forceps delivery prior to caesarean. The doctor had not deviated from accepted practice. Lord Denning made it clear that, so long as the clinician (the doctor) had acted with reasonable skill and care, then he should not be held responsible for an adverse outcome. The standard is: you must take reasonable care to avoid acts or omissions which you can reasonably foresee would be likely to injure your neighbour. (Neighbours are people directly affected by such acts.) Within the law, actions would usually be deemed negligent only if care had *not* been taken to guard against *reasonable known* risks. These are risks that would be known *at the time of the incident*, and not in the future when the case may be heard.

As well as being reasonably foreseeable, a successful claim of negligence must also demonstrate a *causal link* between the breach of duty of care by the midwife and the damage suffered by the mother or baby. This causal link is sometimes difficult to prove, as in Case study 6.1 (*Wilsher v. Essex Area Health Authority* [1988] 1 All ER 871 (HL)). In this case a junior inexperienced doctor mistakenly inserted the umbilical catheter into the umbilical vein instead of the artery. The senior registrar was asked to check and failed to notice the mistake. The baby was

Case study 6.1

Wilsher v. Essex Area Health Authority [1988] 1 All ER 871 (HL)

A premature baby was negligently given excess oxygen (increasing the risk of retrolental fibroplasia). The plaintiff alleged that the subsequent blindness was as a direct result of the excessive oxygen but as there were up to five possible causes of the blindness The House of Lords held that the burden of proof lay with the plaintiff and the plaintiff must demonstrate that on the balance of probabilities that the defendant's breach of duty was at least a touchable factor in the harm caused.

subsequently given excessive oxygen and suffered retrolental fibroplasia. Whilst it might appear that the senior registrar was negligent, there were different concurrent problems that may have caused the baby's blindness associated with prematurity. The plaintiffs therefore failed in their claim. Despite the negligence it could not be demonstrated that that one specific act caused the harm.

Early cases of claimed medical negligence resulting in cerebral palsy often involved a difficult delivery and apparent trauma to the baby. Nowadays cases often tend to hinge on the interpretation of the cardiotocograph (CTG) and the causation between a misinterpreted CTG and an allegation of preventable asphyxia, though Gaffney et al (1995) suggest that only a small proportion of all children with cerebral palsy (3–13%) showed signs of intrapartum stress. Misinterpretation of CTG traces can be minimized by a multidisciplinary approach to the creation of standards within the hospital or trust. National or international standards and guidelines may be an even better tool to measure whether reasonable care was given. This would also reduce disputes that may arise as to the definition of the competence of the practitioner involved in interpretation of the CTG trace. This is important when claims involve students and junior staff. It is clear and long established that the minimum standard of care expected from a trainee or inexperienced practitioner is no lower than that expected of an experienced one (*Wilsher v. Essex Area Health Authority* [1988]) as adequate supervision should be given.

Although clinical practice standards are not addressed by the UKCC it is clear that the ultimate responsibility of the midwife to maintain her competence lies with her, and that lack of skill, delegation, or inexperience will not be considered a defence in the eyes of the professional witness or the law, which was also demonstrated in the case of Wilsher (Case study 6.1).

Supervision whilst gaining competency is essential and any limitations in knowledge or competency must be acknowledged and addressed by the individual practitioner. The Code of professional conduct (UKCC 1992b para. 4) states that

'a practitioner should decline to perform any duties or responsibilities unless able to perform them in a safe and skilled manner.' Risk management has advocated that procedures be in place for prompt reporting of incidents, particularly when there is an adverse outcome. A point of good practice would be that any investigations of the cause of any injuries sustained by mother, baby, staff or visitors is well documented at the time. These procedures are instrumental in reducing risks of litigation as well as giving the practitioner evidence to discuss with aggrieved parents if needed (see Ch. 9).

Vicarious liability

Obstetric claims may actually cost more than supplying the maternity service as litigation in the maternity services is extremely expensive. Recent figures from the Clinical Negligence Scheme for Trusts demonstrate that up to 80% of contingent money is for obstetric claims, with the most expensive claim being for children who have subsequently developed cerebral palsy. To minimize risks, insurance companies are asking for specific protocols and guidelines for any high risk or unusual practice. Policies addressing management of eclampsia, waterbirth and ruptured uterus, amongst others, will ensure a discount on insurance premiums. Currently over 400 NHS Trusts use the Clinical Negligence Scheme for Trusts, which would offer the protection of vicarious liability in most reasonable situations a midwife may find herself. This view is supported by Jenkins (1995) who states that vicarious liability is established on the basis of the relationship between the employer and the employee, and concludes that the employer is almost always liable for the acts or omissions of the employee. Lack of understanding of the concept of vicarious liability may be the cause of certain barriers to midwifery practice. For most midwives working within the NHS, their employer will be vicariously liable. If, however, a midwife does something negligently that is obviously outside her contractual duty or acts beyond her skills and competence then she may find herself vulnerable.

The term 'vicarious liability' means that the liability, or the need to account, falls on one person as the result of an action, or the damage caused by the tortious action of another person. NHS Trusts can sue or be sued in the corporate name; they are artificial 'legal persons' or legal personalities. These legal persons are created by statutory procedures which result in vicarious liability or strict liability (i.e. liability but not fault). Certain conditions do have to be met for this situation to arise: there must be an employee–employer relationship and the act for which the employee is personally liable must have been committed during the course of that employment. It would be a mistake to generalize as each case would be examined individually. Insurance is a particular issue for independent midwives who must negotiate vicarious liability when practising in hospitals. There are a small number of midwives who are self-employed or who employ other midwives, but most midwives in the UK are employed in the NHS. It is essential that midwives are aware of both the legal rights and the obligations they have as employers and as employees. Failure on their part to comply with the contract terms may result in a breach of contract. Employees are bound to exercise reasonable care and skill in exercising their duty.

Though a midwife's employer is usually vicariously liable for any negligent actions of the employee, employers can also be held in breach of contract as employees are protected by the law by various statutes including the Employment (consolidation) Act, Employers Liability Acts, Employment Acts, and Health and Safety Acts. An employer may be directly liable in negligence for allowing an inexperienced employee to undertake tasks for which they are not competent to perform without proper supervision (*Jones v. Manchester Corporation* [1952] 2 QB 852, *Wilsher v. Essex Area Health Authority* [1986] 3 All ER 801, 833).

In *Johnstone v. Bloomsbury Health Authority* [1991] it was alleged that expecting junior doctors to work long hours was injurious to health and that the employers were in breach of contract. A definitive case has not yet addressed the contentious issue of junior doctors' hours as a ruling was not given. Employers are under a duty to take reasonable precautions for their employees' safety and to regard statutory provisions. Employers are also responsible for providing adequate training and experience and may be liable to employees in respect of harm suffered at work (HSE 1994). Generally an employer is not liable for harm inflicted on workers by fellow employees.

Consent and trespass to the person

The law can also be empowering for women should they need to assert their rights. Consent means *informed* consent, in that a client or patient must have enough information to make a choice; the consent must be given knowing the risks and benefits (see Case study 6.2). It is an assault in civil law and may also be a criminal offence to subject a pregnant woman (or any patient) to any kind of examination, intervention or treatment without their consent. Nowadays there is no such thing as 'implied consent' and therefore all women must be given sufficient information to make an informed choice. The mentally competent (adult) woman is free to decline the advice or treatment suggested regardless of whether this decision is rational or irrational or for no reason at all. The woman has this basic human right even if as a consequence of declining the treatment or advice she or the fetus, or both, may die. There has been some controversy surrounding the rare cases where

 Case study 6.2

Sidaway v. Bethlem Royal Hospital Governors [1985] 1 All ER 643 (HL)

The plaintiff gave consent to undergo an operation on her spine to relieve shoulder and arm pain; however, she was not made aware of the risks (less than 1%) that the spine may be damaged.

The operation was carried out without negligence but unfortunately the risk materialized and the plaintiff was severely disabled with spinal damage.

The House of Lords held that the surgeon had followed the normal practice of not disclosing the risk and was therefore not negligent.

women have been ordered to undergo non-consensual obstetric intervention. In Re MB [1997] and Re S [1998] it was affirmed that a pregnant woman who has competent mental capacity can refuse treatment for reasons that are rational, irrational or no reason at all, even when the refusal endangers her own life or that of her fetus.

If the woman lacks capacity and this is the opinion of two medical practitioners (preferably one being a psychiatrist) the doctor, through a lawyer, may apply to the court. In such cases the intervention may be deemed not unlawful by the court.

Avoidance of this situation can be achieved to some extent by dealing with potential refusal well before labour in the antenatal period by in-depth discussion regarding the likelihood of intervention, particularly for women with known apprehensions regarding childbirth. Effective communication is the key.

To help practitioners decide if a woman has capacity which is defined as 'some impairment or disturbance or mental disfunctioning', a position statement by the UKCC guides practitioners in such situations and suggests that the three questions that need to be answered in determining whether or not a person has the mental capacity are;

1. Is the patient capable of comprehending and retaining information about the proposed treatment?
2. Is she capable of believing the information given to her about the treatment?
3. Is she capable of weighing up such information to make a choice?

(*Thameside and Glossop Acute Services Trust v. CH [1996]*). Only if the answers to any of these three questions was 'no' would lack of capacity be considered.

In law a fetus becomes a child only at birth, and only at birth acquires legal status and rights. This could be a particular problem if a surgical abortion resulted in a live birth as there is no provision for this situation.

Prior to recent cases and despite the legal principle that an unborn child has no rights there appears to have been confusion, though

Lord Justice Balcombe did uphold this legal principle in Re F (in utero) [1988] Fam 122 when he stated:

'If parliament were to think it appropriate that a pregnant woman should be subject to controls for the benefit of her unborn child, then doubtless it will stipulate the circumstances in which such controls may be applied and the safeguards for the mother's protection. In such a sensitive field effecting, as it does the liberty of the individual, it is not for the judiciary to extend the law.'

The cases of MB (Re MB [1997]) and S (Re S [1998]) also confirms this principal.

Knowledge of such legal principles is important to recognize the lawful boundaries applicable to difficult situations, particularly as time is usually of the essence.

There are a number of situations where midwives are faced with conflicting expectations. For example, the trust policy might be for all women to undergo CTG monitoring whereas the woman declines to undergo it having made an informed decision. Or a woman might wish a pool delivery but the midwife's employer does not support this practice. In both these situations the midwife is under a legal and moral obligation to attend and provide midwifery care. Failure to respect women's rights and choice may result in a woman claiming trespass to the person. Women are becoming more aware of their rights and less susceptible to paternalistic attitudes. Midwives need therefore to be increasingly aware of the legal issues that relate to accountability and responsibility in the clinical practice situation. There have been well-documented cases where employment issues have been in conflict with the rights of the woman or Midwives rules, or both (Hewson 1997).

Most claims of medical (midwifery) negligence are not notified to the hospital for some years unless it concerns the woman herself, when it will be governed by the statute of limitations and therefore must be made within 3 years. It is unrealistic to expect all midwives to maintain their contemporaneous notes as if each case will end in litigation, but to demonstrate competence is essential. Poor record keeping, lost CTGs and fatigued memory have been the cause of successful claims even when the standard of care has been reasonable and clinical competence was likely. The evidence available must show what actually happened, including the way the decisions were approached and consent obtained, as in some cases it could be nearly 25 years before a case is heard in court.

Summary

The primary and secondary legislation that govern the practice of midwives highlights a dichotomy. Whilst it might be argued that it curtails the accountability of a midwife, it also allows enhancement of the role through expecting competency in new skills to meet contemporary practice. Requests by the consumer for increased choice, control and continuity of care challenges midwives to become more flexible within their sphere of accountability. These new patterns of care which offer the consumer more choice also offer the midwife a wider role and increased accountability and responsibility.

Midwives need to be fully aware of the standard of care they are legally bound to provide and the consequences of not doing so both in the professional and civil fields if they are to embrace this wider and possibly more responsible and challenging role.

REFERENCES

Batey M V, Lewis F M 1982 Clarifying autonomy and accountability in nursing service part 1. The Journal of Nursing Administration September:13–18

Bergman R 1981 Accountability—definition and dimensions. International Nursing Review 28(2):53–59

Bolam v. Friern Hospital Management Committee [1957] 1 Weekly Law Reports 582

Bradshaw G, Bradshaw P 1997 The professionalisation of midwifery. Modern Midwife 7(12):23–25

Burton v. Islington Health Authority [1992] 3 All England Law Reports 833 (CA)

CMB (Central Midwives Board) 1919 Midwives rules. CMB, London

Clarke E, Renfrew M 1992 Research awareness and the midwife. Module 9 in the Midwifery Update series. Distance Learning Centre, South Bank University, London

Clarke R 1995 Midwives, their employers and the UKCC. An eternally unethical triangle. Nursing Ethics 2(3):247–325

Colditz, PB, Henderson-Smart DJ 1990 Electronic fetal heart rate monitoring during labour: does it prevent perinatal asphyxia and cerebral palsy? Medical Journal of Australia 153(2): 88–90.

Copp G 1988 Professional accountability the conflict. Nursing Times 84(43):42–44

Cross R 1996 Midwives and management. Books for Midwives, London, p 5

Dimond B 1994 Legal aspects of midwifery. Books for Midwives, Hale

DoH (Department of Health) 1993 Changing childbirth part 1. Report of the Expert Maternity Group. HMSO, London

Ennis M, Vincent C 1990 British Medical Journal 300(May): 1365

Entwhistle F 1993 Extend with care. Nursing Times 89(28) July 14:66–68

Fraser D 1995 Client centred care—fact or fiction. Midwives 108(1) June 289:174–177.

Fraser D, Murphy R, Worth-Butler M 1997 An outcome evaluation of the effectiveness of pre-registration midwifery programmes of education. ENB, London

Gaffney G, Flavell V, Johnson A, Squier M, Sellers S 1995 Model to identify potentially preventable cerebral palsy of intrapartum origin. Archives of Diseases in Childhood 73:F106–F108

Hartley J 1997 'Normal pregnancy and labour'—is it limiting midwifery practice? British Journal of Midwifery December 5(12):773–776

HSE (Health and Safety Executive) 1994 COSHH, the general approved code of practice. HSE, London

Hewson B 1997 Court ordered obstetric intervention: the Last Word? Healthcare Risk Report June:9–11

HMSO 1902 Midwives Act. HMSO, London

HMSO 1951 Midwives Act. HMSO, London

HMSO 1979 Nurses, Midwives and Health Visitors Act. HMSO, London

HMSO 1992 Nurses, Midwives and Health Visitors Act. HMSO, London

HMSO 1997 Nurses, Midwives and Health Visitors Act. HMSO, London

House of Commons (1992) Health Committee second report on maternity services. HMSO, London

Hunt J M 1984 Research—why don't we use these findings? Nursing Mirror 158(8) February 22:29

Hutton I 1994 What women want from midwives. British Journal of Midwifery, 2:608–611

Jenkins R 1995 The law and the midwife. Blackwell Science, Oxford

Johns C 1989 Accountability and the practice nurse. Practice Nurse 2(7):303–304

Johnstone v. Bloomsbury Health Authority [1991] 2 All ER 293

Jones v. Manchester Corporation [1952] 2 QB 852

Jones M 1996 Accountability in practice. A guide to professional responsibility for nurses in general practice. Mark Allen, Wiltshire

Kendrick K 1995 Codes of professional conduct and the dilemmas of professional practice. In: Soothill K, Mackay L, Webb C (eds) Interprofessional relations in health care. Edward Arnold, London

Kitson A 1993 Accountable for quality. Nursing Standard 8(1):4–6

Lewis F M, Batey M V 1982 Clarifying autonomy and accountability in nursing service: part 2. The Journal of Nursing Administration October:10–15

McCourt C, Page L 1996 Report on the evaluation of one-to-one midwifery. Thames Valley University, London

McKay 1997 The route to autonomous practice. Nursing Times 93(46):61–62

Mander R 1995 Where does the buck stop? Accountability in midwifery. In: Watson R (ed) Accountability in nursing practice. Chapman Hall, London, pp 95–106

Page L 1995 Effective group practice in midwifery working with women. Blackwell, London

Pearson A, Vaughan B 1986 Nursing models for practice. Heineman, London

Pope R, Cooney M, Graham L, Holliday M, Patel S 1997 Aspects of care provided by midwives—part one: an overview. British Journal of Midwifery 5(12):766–770

Ramsay B 1997 When midwives perform obstetric tasks at night, trainees spend more time in clinic. British Medical Journal 314(7036) June 21:1830

Re F (in utero) 1988 Fam 122

Re S 1998 St George's Healthcare National Health Service Trust v S (1998) 2 FLR 728

Re MB, The Times LR, 18 April 1997

Reid T 1993 Welcome to change. Nursing Times 89(11):26–30

Reid T 1994 Waterbirth. Nursing Times 90(11):26–30

Robinson S, Golden J, Bradley S 1983 A Study of the role and responsibilities of the midwife. Nursing Education Research Unit. Report to King's College, University of London

Schott J 1993 Changing ourselves. British Journal of Midwifery October 5:230–231

Sidaway v. Bethlem Royal Hospital Governors [1985] 1 All England Law Reports ER 643 (HL)

Soothill K, Mackay L, Webb C 1995 Interprofessional relations in health care. Edward Arnold, London

Thameside and Glossop Acute Services Trust v. CH [1996]

Tschudin V 1989 Ethics in nursing: the caring relationship. Heineman Nursing, Oxford

UKCC (United Kingdom Central Council) 1992a Scope of professional practice. UKCC, London

UKCC (United Kingdom Central Council) 1992b Code of professional conduct. UKCC, London

UKCC (United Kingdom Central Council) 1993 Midwives rules. UKCC, London

UKCC (United Kingdom Central Council) 1996 Guidelines for professional practice. UKCC, London

UKCC (United Kingdom Central Council) 1997 Handbook—protecting the public through professional standards. UKCC, London

UKCC (United Kingdom Central Council) 1998a Midwives rules and code of practice. UKCC, London

UKCC (United Kingdom Central Council) 1998b Guidelines for records and record keeping. UKCC, London

Whitehouse v. Jordan [1981] 1 Weekly Law Reports 246 (HL)

Wilsher v. Essex Area Health Authority [1988] 1 All England Law Reports ER 871 (HL)

Wraight A, Ball J, Seccombe I, Stock J 1993 Mapping team midwifery IMS Report Series 24-2. Institute of Manpower Studies, Brighton

FURTHER READING

Pyne R 1998 Professional disciplines in nursing, midwifery and health visiting. Blackwell, Oxford

Watson R (ed) (1995) Accountability in nursing practice. Chapman Hall, London

7

The scope of professional practice

Nicola J Dunn   Carol Newton

This chapter aims to clarify the role and responsibilities of the midwife within the scope of professional practice. It considers the debate surrounding post-registration education and practice, specialist and advanced practitioner principles and their application to midwifery. It discusses the more common developments of the midwife's role and applies the scope of professional practice to them.

INTRODUCTION

The midwife's role is clearly defined in the Midwives rules and code of practice (UKCC 1998a). Additionally, the midwife's responsibilities and scope of practice are explicitly stated in Rule 40 (UKCC 1998a). There may, however, be occasions when a midwife wishes to add to her existing scope of practice, and therefore the principles and framework for incorporating a new skill into her role become relevant. To reiterate the Midwives code of conduct (UKCC 1994), the supervisor of midwives must be consulted prior to any adjustment to the midwife's role with regard to preparation and experience needed.

Those aspects of a midwife's role which require additional knowledge and skills are many. The aim of this chapter is to discuss the more common developments of the role, and apply the scope of professional practice to them, with the view that any new skill or development could be ascribed to similarly.

The scope of professional practice

The scope of professional practice has existed as a concept for nursing, midwifery and health visiting since June 1992 (UKCC 1992a). Following the UKCC 1992 publication of the Scope of professional practice for nursing, midwifery and health visiting, accountability and professional judgements have been the bedrock that have underpinned the practitioners responsibilities beyond the traditional boundaries of practice.

The six principles of the scope of practice

The six principles of scope were conceived to assist practitioners to be more flexible and professionally challenging in their practice, their aim being to provide innovative solutions in meeting the needs in a health service that is constantly changing (UKCC 1997a).

The six principles require the midwife to:

1. be satisfied that patient and client needs are uppermost
2. keep up to date and develop knowledge, skills and competence
3. recognize limits to personal knowledge and skill and remedy deficiencies
4. ensure that existing practice is not compromised by new developments and responsibilities
5. acknowledge personal accountability
6. avoid inappropriate delegation which might compromise patient or client interests.

These UKCC principles should enable practitioners to decide themselves what skills and additional knowledge they need, and define the limits of their own practice without the need to acquire certificates demonstrating the licence to do so. The onus is on the individual practitioner to take responsibility and accountability for her practice and conduct. From the point of registration, each practitioner is subject to the Council's Code of professional conduct (1992b) which provides a statement of the values of the professions and establishes the framework within which practitioners practise and conduct themselves. Each registered practitioner is accountable for their actions and omissions to the Council, and this position is regardless of employment circumstances.

Extended practice

Extended practice is a notion that has existed traditionally within nursing working on the premise that pre-registration education equips the nurse to perform at a certain level, and that increasing the range of nursing duties following registration requires 'official' extensions by certification. This practice is deemed no longer suitable as it is the Council's view that principles for practice should form the basis for the scope of practice not certificates for tasks.

Within midwifery, practice is set out in the Midwives code of practice (UKCC 1998a). The code categorically states that: 'As a practising midwife you are accountable for your own practice in whatever environment you are practising' (UKCC 1998a p. 25). This is further expanded upon by stating that: 'In all circumstances, the safety and welfare of the mother and her baby are of primary importance' (UKCC 1998a p. 25).

Midwives have a defined sphere of practice, and are accountable for that practice. The emphasis is placed on 'appropriate preparation', and being 'clinically up to date'. The responsibilities of the midwife and the registered medical practitioner are complementary and closely interelated; however, each practitioner retains clinical accountability for her own practice. The settings in which the midwife practises may require a midwife to acquire new skills; therefore it is recognised that some developments in midwifery practice can become an integral part of the role of all midwives, and other developments may become part of the role of some midwives. The UKCC recognized that midwives have always had a clear framework for developing their scope of practice (UKCC 1992a pp. 8–9). The publication the Scope of professional practice (UKCC 1992a) provided important key principles to supplement the midwife's regularly updated Midwives rules (e.g. UKCC 1993, updated UKCC 1998a) and code of practice.

However, the Council believes that the Midwives code of practice (UKCC 1998a) and the Midwives code of conduct (UKCC 1994) together provide the key principles for the scope of midwifery practice, which are also clearly detailed alongside the midwife's responsibilities in rule 40 of the Midwives rules (UKCC 1998a).

New skill acquisition

Where new skill acquisition may not necessarily become an integral part of the role of all midwives each employing authority should have locally agreed policies which observe the Council's requirements which the midwives should familiarize themselves with. In addition, consultation with the supervisor of midwives regarding appropriate preparation and experience should also be sought in these instances.

However, before any future developments or skill additions are made, the practitioner's current scope of practice should be reviewed. This can be undertaken through the personal profile, and discussed as part of the practitioner's appraisal, or through the statutory annual supervisory review. If a practitioner is currently and regularly undertaking a particular skill competently, this is already part of that practitioner's scope of practice, and training does not have to be repeated unless so required to maintain standards.

The Midwives rules

The UKCC Midwifery Committee have been considering the plight of midwives in clinical practice when the requirements of the Midwives rules conflict with the policies of their employers. An example of this is evident with resuscitation of the newborn. Rule 40 of the Midwives rules (UKCC 1993) required the midwife to call for medical aid when deviation from the norm occurs either with the mother or baby. However,

many maternity units have policies that require a midwife to summon a neonatal nurse practitioner if any deviation from the norm occurs in the health of the baby. This places the midwives in a vulnerable position, because whether it be a medical or neonatal nurse practitioner that the midwife chooses to call for assistance this could be contravening either the local policy or rule 40 of the Midwives rules (UKCC 1993). This has been previously highlighted with waterbirths (UKCC 1997b), and midwives have been placed in a 'no win' situation. This obvious mismatch between practice and legislation prompted the amendments to the Midwives rules to ensure midwives were supported through legislation to the changing needs of women and the maternity service. The issue with neonatal resuscitation will be resolved, as the second paragraph of the 1993 rule 40(1) which explicitly demands a midwife to summon a registered medical practitioner has now been amended. It now forms rule 40(3) (UKCC 1998a), and states that in an emergency:

'... a practising midwife shall call a registered medical practitioner or such other qualified health professional who may reasonably be expected to have the requisite skills and experience to assist her.'

The word 'practitioner' has been avoided in keeping with the Council's principal rules. The inclusion of 'other qualified health professional' as has relevant skills and experience enables the midwife to use her discretion in determining who she will call depending upon the severity of the problem. This will serve to enhance the midwife's autonomy and accountability. The responsibility will now rest on the midwife to discern the nature of the problem and the appropriateness of the person she chooses to summon, as this will apply to calling for necessary assistance to either mother or baby. However, Meah (1998) warns midwives not to confuse flexibility with ambiguity, and to negotiate, at local level, clear guidelines promoting common understanding.

The final paragraph of rule 40(1) (UKCC 1993) has been deleted largely owing to the changes in structures and work practices within the maternity services making this section obsolete.

Additionally rule 40(2) (UKCC 1998a) has been adjusted to read: 'Except in an emergency, a practising midwife shall not provide any midwifery care, or undertake any treatment which she has not, either before or after registration as a midwife, been trained to give or which is outside her current sphere of practice.' The inclusion of the word 'or' allows the midwife to seek assistance if she has not had appropriate training, or if the care/treatment is outside her current sphere of practice. The use of the word 'current' permits developments in practice in response to new innovations in care.

What continues to be paramount is that practitioners' knowledge and practice remain up to date and their competency is maintained. Changes and developments of a midwife's scope of practice may be a response to:

- advances in research
- alterations in the provision of health care services
- changes in local policy
- new approaches to professional practice.

With changing and complex demands from contemporary health care, the need for more specialist skills and knowledge becomes obvious. Education and experience naturally develop and refine, and, to build on from pre-registration education that has prepared practitioners for safe practice, post-registration education provides the medium for practitioners to develop their expertise and expand their range of skills. This expansion is based firmly on the six key principles outlined on p. 112 and re-emphasized by the UKCC more recently: 'These principles recognise that every registered practitioner is accountable for their own practice and that their own professional judgement can provide creative solutions to meeting the needs of patients and clients' (UKCC 1997b).

Post-registration education and practice—specialist practitioner

The Post-registration education and practice project (PREPP) (UKCC 1989) was developed by the UKCC to raise standards of post-registration education and practice to contribute to the maintenance and development of professional knowledge and competence. The need for some practitioners practising within a speciality to possess the UKCC recordable qualification to become specialists has been identified, with specialist practitioners 'exercising higher levels of judgement, discretion and decision making in clinical care' (UKCC 1998b p. 1). Programmes leading to specialist qualifications approved by the national boards have been available in the UK since Autumn 1995. These courses are currently operating a transitional arrangement in order to use the title 'specialist practitioner'. The practitioners must have a post-registration clinical recordable qualification following a course of 4 months or more relevant to the area of practice; have on record that they and their employer are confident in their skills and knowledge to practise safely and effectively; and have consolidated their pre-registration recordable qualification. It is acceptable in this instance for the programme to be at diploma level. Since November 1998 the programmes should be at no less than first degree level, nor less than 32 weeks full time, and be comprised of 50% theory and 50% practice.

Midwifery has opted out of using the title 'specialist' as the draft learning outcomes encompassed many of the requirements of pre-registration midwifery programmes. However, the recently published UKCC document detailing the standards for specialist education and practice (UKCC 1998c) states that practitioners on part 10 of the professional register wishing to record the qualification of specialist practitioner can do so providing they have completed a sufficient period of experience to have consolidated the pre-registration outcomes. Additionally, they must provide evidence that the specialist practice qualification is necessary for 'higher order responsibility in clinical care and that it is relevant, required and responsive to health needs' (UKCC 1998c p. 3). Unfortunately it appears from the programmes available that 'specialist community nursing education and practice—public health nursing/health visiting' is the only programme where those registered on Part 10 of the professional register are eligible to apply. This paradoxically permits a non-nurse midwife (direct entrant) to record a nursing qualification.

Although, essentially, midwives have rejected the road of specialist practice as cited earlier in view of the requirements of the pre-registration midwifery programmes, there is a small number (mostly midwives on neonatal units) who want to be specialist practitioners. The current situation allows more opportunities for the nurse or midwife on part 1 and 10 of the Professional Register to record a qualification as a nurse specialist, but not as a midwife specialist specifically. However, according to the UKCC, specialist programmes must consolidate the pre-registration learning outcomes. This in effect, means that only children's nurses are able to become specialist practitioners in neonatal nursing, and not midwives. This absurdity generates the situation where general nurses and midwives would say they are equally qualified, but in professional terms this is not the case (Whyte 1998).

ADVANCED PRACTICE OR EXPANDED PRACTICE?

There was, and still remains, some confusion surrounding the concept of advanced practice initially voiced in the original PREPP document (UKCC 1989), and the expansion of role cited within the Scope of practice. The confusion concerns titles, roles and responsibilities. The UKCC did not at its inception see 'advanced practice' as an additional layer of practice to be added to 'specialist practice', but as an important field of professional practice concerned with the continuing development of practitioners in the interests of the clients and the health services. Again, midwifery is currently considering the role and title of 'advanced practice', with a debate going on regarding the title and whether it should be recordable. In March 1997, the UKCC made the decision not to set standards, with an acknowledgement that all practitioners have the opportunity of advancing their practice. Therefore there are no standards set for advanced practice (UKCC 1998b). The following sets out the

UKCC's vision from the original PREP document (UKCC 1989):

Advanced midwifery practice is concerned with:

- adjusting the boundaries for the development of future practices
- pioneering and developing new roles which are responsive to changing needs
- advancing clinical practice, research and education to enrich midwifery
- contributing to health policy and management and the determination of health needs
- continuing the development of midwifery in the interests of the mother, the baby, the family and the health services.

Advancing midwifery practice in this way will lead to:

- innovations in practice
- an increase in midwifery research and research-based practice
- the provision of expert professionals who will have a consultancy role
- a high level of professional leadership
- increased political and professional influence in respect of the development of maternity services
- expert resources for, for example, education, supervision and management.

Since 1996, the UKCC have held several meetings discussing the history of PREP, and how advanced practice fits in with this. The main points to emerge from these meetings are that the title of 'advanced practice' is not seen as a particularly helpful descriptor, and the term 'consultant midwife' may be adopted. There appears to be agreement that advanced midwifery practice is concerned with role expansion, but in all aspects of midwifery practice as opposed to being merely an adoption of particular clinical skills. It should be peer awarded, and explicitly practice focused. It has been envisaged that advanced midwifery practitioners will be few, and their prime function would be to move the profession forward (i.e. advancing midwifery practice as a whole). Advanced practice is perceived currently to require a high level, eclectic knowledge base, the ability to question practice constantly, high motivation and commitment, maturity, confidence and self-awareness. Advanced practitioners are to be grounded in practice, and have research, education and consultancy functions. They will be innovators, at the forefront of developments, influencing local and national policy. However, the progression of this tenet is at present still being explored by Council and the profession as a whole.

Advanced midwife practitioners

A strong argument in favour of advanced midwife practitioners is presented by Charlton (1996) as being composed of those midwives with a high degree of skill and experience in different areas, an obvious area being in the delivery suite. He places great value on the support and advice that knowledgeable and experienced midwives offer to junior members of staff, and fears for their survival in the current climate of continuity of carer, with midwives on the first day of registration being entitled by law to practise their profession. Although knowledge is deemed important for advanced practitioners, he questions the validity of the argument for education to be at master's level. He stipulates that midwives need to have a sound understanding of the basics behind clinical conditions to provide true advocacy. This appears to resemble the state of play in many labour wards today, with midwifery coordinators assuming a supportive and advisory role for junior midwives, as well as being an additional knowledge resource. It could therefore be argued that experience is more effective in determining advanced practitioner status for which, as yet, there is no academic recognition at that level in clinical practice.

Sisto & Hillier (1996) also acknowledge that this concept of 'mastery' is problematic, as midwifery experience is relatively uncharted, and question whether advanced midwifery practice can be a reality. They accept that if midwives with advanced knowledge and skills operate their care at a 'sophisticated level of intellectual synthesis' (p. 179) then the concept is a valid

one. They provide another point of view: that of expert midwife as opposed to advanced practitioner. To this end they propose that expert midwives possess enhanced diagnostic skills to discern the boundaries between normal and abnormal. They innovate and develop theory in practice. The advanced practitioner in midwifery influences policies and the organization of practice, and would assume a role of team leader, supervisor of midwives or manager. The expert midwife, on the other hand, is concerned with the 'how' and 'why' of practice, and is not organizationally bound. The advanced practitioner in midwifery is primarily concerned with the 'why' first and then the 'how'; she is also embedded within an organizational structure. Sisto & Hillier propose that both expert and advanced practitioners are likely to demonstrate mastery, but from different perspectives. They expand further to say that an advanced practitioner of midwifery may not be in current practice but will utilize the knowledge and expertise of other midwives to act as a catalyst to drive the service forward.

Noble (1996) disagrees with the notion that expert midwives specialize in one area of practice as this contravenes the ethos of the Midwives rules (UKCC 1998a), and smacks in the face of continuity of care or carer. Additionally she refutes the notion that a midwife not in current practice can be an advanced practitioner, as 'they are the experts of all-round clinical midwifery, continually advancing their evidence-based practice' (p. 176).

Advancement can also imply progression, which generally requires new learning, therefore rendering the advanced practitioner a learner again with a return to basics from time to time, which engenders 'lifelong learning' (Allen 1996). This supports the view that all midwife practitioners given the education and opportunity can become 'advanced'.

Walsh (1996) welcomes the prospect of a career pathway above the level of grade G, and endorses the opinion already expressed that clinical practice would constitute a major part of the role. Walker (1996) sees the advanced practitioner as one who encompasses the 10 key characteristics as defined by the English National Board (ENB 1993). In this instance all midwives in possession of the Higher Award in Midwifery Practice are advanced practitioners, which could be a useful spin-off if utilized in this way.

Boden & Pritchard (1996) suggest that the advanced midwife practitioners should be facilitators in 'educating junior staff and trainees', and be: 'prepared to extend their clinical role beyond the currently accepted "normal" sphere of practice, taking responsibility for duties currently undertaken by junior doctors e.g. admitting and clerking patients, assessing needs, ordering scans and blood tests' (p. 176).

This is echoed by Walker (1996) who feels advanced midwifery practitioners should be involved in teaching programmes for student midwives, midwives, GP trainees, junior doctors and medical students. This Walker (1996) argues will inculcate a trusting relationship and enhance role awareness. Page (1996) likens the role as both companion and clinician to the family with the view to their long term well-being. This appears to encompass a significant portion of the GP role remit.

Credibility

Credibility as viewed by the midwifery profession, the medical profession and the women who will receive the care either directly or indirectly has to be a consideration when debating the role and responsibilities of the advanced midwifery practitioner. Does academic qualification or practical experience promote credibility? The debate surrounding education to at least master's level is a valid one, as is the requirement of appropriate experience. Jones (1996) adds a further dimension: that of management ability. Jones (1996) also poses a very real concern for the profession should midwifery choose to go down this line, and that is that 'the advanced practitioner', who is educated to master's or doctorate levels, is unlikely to remain in clinical practice for low clinical grading. This must force the decision to be made at some point as to the purpose of this position, and to ensure midwifery is itself advanced by

this proposal, and not merely the practitioners themselves.

Activity 7.1 considers the matter of the advanced practitioner.

Activity 7.1

Consider the debate of advanced midwife practitioner. What aspects still need to be explored before a conclusion can be reached?

Role expansion

Role expansion by the midwife has been affected by the need to reduce junior doctors' hours, the effects of which need to be closely monitored. The UKCC have identified that changes made to local policies impacting on a midwife's clinical practice subsequently causing professional and employment conflict are partly in response to this (UKCC 1998b). Woodrow (1996) asserts that tasks are not unique to specific professions, claiming that everything a doctor or other health care worker undertakes is at some time undertaken by someone else. Anecdotally, it could also be said that it was not uncommon to witness junior doctors performing some tasks which they did not know how to do, under the verbal instruction of a midwife who did know how to do it but was not allowed to within current definitions of her sphere of practice.

Role expansion or extension is an ongoing deliberation. However, for the ease of the reader in this instance, extension implies additional duties being delegated, with indirect supervision from medical staff. This has led to problems with both autonomy and accountability, yet has remained unchallenged (Scholefield, Viney & Evans 1997). Expansion does not discount skills undertaken as extended roles, but permits the boundaries of practice to be defined reflecting the client population need. Greater autonomy and satisfaction have been reported since its introduction, as it has enabled decisions to be made at a local level close to the client and has provided a greater degree of professional accountability (Scholefield, Viney & Evans 1997).

Delegation of care

When considering neonatal resuscitation, following an audit of the paediatricians' involvement at delivery at one large maternity unit (Newton 1997), all midwives employed by the trust have since attended a programme on basic life support and advanced resuscitation methods. Paediatricians no longer attend elective caesarean sections unless there is a problem or meconium staining is present, and a formal protocol for the attendance of paediatricians at delivery has been discussed. This maternity unit has adopted a policy where all midwives rotate onto the labour ward and, as midwives are on site 24 hours a day, availability and response time to carry out neonatal resuscitation does not pose a problem. As all midwives do rotate onto the labour ward, it was feasible to train all midwives as they would easily maintain these skills. In some areas it may be appropriate to train only 'core staff'.

Fears have been expressed that existing elements of care would be compromised, or inappropriate delegation of care would occur which would not be in the best interests of the client or the profession (Copp 1988, Scholefield, Viney & Evans 1997). However the Scope of professional practice document (UKCC 1992a) explicitly states that any adjustment to practice must not compromise the existing elements of care or result in inappropriate delegation. Bick (1996) argues that postnatal care is already neglected, and that improvements in this area should be considered before the introduction of the advanced practitioner, with all midwives needing to advance their own practice before supporting selected individuals to undertake additional responsibilities.

Midwives need to utilize the Midwives rules (UKCC 1998a) in conjunction with the Scope as the rules clearly define the role and sphere of practice. Without these restrictions on what a midwife can do within her practice the possibilities would be that a midwife could make decisions that were beyond her role (even though she may be competent). The most extreme scenario could be a midwife performing a caesarean

section when needed in an emergency. Though this may be possible within the Scope, it would not be possible within the rules as a midwife. Most will recall the recent media coverage of a doctor delegating part of a surgical operation to a theatre sister. Although the doctor delegating felt the nurse to be competent, as did the nurse herself, it was outside her role and sphere of practice as depicted by the UKCC, hence the inevitable disciplinary aftermath.

Activity 7.2 considers this incident further.

Activity 7.2

In light of this incident, in what other aspects of midwifery practice could this situation reoccur if the midwife is governed by the Midwives rules and code of practice?

INCORPORATING THE SCOPE OF PRACTICE INTO PRACTICE

It has become apparent that midwives are effective change agents with practice providing a more integrated and holistic approach. It is essential that it is constantly being evaluated. Two main examples of where this is evident are perineal suturing and epidural top-ups by midwives. The Midwife's code of practice (1998a p. 29) states: 'Developments in midwifery care can become an integral part of the role of the midwife and are then incorporated in the initial preparation of the midwife'.

It is estimated that 40% of women choose to have epidural analgesia, and with the development of highly technological approaches to midwifery care there has been a simultaneous increase in the incidence of perineal trauma. It seems reasonable therefore that the need to master the art of epidural top-up and perineal suturing should form an integral part of student midwives' education and training, despite the continuing evidence that the incidence of episiotomy is declining (Draper & Newell 1996). Perineal suturing was traditionally delegated to the junior doctor whose training in repair was probably minimal; this was compounded by the regular rotation of junior doctors (Draper & Newell 1996). However, since the early 1980s, midwives have been educated to suture the perineum, and the numbers of midwives repairing the perineum after delivery is increasing. It is now considered part of the continuing care that the person performing the delivery should repair or decide not to repair the perineum (Lewis 1996). This serves to eradicate the problem of often inexperienced junior doctors undertaking perineal repair on a vulnerable client group.

There are other aspects of care that are currently under review and in some areas already introduced into the midwife's role. These will now be considered in detail and are: intravenous cannulation, midwife prescribing and the initial examination of the healthy newborn.

Intravenous cannulation

The RCM recommended (1994) that, in view of the responsibilities placed upon a midwife in the management of emergencies such as eclampsia, haemorrhage and obstructed labour, midwives should be competent in the skill of intravenous cannulation.

The procedure of cannulation is now becoming routine for many nurses in different specialities of their profession (Dougherty 1996a). It seemed reasonable therefore that McCall (1997, unpublished work) asked the question 'Should midwives perform this task?' With the reduction of junior doctors' hours and the expansion of midwifery tasks, McCall investigated the opinions of two groups of midwives and doctors: one group at a maternity unit where intravenous cannulation was routinely performed by midwives, and one group at a unit where midwives do not cannulate. Her objectives for the study were to:

1. find out whether cannulation currently being performed by midwives is successful
2. assess the willingness of midwives and doctors to having the role of cannulation being taken on by midwives.

The results demonstrated that those midwives already cannulating were happy to do so and felt it a valuable skill to have, and those midwives who were not would like to see cannulation incorporated into their role. The doctors were generally happy with this, with none being actively opposed to it. They stated that they wanted the midwives to have adequate training and supervision but did not clarify this further (McCall 1997, unpublished work).

Jackson (1997) warns practitioners of their accountability when taking on an 'advanced practice skill', and stresses they must take responsibility for ensuring they have sufficient theoretical knowledge and practical skill for their safe practice. He argues that the previous fragmented approach with certain health care professionals undertaking only certain health-related tasks has changed with the Scope of professional practice (UKCC 1992a) enabling roles and skills being adopted to suit the needs of the clients in their care. However this professional development must not compromise professional integrity, nor disregard their level of accountability. Team liability does not exist in law (Dimond 1994). For cannulation to be successfully incorporated into practice, the organization and management need to be fully committed.

Cannulation should not fragment existing aspects of care, and should be introduced as an holistic care package and not a task (Jackson 1997). Methods of introducing cannulation within an organization vary from educating designated appropriate individuals, a cannulation team approach, to a combination of these. Dougherty (1996b) describes the benefits of an i.v. team in hospital practice at the Royal Marsden Hospital in London, which provides a full hospital-wide service following the reduction in junior doctors' hours. Jackson (1997) feels that this system deprives staff who are ward or department based, and thus responsible only for those patients within that setting. Additionally it makes cannulation a task. Dougherty (1996b) argues that if ward staff are expected to acquire this skill to the proficiency of the i.v. team, they need to be supported by a clinical i.v. expert (member of the team); also, extra valuable care-giving time could be wasted by the ward-based practitioner owing to lack of skill and expertise. Maintaining the competency of this skill could additionally be questioned in view of the number of clients under the care of that practitioner needing intravenous cannulation. Statistically, Dougherty (1996b) cites an 83% accuracy rate for the i.v. team as opposed to 50% with the non-i.v. team, and an 80% reduction in phlebitis rates since the i.v. team's introduction. This serves to reduce client pain and suffering, and the costs incurred with treating phlebitis, which could include increased lengths of stay.

In McCall's study (1997, unpublished work), none of the midwives currently undertaking intravenous cannulation were performing it very regularly. The majority were siting a cannula less than once a week, with a minority cannulating between one and five times a week. The main problem identified was a poor success rate of correct insertion of the cannulae. This appears to support Dougherty's (1996b) argument.

Maintenance of the competency of this skill is an obvious area of concern. How often it should be performed to maintain competency is a good question. Also, should cannulation by midwives be undertaken routinely or just in emergency situations? The type of emergencies midwives might be faced with include haemorrhage and severe pre-eclampsia, both of which require immediate cannulation as an emergency procedure. This could be in either the hospital or the community setting, therefore it is reasonable to prepare all midwives to deal appropriately with the emergency until medical assistance arrives. However, as emergencies tend to occur infrequently, proficiency could be lost if a required number of cannulations inserted within a set time scale is perceived as competence.

It could be argued therefore that there is justification for all midwives to undertake cannulation in both routine and emergency situations, as non-routine cannulation would serve to increase the numbers performed by midwives attempting to conserve their proficiency in this skill. Non-emergency cannulation is most likely to be undertaken prior to an epidural anaesthetic, or to the commencement of a Syntocinon infusion to augment labour. The benefits of midwives undertaking this are quite obviously a reduction in the time spent waiting for a doctor, and it fulfils the continuity of carer concept. It does, however, lead onto another two aspects of role expansion: that of midwife prescribing and intravenous drug administration.

Midwife prescribing

The UKCC Midwifery Committee in March 1996 convened to discuss the supply and administration of intravenous fluids by midwives in an emergency. They concluded that in this circumstance it would be in the best interests of the woman to receive intravenous fluids as soon as possible from the midwife. The midwife was unfortunately prevented from initiating intravenous therapy under the restrictions imposed by the Medicines Act 1968. It was therefore considered appropriate for an application to be made to amend schedule 3(II) which would incorporate an approved i.v. fluid to be added to the list of parenteral medicines which midwives are able to supply and administer.

Midwife prescribing has also been deliberated by the UKCC Midwifery Committee. The relevant legislation includes:

- the Medicines Act 1968
- the Misuse of Drugs Act 1971
- the Misuse of Drugs Regulations 1985
- the Medicines (Products Other than Veterinary Drugs) (Prescription Only) Order 1983.

Further guidance is contained within:

- the Midwives rules and code of practice (UKCC 1998a)
- the Midwives code of practice (UKCC 1994a)
- Standards for the administration of medicines (UKCC 1992c)
- Guidelines for the Safe and Secure Handling of Medicines (the Duthie Report) 1988.

Following a survey from all LSA responsible officers in the United Kingdom, it was established that there was a lack of clarity concerning some aspects of drug use in midwifery practice.

Following on from this the committee are currently considering two aspects:

1. clarification of current arrangements
2. a midwife prescribing initiative.

Included within the survey a list was formulated of all drugs used throughout the UK that are contained in standing orders for use by midwives (UKCC 1997c). It includes the following i.v. fluids:

- Hartman's solutions
- dextrose 5%
- normal saline
- compound sodium lactate (1 unit only).

Standing orders are generally for prescription only medicines including controlled drugs in hospital practice only. It therefore questions whether midwives attending emergencies in the community or home confinements are discriminated against midwives working in the hospital.

The administration of Syntocinon has also become an integral part of the role of the midwife in augmenting labour. Both of these prescriptive aspects of care highlight the fact that intravenous cannulation is not in isolation, but often requires actions that follow on from it that also demand knowledge and competence.

It would be a naive practitioner who accepted at face value additional skills to her current scope of practice without acknowledging the wider ramifications of her actions. What needs to be considered is the added knowledge, responsibility and accountability that will inevitably accompany it. In addition once a midwife accepts this role, she has a responsibility to perform it, and to reiterate McCall (1997, unpublished work), she may be found negligent if she fails to attempt to perform the task should she be required to do so. None of the midwives in McCall's study had attempted to insert a cannula in an emergency; the reason for this is unclear. It could either be that an emergency had not occurred when it necessitated a cannula to be inserted, or that the midwives simply declined. This is worthy of note, as some midwives had been allowed to perform intravenous cannulation for 15 months (the mean length of time being 4.1 months).

The issues with intravenous cannulation and prescribing appear to be:

1. the scope of professional practice
2. an adequate knowledge source
3. skill acquisition
4. skill proficiency
5. supply and administration of intravenous fluids
6. midwife prescribing.

Activity 7.3 considers the issue of intravenous cannulation.

 Activity 7.3

What theoretical and practical knowledge base is required for midwives to extend their scope of practice in intravenous cannulation?
   What previous training and competencies must the midwife already possess?

Examination of the healthy neonate

Who should examine the 'normal' neonate is a legitimate question. It seems logical that, as midwives increasingly become the lead professionals for women deemed at lower end of the continuum of risk, they should also take responsibility for assessing the health and well-being of normal neonates. Yet, as MacKeith (1995) recounts, there is an assumption that the neonatal examination should be undertaken medically for the detection and prevention of problems, and to assure the parents of their baby's well-being.

In today's current practice the norm is for the neonate to undergo two examinations: one immediately after delivery, generally performed by the midwife, the second by a medical practitioner within a specified time scale according to local policy, usually 24–48 hours after delivery. The main differences between the two examinations are that the doctor listens to heart and lung sounds, palpates the abdomen, feels the pulses, checks the fundi and performs hip dislocation test (the Ortolani or Barlow's test). If midwives were to combine and undertake the two examinations together, the midwife would need to be taught the extra components that the doctors undertake. This is in addition to assuming full responsibility for failure to identify any serious treatable condition. Conversely would medical practitioners be willing to 'let go' of what is currently their only required role in the management of a normal mother and baby?

Rigby undertook an exploratory survey (1997, unpublished work) to ascertain the views of GPs and midwives regarding the newborn examination of a healthy neonate being undertaken by a midwife having had the necessary training and education. The aims were to:

- discover the views of GPs and midwives
- discover if midwives would feel able to carry out the newborn examination, and if not why?
- identify the training and education needs midwives feel they would require
- identify the experience of the midwives surveyed
- find out the GPs feelings about midwives undertaking the newborn examination
- discover the reasons why GPs would not want midwives to carry out the newborn examination
- discover the experience of the GPs surveyed.

The results showed a 60:40 split with 60% of midwives on average willing to undertake the examination of the newborn. Reasons cited for not feeling able to undertake the examination were:

1. increase in workload and responsibility
2. the Paediatrician has greater knowledge
3. no monetary reward for extra skills
4. legal implications if a problem were missed
5. the large amount of training and education that would be involved
6. the examination is not in the Midwives rules or code of conduct
7. it is the responsibility of the doctor.

Interestingly the results showed no significant difference in response between the location or the clinical area where the midwives worked, or between those midwives with greater than 2 years' experience.

The response from the GPs demonstrated almost 75% in favour of midwives carrying out the newborn examination. Of the 25% who felt they were not willing to allow midwives to undertake the newborn examination, the reasons cited were:

1. It is the responsibility of the GP.
2. Midwives may have difficulties in detecting abnormalities such as heart murmurs.
3. The newborn examination is an ideal opportunity for the GP to meet the new infant and family.
4. The GP may miss out on the postnatal examination of the mother owing to poor communication between themselves and the midwives.
5. Who will take responsibility if a problem is not detected?
6. The GP would be willing only if hospitals implemented midwives carrying out the newborn examination.

There was again no statistical significance to the year of qualification and the response that GPs gave. Of interest was the compulsory vocational training, which began in 1979: of those GPs who qualified prior to 1979 less than 25% had a postgraduate qualification, unlike those GPs qualifying after 1979, where the majority possessed at least two postgraduate qualifications. However, this observation was not reflected in differences in the results of the study.

The training and education needs identified by the midwives to enable them to feel competent in carrying out the newborn examination were:

- training on the examination of the hips, heart and reflexes
- study days or courses with assessment
- working with the paediatrician on the wards
- how to perform the examination and refer if a problem detected
- anatomy and physiology of the neonate
- counselling skills.

Prior to the introduction of role expansion, it is necessary to ascertain its need, justification and whom it will affect. Using the framework of the

Scope in professional practice, the newborn examination is a prime nominee. However, midwives must be familiar, as already stated, with the contents of the Midwives rules and code of practice (UKCC 1998a). Despite the reason stated by midwives in Rigby's survey (1997, unpublished work) for not undertaking the newborn examination because it is not in the rules or code of conduct, the Midwife's code of practice (UKCC 1998a) explicitly states that they are entitled to 'examine and care for the newborn infant' (p. 26).

On the other hand, the view proposed that midwives may have difficulties in detecting abnormalities such as heart murmurs is a valid one. Congenital heart disease affects just below 1% of newborn babies, and only a small percentage of these show signs of ill health (Fowlie & Forsyth 1995). However, some conditions are difficult to detect immediately after birth, in particular ventricular septal defects. Fowlie & Forsyth (1995) even question the importance of detection prior to clinical presentation. Congenital dislocation of the hips may also be overlooked owing to relaxation of the baby's ligaments from maternal hormonal influences. The incidence of unstable hips is 15–20:1000, but only 10% of these become dislocated, with another 10% possibly exhibiting signs of subluxation or dysplasia (MacKeith 1995). The incidence of congenital heart disease is 4–10:1000 (Verklan 1997). What also has to be remembered is that often with these babies there are other factors that render them outside the 'normal' neonate category; for example, children of diabetic mothers have an increased incidence of some heart defects. Breech presentations are more likely to have congenital dislocation of the hips. Antenatally, screening is more intensive, with ultrasound being used to detect problems such as those cited, if used it must carry a degree of shared responsibility in their subsequent detection.

The midwife when carrying out total care is perhaps more likely to detect problems in the neonate when taking all the other factors into account, when it could be argued that the paediatrician or GP on meeting the family for the first time may have an oversight. The Medical Defence Union in 1988–1990 dealt with 17 allegations of missed diagnoses of congenital heart disease, and 48 allegations of undiagnosed congenital dislocation of the hip (MacKeith 1995). Abu-Harb, Hey & Wren (1994) undertook a retrospective study of the detection of potentially serious correctable heart defects. Of the 14 cases whose heart conditions were not predictable, only one was detected by the routine postnatal examination. It has been estimated that in the catchment area of a large children's hospital 300 children die each year in the UK from unsuspected congenital heart disease.

As there appears to be no definitive 'missed' problem if the examination is undertaken by a paediatrician or a GP, or if the examination is not undertaken at all, this presents a strong case for the midwife as she is already in attendance. Additional training is required but the question is, how much?

The midwife must have sound knowledge in the normal physiology of the neonate in order to identify normality and recognize any deviation from this. This knowledge is not new to practising midwives, who assume responsibility for the infants in their care when a paediatrician is not present, and will still by statute be required to summon 'a registered medical practitioner or other such registered person as has relevant skills and experience' when obvious signs of ill health (e.g. pallor or cyanosis) are noted.

It could be argued that the midwife is already equipped to undertake the examination of the newborn, combining the examination after delivery undertaken by the midwife with that examination generally undertaken by the paediatrician. This is for individual midwives and their supervisors to agree upon, using the framework which envelops their scope of professional practice.

Activities 7.4 and 7.5 consider the principles of the scope of practice.

As with any new skill acquisition, be it examination of the newborn, intravenous cannulation, epidural top-up or perineal repair, the Midwife's code of practice (UKCC 1998a) states that a midwife must take responsibility for maintaining

Activity 7.4

Consider the six principles of 'scope' and their relevance to the examination of the newborn.
Identify the midwife's needs if required to undertake the examination of the healthy newborn.

Activity 7.5

Describe if and how midwives suturing of the perineum meets each of the six principles of the scope of professional practice.

and developing her competency of skills. At present there does not appear to be any long term follow-up or auditing of practice, yet the Changing Childbirth document (DoH 1993) places research, audit and evaluation of services as the central processes in providing effective and efficient care. As previously discussed, maintaining competency and proficiency is difficult to quantify. However, within many scope of practice documentation for different trusts, the practitioner is required to sign a competency statement, with many trusts asking for evidence of competence to be provided by the practitioner. This declaration by the midwife indicates that she is satisfied with their level of competence and is willing to accept responsibility for undertaking the procedure, which as McCall (1997, unpublished data) pointed out must be undertaken if the need arose, as failure to do so could be construed as negligence.

When considering any future expansions to the midwife practitioner's role, midwives should be encouraged to review their current sphere of practice with their supervisor of midwives. It should be documented in the profile and discussed as part of the appraisal system. If midwife practitioners are currently undertaking, and are competent in additional skills that used to be 'an extended role', and are now part of their scope of practice, midwifery practitioners must ensure that their knowledge and practice remain up to date and their competency is maintained.

The Scope of professional practice document has provided clearer support for midwives to fulfil the role of the autonomous, accountable practitioner (see Chs 6 and 8). By adjusting the boundaries for a midwives' sphere of practice the midwife is individually responsible and accountable for her actions or omissions, and for the development of her own knowledge base (Woodrow 1996). Midwifery practice is constantly being influenced by the changing needs of society, and must respond sensitively, relevantly and dynamically to the changing needs of the individuals and the health care system.

Summary

The midwife's role is clearly defined in the Midwives rules and code of practice (UKCC 1998a). The Scope of professional practice was conceived to allow practitioners to be more flexible and professionally challenging in their practice to meet the needs of a health service that is constantly changing. Within the Scope, practitioners are to define the limits of their own practice and take responsibility and accountability for their own practice and conduct. Extended practice with specialist and advanced practitioner status is still being actively debated within midwifery, as are new skill acquisitions by the midwife in view of the reduction in junior doctor hours. Midwives must consider the wider ramifications of any adjustment to their sphere of practice, and the supervisor of midwives must be consulted prior to any alteration to the midwife's role with regard to preparation and experience needed.

REFERENCES

Abu-Harb M, Hey E, Wren C 1994 Death in infancy from unrecognised congenital heart disease. Archives of Disease in Childhood 71:3–7

Allen R 1996 Discuss, argue, analyse, synthesise and apply findings to practice. British Journal of Midwifery 4(4):177

Bick D 1996 The need for debate on postnatal practice. British Journal of Midwifery 4(4):177

Boden S, Pritchard G 1996 An advanced midwifery practitioner should ... British Journal of Midwifery 4(4):176

Charlton D (1996) What constitutes an advanced practising midwife? British Journal of Midwifery 4(4):174–175

Copp G 1988 Professional accountability: the conflict. Nursing Times 84(43):42–43

Dimond B 1994 The legal aspects of midwifery. Books for Midwives, Hale

DoH (Department of Health) 1993 Changing childbirth. Report of the Expert Maternity Group part 1. HMSO, London

Dougherty L 1996a Intravenous cannulation. Professional Nurse 11(2):47–50

Dougherty L 1996b The benefits of an IV team in hospital practice. Professional Nurse 11(11):761–763

Draper J, Newell R 1996 A discussion of some of the literature relating to history, repair and consequences of perineal trauma. Midwifery 12:140–145

ENB (English National Board) 1993 Framework and Higher Award. ENB, London

Fowlie P, Forsyth S 1995 Examination of the newborn infant. Modern Midwife January:15–18

HMSO 1968 Medicines Act. HMSO, London

HMSO 1971 Misuse of Drugs Act. HMSO, London

HMSO 1983 Medicines (Products Other than Veterinary Drugs (prescription only) order). HMSO, London

HMSO 1985 Misuse of Drugs Regulations. HMSO, London

Jackson A 1997 Performing peripheral intravenous cannulation. Professional Nurse 13(1):21–24

Jones K 1996 Alternative option to management or full-time academia. British Journal of Midwifery 4(4):177

Lewis L 1996 Extending the midwives' role in perineal management. Nursing Times 92(11):39–41

MacKeith N 1995 Who should examine the 'normal' neonate? Nursing Times 91(14):34–35

Meah S 1998 A perspective on the proposed changes to Rule 40. RCM Midwives Journal 1(1):15–16

Newton C 1997 Resuscitation of the newborn: whose role? British Journal of Midwifery 5(4):199

Noble W 1996 Does the profession need advanced midwife practitioners? British Journal of Midwifery 4(4):176

Page L 1996 Combining knowledge and sensitivity to women's needs. British Journal of Midwifery 4(4):177

RCM (Royal College of Midwives) 1994 RCM Standing practice group paper 4. The use of intravenous infusion by midwives. Midwives Chronicle October:394–395

Scholefield H, Viney C, Evans J 1997 Expanding practice and obtaining consent. Professional Nurse 13(1):12–16

Sisto S, Hillier D 1996 Advanced midwifery practice: myth and reality. British Journal of Midwifery 4(4):179–182

UKCC (United Kingdom Central Council) 1989 Post registration education and practice project. UKCC, London

UKCC (United Kingdom Central Council) 1992a Scope of professional practice. UKCC, London

UKCC (United Kingdom Central Council) 1992b Code of professional conduct. UKCC, London

UKCC (United Kingdom Central Council) 1992c Standards for the administration of medicine. UKCC, London

UKCC (United Kingdom Central Council) 1993 Midwives rules. UKCC, London

UKCC (United Kingdom Central Council) 1994 Midwives code of conduct. UKCC, London

UKCC (United Kingdom Central Council) 1997a Scope in practice. UKCC, London

UKCC (United Kingdom Central Council) 1997b Consultation on proposed amendments to the Midwives rules, rule 27 and section B, practice rules 40 and 37 (Registrar's letter) 24/1997. UKCC, London

UKCC (United Kingdom Central Council) 1997c Drugs contained in standing orders for use by midwives MC/97/14. UKCC, London

UKCC (United Kingdom Central Council) 1997d Midwife prescribing Agendum 5.2. MC/97/14. UKCC, London

UKCC (United Kingdom Central Council) 1998a Midwives rules and code of practice. UKCC, London

UKCC (United Kingdom Central Council) 1998b Midwifery Committee specialist practice agendum 8.3. MC/98/02. UKCC, London

UKCC (United Kingdom Central Council) 1998c Standards for specialist education and practice. UKCC, London

Verklan MT 1997 Diagnostic techniques in cardiac disorders. Neonatal Network 16(4):9–15

Walker J 1996 The need for ten key characteristics. British Journal of Midwifery 4(4):177

Walsh D 1996 Radical transformation prompting action. British Journal of Midwifery 4(4):176

Whyte A 1998 Whose baby? Should neonatal units come under the aegis of midwives or children's nurses? Nursing Times 94(20):24–26

Woodrow P 1996 Professional practice: the impact of UKCC practice principles. Nursing Standard 10(49):39–41

FURTHER READING

Brimacombe M 1995 Reaping pain from what others have sewn. The Independent 14 March:21

DoH (Department of Health) 1993 Hospital doctors: training for the future. The report of the Working Group on Specialist Medical Training (the Calman Report). Health Publications Unit, Heywood

Johnson G L 1990 Clinical examination In: Long W A (ed) Fetal and neonatal cardiology. WB Saunders, Philadelphia pp 223–235

Kirkham M 1995 Using personal planning to meet the challenge of Changing childbirth. In: The challenge of changing childbirth. Midwifery educational resource pack. ENB, London

Page L 1995 Putting principles into practice In: Page L (ed) Effective group practice in midwifery—working with women. Blackwell Science, Oxford, pp 12–32

Parker S 1993 Trading places. Nursing Times 89(45):42

Scales K 1996 Legal and professional aspects of intravenous therapy. Nursing Standard 11(3):41–45

Scott S 1996 Doctor's assistant or a Trojan horse? Nursing Standard 10(33):17

Terry J, Baronowski L, Lonsway R A, Hedrick C 1995 Intravenous therapy: clinical principles and practice. W B Saunders, Philadelphia

8

Autonomy and team work

Jayne E Marshall   Sarah Kirkwood

In recent years, government reforms such as The Patient's Charter (DoH 1991) and Changing Childbirth (DoH 1993) have given consumers more scope to become increasingly involved in their own health care and maternity care by sharing partnership within the decision-making process.

This chapter aims to examine issues of autonomy within the complexities of the relationships between the midwife, the woman and the members of the multidisciplinary health care team, in both the hospital and community setting. Emphasis will be placed on the role of the midwife as an autonomous practitioner in empowering women to make informed choices whilst working in collaboration with other members of the multidisciplinary team. Issues of power and control will also be addressed from all perspectives.

Initially, the concept of autonomy will be explored in general terms, in order to establish the meanings that can be attached to the rather abstract word, and why it is regarded as a normative ideal. Its historical roots in political and moral thought will also be considered, as will the relationship that autonomy has with freedom and responsibility, which culminates in accountability.

WHAT IS AUTONOMY?

Origins, definitions and variations of autonomy

Historically, the word 'autonomy' has derived from Ancient Greece, where *'autos'* (meaning self) and *'nomos'* (meaning rule or law), were joined together to refer to political self-governance in the city-state. Words such as self-rule, self-support, self-sufficiency, liberty, freedom, power and authority give an indication of the meaning of autonomy, but nevertheless it is indeed a very complex concept with limited theoretical dimensions.

Personal autonomy

In moral philosophy, personal autonomy has emerged to refer to personal self-governance, self-rule and being in control of one's life (American College of Obstetricians and Gynaecologists 1992, Jones 1995). As this should involve behaving in a rational way and being in control of one's liberty and freedom, it is important to recognize that autonomy and freedom are not synonymous. The concept of freedom can suggest a liberal indulgence of one's desires in order to minimize frustration, regardless of the effect such actions may have on other persons involved, whereas autonomy would expect people to be able to rationalize their actions.

Lee (1986 p. 16) suggests: 'Autonomy is the capacity to think and act on one's reasoning, to determine the course of one's life by oneself ... a capacity which may be achieved to a greater or lesser degree'. This definition further challenges the extent of personal autonomy in respect of the freedom one can have to exercise one's actions because of certain variables, such as the interests of others, societal rules and laws and organizational policies and procedures, in addition to one's personal integrity.

Freedom and autonomy

Feinberg (1973), asserts that real freedom is synonymous with self-discipline and self-restraint, where one becomes free to make real choices concerning a variety of possible courses of action. Considering this further, Feinberg (1973), also states that behaviour which is either impulsive or compulsively driven is both unfree and non-responsible, as persons exhibiting such behaviour are unable to choose to do otherwise. Compulsive behaviour, such as the practice of checking and counterchecking in an effort to minimize mistakes, following step by step guidelines for the performance of various psychomotor skills, etc., not only denotes avoiding responsibility but also an absence of freedom to choose a viable alternative. Similarly, impulsive behaviour that attempts to satisfy one's passionate desires, irrespective of the consequences, is irresponsible conduct, which also inhibits the freedom to choose against the action.

It could therefore be said that impulsive behaviour implies the lack of personal autonomy and the capacity for genuine autonomous action. Holden (1991), suggests this is due to the absence of self-discipline, combined with an inability to prioritize desires in order to minimize potential frustration. Real responsibility therefore involves the exercise of self-discipline and self-restraint, both of which are preconditions for being free to choose an appropriate course of action.

Conscience

Self-discipline also incorporates the ability to act conscientiously and seeking always to do what is right. However, one cannot seek to do what is right without being possessed of the courage to act on one's own convictions in accordance with one's own conscience. Garnett (1969) believes conscience involves both cognitive and motivational or emotive elements. He further draws a distinction between *traditional* and *critical* conscience. It has been suggested that traditional conscience constitutes internalized indoctrinated moral values, whereas critical conscience critically re-evaluates previously held moral values in conjunction with continuous appraisal of the individual person's moral conduct.

In situations where conscience fails to adopt strong convictions as to the morally desirable course of action, persons may act in accordance with their reason or desire. The conscience (or will) is called upon where reason and desire are in conflict. If the will is weak, then desire is favoured, whereas whenever the will is strong then reason will ultimately overrule the desire. The integrity of the personality depends on the strength of the will and the capacity to exercise one's critical conscience, holding beliefs with the courage of conviction and being free to choose alternatives—that is, being free from either impulsively or compulsively driven behaviour. As Holden (1991) affirms, it is only when the integrity of the personality is preserved that the capacity to exercise genuine responsibility is obtained.

Professional autonomy

In defining autonomy within the context of professional practice, Lewis & Batey (1982 p. 15), specify it as being: 'the freedom to make discretionary and binding decisions consistent with one's scope of practice and freedom to act on those decisions'. Discretionary decisions and subsequent actions do not include the mere application of standard protocols imposed by others; neither do they include concrete and routine decisions. Within midwifery, for example, the knowledge required to inform decisions and perform actions can be constantly shifting because of the variability within and across the clientele group. Decisions that are binding are those in which the decision is the practitioner's own and, providing discretion has been exercised by the practitioner, no other person has the rightful power to change the decision.

A practitioner's scope of practice should clearly denote the work-related boundaries within which decisions and actions occur; by including scope of practice within the definition, Lewis & Batey (1982) distinguish autonomy from absolute independence. However, Lewis (1998) argues that, within the midwifery context, the boundaries of the midwife's practice are not entirely clear, despite the existence of the Scope of professional practice (UKCC 1992), the Midwives rules and code of practice (UKCC 1998) and the RCM guidelines on normal midwifery (RCM 1997), since the

many different and divergent ways in which midwives presently work can effect their autonomy, independent thought and decision making. Autonomy is confined to that for which the practitioner holds authority derived from expert knowledge and position. An autonomous practitioner both decides and acts on the decision; therefore autonomy cannot be decision making alone: the decision is the basis for determining a specific course of action, or no action at all.

Autonomous practice and accountability

Autonomous practice is a hallmark of professional practice that involves both personal and professional responsibility, according to Johns (1990) and Holden (1991). This responsibility involves ethical conduct and, for the midwife, the exercise of discretionary powers for the benefit of the mother and her family. By accepting responsibility and being given the authority to act and autonomy to exercise that authority, the midwife can be held *accountable* for her actions. Lewis & Batey (1982) conclude from many definitions that accountability is a formal obligation to disclose aspects of performance for which the practitioner has authority. For example, a midwife has pluralistic accountability by being responsible to the organization for fulfilling her job description and to the client for outcomes of care, accountable to herself in working to the best of her ability and seeking new knowledge through learning opportunities, accountable to her colleagues for support and collaborating with them to ensure optimum client care, and finally accountable to the midwifery profession for acting in accordance with the Midwives rules and code of practice (UKCC 1998). Within the context of autonomous practice, the midwife should also ensure that the mother has autonomy and is able to express her opinion freely, being part of the decision-making process within the planning of her care.

Client or patient autonomy

An individual client or patient-centred approach to health care should rightfully acknowledge client autonomy, treating each individual with respect, dignity and privacy at all times. This is considered to be the humanistic perspective of health care. Client autonomy has been emphasized in the report of the Expert Maternity Group: Changing Childbirth (DoH 1993 p. 8): 'the woman should be able to feel that she is in control of what was happening to her and able to make decisions about her care, based on her needs, having discussed matters fully with the professionals involved'.

It is so important to recognize that knowledge gives an individual control. Retaining this knowledge to oneself is a way of maintaining control over another individual, whereas, in comparison, imparting knowledge to others results in empowering them.

From the late 1970s, the National Health Service (NHS) has undergone many reforms culminating in the internal market as enshrined in the NHS and Community Care Act 1990 (DoH 1990), in which the commitment to quality and consumer choice and participation was evident throughout. Directives such as Patients First (DoH 1982), The Patient's Charter (DoH 1991), The Health of the Nation (DoH 1992) and The Patient's Charter and the Maternity Services (DoH 1994) further emphasized this commitment. However, there may be some situations in which the wishes of the client conflicts with that of the practitioner as such choices would be totally inappropriate, and the clients's well-being (and possibly that of the fetus in the situation of maternity) may well be put at risk. This situation challenges the midwife in terms of both the legal and ethical implications of her professional responsibility to the client (and the fetus) conflicting with her respect for the autonomy of the client to make such choices. It would be difficult for the midwife's autonomy to supersede that of the client in this instance, as doing so would be seen as going against the client's wishes. Nevertheless, it is also important to consider that the formation of a good working partnership, in which the autonomy of each individual is respected, should lead to a more positive experience for both client and professional.

Autonomy as an ethical principle

It was Appelbaum, Lidz & Meizel in 1987 who stated that the principle of autonomy in general ethics refers to the respect for the autonomy of others, in comparison to bioethics where it relates to the obligation of health professionals to respect the rights of clients to make their own decisions about their care and treatment: the basis of informed consent. It is one thing to be autonomous and another to be respected and autonomous. To respect an autonomous person is to recognize and appreciate the person's capacities and capabilities, including the right to hold certain views, to make certain choices and to take certain actions based on personal values and beliefs. Such respect for autonomy is an intrinsic value of deontology (see Ch. 5), where autonomy is always a priority and follows Kantian philosophy where people are seen as ends in themselves rather than being treated merely as means to the ends of others (Benjamin & Curtis 1986). The moral justification would therefore rest on those who would restrict or prevent a person's exercise of autonomy. In comparison, autonomy would be seen as an extrinsic value of utilitarianism and therefore non-essential if the consequences are such that, by respecting the principle, less good is achieved than by not respecting it: thus ignoring the principle of beneficence.

There are two basic approaches to autonomy according to Jones (1995). The first is adapted from a libertarian perspective that assumes anyone older than a toddler is autonomous, unless either mentally impaired or possibly emotionally distressed. It would seem that this is an obvious generalization, as there is no acknowledgement of the assessment of individual capabilities and understanding, although it is considered that autonomy can be lost with age, as in degenerative senility. This approach would suggest that a person's view must be accepted even in the absence of any acceptable reason or rationality, thus allowing the freedom to make a mistake. Such an approach would be totally inappropriate for an accountable health professional to adopt when dealing with the lives of others.

The second approach to autonomy, which is more rigorous than the libertarian perspective, features the ability to rationalize, reflect and make clear judgement, and considers autonomy to be a matter of *degree* rather than an *all or nothing* capacity. It would therefore seem that the more rational and deliberate an individual's actions are, the more choice they are allowed.

However, if these factors are weak or even absent, then it is questionable as to whether or not the decisions should be overridden. Furthermore, it could also be argued that someone making a decision based on fear or whilst affected by sedation (such as a woman during intrapartum care), may be using an irrational basis and therefore not acting entirely autonomously. As a result, decisions may be made for that individual by others, such as health professionals. It is therefore important that these clients be afforded the same respect for autonomy as any other rational person by being fully informed at all times of the options to care available that are pertinent to their individual circumstances.

HOW AUTONOMOUS IS THE MIDWIFE?

Midwives are often referred to as *practitioners in their own right*, inferring that they are autonomous (Gillen 1995, McCrea 1993, Mander 1993, Rogers 1991, Symon 1996). However, many factors may prevent or limit professional autonomy, whilst others may enhance it. In order to examine these factors, an historical perspective of the role of the autonomous midwife practitioner will first be presented.

An historical perspective of the autonomous midwife

The role of the midwife has evolved historically from a genuine concern to care for childbearing women through help and assistance (i.e. to be *with woman*). This helping act, according to McCrea (1993), forms the philosophical basis for midwifery practice and rests on a number of values, the most important being that childbirth is a normal physiological process to be assisted by midwives in their role as providers of normal maternity care. However, the last two centuries in particular have witnessed a struggle between the male-dominated medical profession and female midwives for the control and care during pregnancy and birth alongside the attempt to gain professional status for midwives. It has been the medical profession that has been the role model for other aspiring occupations, such as radiographers, physiotherapists, chiropodists etc., to seek professional status. Considering its traditionally male characteristic, it is questionable as to whether or not it is one for midwives to copy, as to do so would be reaffirming the established position of male control over childbirth, which would be inappropriate in the context of ensuring the pregnant woman has genuine choice and control.

It has been postulated that because professional groups are dominant groups, they are essentially male, since they are primarily concerned with maintaining control. According to Symon (1996), this line of reasoning would accept the Weberian principle of occupational closure and extends the Marxian analysis which claims that control is class centred, as well as gendered. Medicine, in addition to law and theology, had long been recognized as one of the learned, male-dominated professions produced by the medieval universities of Europe. It was not until some time in the 19th century that a minority of women actually managed to break down the barrier of gender prejudice and exclusion and achieve status in medicine, although this was usually at some cost: through conforming to the requirements of male detachment and objectivity.

At this time the Medical Act of 1858 set up the GMC, who subsequently abolished apprenticeship entry into medicine and the employment of unqualified assistants. In addition, as health care developed with medical and scientific discoveries in the late 19th century, doctors found themselves in a very powerful position of control—not only in respect of their own professional control, but also of others who worked within the area of health care. The emerging groups of health care providers therefore had to negotiate their respective areas of influence and responsibility with the medical profession.

The varied social and clinical status of the midwife throughout history has been well documented, particularly by Towler & Bramall (1986). Midwives have generally occupied a humble and often despised position in society until the turn of the 20th century, despite certain Greek midwives around 500 BC having social recognition being of an honoured class, for example, Phainarete the mother of Socrates. This relegation could be attributed to the low societal status of women and to their exclusion from learning. To assist women in childbirth, self-appointed midwives used herbal remedies and became the unofficial healers of the lower classes. As a result they were outlawed by the Church and classed as witches. By the 14th century, university-qualified physicians began to challenge the faith of the people in the traditional midwives and their remedies, and gradually assumed authority and power.

It was around the 18th and 19th centuries that the male 'midwives' (accoucheurs), who originally attended the labours of women when complications developed, first began to attend normal labours of the wealthy. Nevertheless, despite fierce competition for clients and fees, the time-consuming and financially unrewarding work which constituted most of midwifery practice remained with women. According to Donnison (1977), in the mid 1870s, it was estimated that 70% of all births in England and Wales were attended by midwives and took place in the home. However, none of these midwives had received any formal training and, whilst the most able were extremely skilled in their work, there were many who were ignorant, slovenly and cheap (Smith 1979).

Men-midwives also lacked training and it was not until the late 19th century that a few doctors of higher status took an interest in maternity care. Also at this time a small group of women, concerned about the general health of women and children and the quality of maternity care, as well as the potential demise of the midwife, recognized that she too must become politically and professionally organized, and above all educated. As a result they founded the Matrons Aid Society, which later became the Midwives Institute. Midwives were not in a position to train each other, and were dependent on the few enlightened doctors to set up training schemes for them. Following the Medical Act of 1886, medical practitioners were required to have a qualification in medicine, surgery and midwifery, which at least regulated the attendance of male midwives.

At this time the GMC was particularly concerned at the suffering caused by the little training of the female midwives who attended the many who could not afford medical fees. In addition, the high maternal and perinatal mortality rates also gave cause for concern, therefore in 1889 several committees were formed to investigate the training and registration of midwives. Although some nurses, such as Florence Nightingale, supported the registration of midwives others, who included the founder of the British Nurses Association, Mrs Bedford-Fenwick, actually opposed it. Mrs Bedford-Fenwick had in fact hoped that midwives would join together with nurses to campaign for registration, but the Midwives Institute took the view that midwives were independent practitioners in their own right and their registration should be dealt with separate to that of nurses, much to her displeasure. After much opposition from both nurses and doctors groups, as well as some militant midwives such as the Manchester Midwives Association, who feared registration would entail midwives coming under medical control with a subsequent loss of their autonomy, the first Midwives Act was passed in 1902. (The first Scottish Midwives Act was passed in 1916.) The Midwives Act acknowledged clinical features of professionalism and hallmarks of a profession: the requirement for specified training and the maintenance of a register that serves to monopolize the legal use of the term 'midwife'. By 1905, 50% of births in England were attended by midwives whose names were on the Roll of Midwives.

The Central Midwives Board (CMB) for England and Wales was set up as a consequence of the Midwives Act, and Cronk (1990) makes an interesting observation: that for 70 years the chair of the CMB had belonged to male obstetricians, until 1973 when Margaret Farrer became the first Midwife Chairman, thus reiterating medicine's control over midwifery training and practice for the majority of this century. However, the professional identity of the midwife was further subsumed with the demise of the CMB to a single statutory organization of the United Kingdom Central Council (UKCC) for Nursing, Midwifery and Health Visiting, as result of the Briggs Committee's recommendations in 1972 (Committee on Nursing 1972). In addition, legislation in the form of the Nurses, Midwives and Health Visitors Act 1979 (HMSO 1979) procured the provision of midwifery practice becoming enshrined in a predominantly non-midwifery legal framework of reference. This has further restricted the autonomy of the midwife as it failed to recognize the independent nature of their role that distinguishes them from nursing and medical colleagues.

The medical profession has also eroded midwives' autonomy in other ways. The policy of institutionalized confinement, which has developed throughout this century as a means of attempting to reduce the mortality among childbearing women and their babies, was initiated in 1924 at a time when the home birth rate was 84% (Campbell 1924). This policy culminated in the Peel Report of 1970 (Maternity Advisory Committee 1970), which, despite the lack of any substantial evidence, recommended that there should be provision for a 100% hospital birth rate and that small isolated obstetric units be phased out and replaced by consultant and GP units in general hospitals. Not only would there be no choice for women regarding place of birth, but also the midwife's autonomy would be eroded even further.

Following the inception of the NHS in 1948, maternity care along with general health care was to be provided free at the point it was delivered, and so a more rapid shift towards births in hospitals and maternity homes was experienced as a consequence. By 1958, the home birth rate had fallen to 34%. In addition, free antenatal care was made available to all women, resulting in the GP becoming the first contact for the pregnant woman. It was probably at this point that the medicalization of childbirth really began.

The role of the midwife in the 1970s was constantly under the threat of continuing technological advances and increasing obstetric intervention that subsequently affected the woman's control, particularly in labour: induction of labour, artificial rupture of the membranes, cardiotocography, epidural analgesia, to highlight but a few. As Towler & Bramall (1986 p. 259) state: 'So great was the change in hospital practice that the midwife who trained during this period was conditioned to seeing her role as that of assistant to the doctor, a machine minder or technological handmaiden'. Midwifery was therefore becoming visualized in a highly sophisticated, controlled environment where women were merely the recipients of care provided by specialists, who in turn would have control over the whole process (Walton & Hamilton 1995). What was not being taken into consideration at this time was the opinion of women both as mothers and as midwives. Apprehension about the vision of childbirth into the 21st century led to voices of dissent from individuals and representative groups from both consumer and representative organizations, such as the Association for the Improvements in Maternity Services (AIMS), the National Childbirth Trust (NCT), the RCM and the Association of Radical Midwives (ARM).

In addition, a small number of midwives decided to opt out of the state system and return to a style of independent practice that they hoped would allow greater autonomy and job satisfaction. Hunter (1998) argues that in the early 1980s only independent midwives were fulfilling the complete role of the midwife and working as practitioners in their own right. Now, in the 1990s, although the number of independent midwives remains small in comparison to the total number of practising midwives, probably because of the issues of financial insecurity and insurance cover (Cassidy 1994, Tyler 1996), their approach to a more holistic woman-centred model of care provides their peers with a working role model for ideal practice.

Since the mid 1980s, the driving force to normalize maternity care for the majority of women classed as low risk has become increasingly evident in the form of innovative developments—for example, team midwifery, midwives' clinics and midwife-led units within consultant unit—and these have led to some midwives reasserting their autonomous role. This increasing profile of midwifery has also been supported by the Winterton Report (House of Commons Health Committee 1992) and the report of the Expert Maternity Group (DoH 1993), in Changing Childbirth, both of which have further encouraged midwives to regain some of the territory of normal midwifery which many feel was taken over by the medical profession in the 19th century.

The report of the Expert Maternity Group (DoH 1993) identified that each woman should have 'choice, control and continuity of care' during childbirth, that the care be 'woman centred, appropriate and accessible' and the service be 'effective and efficient', and so have the potential to change basic midwifery practice. However, Hunter (1998) endorses the belief that the issue of power and control is crucial to any analysis of the history and future of midwifery in which the focus of debate has been the midwife's autonomy. Whilst the report of the Expert Maternity Group (DoH 1993) has created a climate in which midwives can achieve autonomous practice, it also challenges them to share power with clients. Furthermore, the Government's recent white paper: The New NHS: Modern—Dependable (DoH 1997) is offering midwives further opportunity to adopt ways of working within the primary health care team and provide the kind of care women want. As Lewis (1998 p. 60) affirms: 'It (the White Paper) may also help midwives obtain the clinical expertise, professional freedom and self-governance which will truly make us the practitioners of normal childbirth that we continually claim to be'.

It is at this point that the factors that affect the autonomy of the midwife in present day maternity care will be discussed. .

Factors affecting the midwife's autonomy

Health professionals such as midwives have dual autonomy as people in their everyday lives and as practitioners in their working lives. The national boards for nursing, midwifery and health visiting, in their guidelines leading to entry to part 10 (registered midwife) of the professional register, state that a midwife is a person who is: 'Qualified and accountable for their sphere of practice. The midwife has responsibility and authority to practice as an autonomous, accountable practitioner with mothers during antenatal, intranatal and postnatal periods, and with the neonate' (ENB 1991).

This infers that the midwife can utilize the knowledge skills and attitudes acquired during training and subsequent practice, in order to achieve the best possible outcome for both the client as well as the practitioner. In practice, however, it may be difficult to utilize professional autonomy to its full extent, partly as result of maternity unit policies and procedures, many of which can affect the woman's freedom of apparent choice or movement, and the midwife's practice, and partly because of the statutory legislation defining the midwife's practice.

Few professionals would argue against the formulation of policies and procedures for the safety of those receiving and providing care, particularly in an emergency or when new staff are employed, but one must consider how and by whom such standards of practice may have been determined. It has been the norm in most British maternity units for policies and guidelines to have been drawn up by senior midwives in conjunction with senior obstetricians and, as Rothman (1984) asserts, midwives do not have a reciprocal right to determine medical practice. It must therefore be argued that policies should be flexible, based on current research and formulated by a representative group of professionals. Inflexible, obstetric and litigation fearing policies can but create a conflict between the midwives, the obstetricians and the women.

At the present time, the ethos of the midwife's statutory control is maintained by the UKCC, whose membership is predominantly from the nursing profession. This has resulted in a statutory body whose interests do not always lie in the developments within the midwifery profession, let alone with the role of the midwife. The autonomous nature of the midwife's practice and her role in prescribing and administering certain medicines, have been recognized for most of this present century as a need for midwives to press for their own specific regulatory framework, which has been established in the form of legislation: the Nurses, Midwives and Health Visitors Act 1979. However, this Act further erodes the autonomy of midwives as it actually requires them to work within a non-midwifery legislative framework of reference. On the other hand, the existence of the Midwives rules and code of practice (UKCC 1998), which relate to clinical care as well as disciplinary procedures, including cases of professional misconduct, further distinguishes midwives from other health professionals, including nurses and doctors.

As a newly qualified practitioner, according to the UKCC (1998) and the RCM (1992), the midwife is expected to be autonomous and accountable from the point of registration, and could quite legally set up in independent practice from the day she qualifies (Jackson 1994). However, Fraser, Murphy and Worth-Butler (1997), in a study commissioned by the ENB, found that 3 year pre-registration midwifery programmes do not always equip student midwives with the confidence needed for autonomous practice. Whilst these new students were committed to women-centred, midwifery-led caseload practice in the community, the realities of practice in their first midwifery post upon qualification meant that they were more likely to work in busy, often short-staffed hospitals. Here they were expected to have ward management skills and be able to participate in caring for women with complications and pre-existing medical conditions. The newly qualified midwife therefore found herself requiring considerable support in her first post (particularly in the provision of intrapartum care). New midwives are now being encouraged, along with their counterparts in nursing and health

visiting, to undergo a period of supervision under a preceptorship scheme in order to broaden and deepen their competence and ability. Being supervised in this way could imply that the midwife's training has been incomplete and would appear to conflict with the concept of the autonomous, accountable practitioner. In addition, in order to ensure that good standards of care are maintained, the practice of all midwives, regardless of experience and type of employment, is under the control of LSAs. In practice, the function of supervision is usually undertaken by an experienced practising midwife. Again this act of supervision may be seen by some midwives, such as McKay (1997), as a means of inhibiting their autonomy from above, but one could equally argue that it is also a means of midwives retaining control of the midwifery profession and should therefore be safeguarded from other professions (see Ch. 10).

Now undertake Activity 8.1.

Activity 8.1

Sally is a newly qualified midwife who has been allocated a preceptor for the first 6 months of her appointment. She is employed within the local hospital's maternity unit.

In light of the recommendations for preceptorship for all newly registered practitioners, discuss the extent of Sally's autonomy, highlighting the factors influencing your deliberations.

The involvement of other health professionals, such as physiotherapists, dieticians, health visitors and practice nurses, and more recently the introduction of health care assistants in some maternity units, could be considered as further encroachment on the midwife's role, eroding her autonomy. Conversely, in some areas the role of the midwife is developing or expanding, probably, as Bradshaw & Bradshaw (1997) speculate, as a result of the reduction in junior doctors' hours—for example, the midwife ventouse practitioner, the midwife in the high risk obstetric team, the midwife operating department assistant. Whilst some midwives would view such developments as leading to greater autonomy for the midwife others feel they could transform midwives into low class medics (McKay 1997). The appropriateness of such developed skills therefore does need questioning with reference to the fundamental role of the midwife in normal midwifery, when by taking on such highly specialized roles could inadvertently reduce the number of midwives available to care for women in normal labour. Therefore midwives need to seriously consider their own boundaries of practice and what specific aspects of their work they value most, both on a personal level and by those for whom they care. By doing so, as Lewis (1998 p. 61) states: 'We might put into focus the strengths of our profession and reawaken the hearts and hands of all midwives to become truly skilled and autonomous practitioners in childbirth'.

Ultimately midwives must be willing to assume greater responsibility and acknowledge the accountability that comes with power. Education and training (that is controlled by midwives), both initial and continuing, as well as research awareness, are extremely valuable tools to enable the midwife to assume with confidence the role of an autonomous and accountable practitioner within her scope of professional practice alongside medical colleagues. It is also important for midwives to be involved in budget control, standard setting, quality assurance, auditing and peer review in order to ensure the control of midwifery practice and the maintenance of high quality care.

Now undertake Activity 8.2.

Activity 8.2

You are busy looking through one of the midwifery journals and come across an advertisement in the situations vacant section for independent midwives, which sparks some interest. The advertisement states that: 'We are seeking confident, autonomous practitioners who are committed to providing high quality care and contemporary midwifery care in partnership with childbearing women'.

Compile a letter supporting your application for this position, giving evidence of your practice that would fulfil the description specified in the advertisement.

Needless to say, except for independent midwives, the autonomy of midwives employed within the state system in either the community or hospital will to a certain degree be affected by the respect for the autonomy of not only their clients, but also medical colleagues, as the autonomy of midwives cannot be discussed in a vacuum divorced from the reality of the close proximity in which they practise with fellow health professionals and interact with clients. The extent and degree in which the midwife's autonomy can be limited or extended by the relationship between health professionals and the client will now be discussed and the potential conflicts and areas of cooperation explored.

The midwife as a member of the primary health care team

Whilst McKay (1997) has explored a view that the involvement of other health care workers in maternity services, such as physiotherapists, dieticians and health visitors, may have played a part in the erosion of the midwife's role and autonomy, Zander (1994) supports the concept that care provided by a group of professionals with differing training and perspectives working together and in cooperation enables individuals to achieve objectives they would be unable to by working individually. Silverton (1998), when discussing the impact of the NHS white paper (DoH 1998), goes further to support the notion that the involvement of midwives with community nurses and GPs in the commissioning of services from the secondary sector will give a boost to patterns of care promulgated under Changing Childbirth (DoH 1993). This would result in opportunities to influence the provision of maternity care locally. This influence, she goes on to assert, would enable choice, ranging from midwifery-led care to care necessitating higher levels of medical intervention. Collaboration is seen as a means to promote all interested parties' aims and objectives, which is commendable in theory.

How much this is achievable in reality can be explored further by looking at the key member of the primary health care team who is most likely to impact on the midwife's autonomy: the GP.

The midwife and the GP

GPs rest their claim for autonomy with regard to the childbearing woman on their responsibility for providing personal, continuing and comprehensive medical care to individuals and families throughout their lives. Zander (1994) further suggests that the GP, having an extensive knowledge of and the most personal relationship with individual families, is probably the most appropriate member of the primary health care team to make decisions on the management of a woman's pregnancy. However, the Changing childbirth report (DoH 1993) states that women should be able to choose for themselves the lead professional providing maternity care. In many instances there is no medical reason why that lead professional should not be the midwife, who specializes in normal midwifery care, rather than the GP.

Some GPs are unwilling to relinquish their control over the maternity services and over the midwife and still see their main role and focus to be the provider and supervisor of antenatal and postnatal care (even when the woman would prefer to choose the midwife). In this, many GPs see themselves as the lead professional, offering valuable continuity of care as well as ensuring that services are properly coordinated. By this, continuity of care is not just seen as a relevance for the pregnancy, but is seen as part of a continuity of care that extends throughout the whole of a woman's life. This view of GPs that they should retain a central role in the provision of maternity care is therefore seen as a potential threat to the midwife's autonomy, especially in the area of antenatal and postnatal care. It is here that there is most danger of duplication, inconsistency and conflict between midwife and GP, as there is little demarcation of role and responsibility. Spencer (1994) actually rebukes health professionals for getting involved in power struggles which mitigate against the well-being and interests of the

woman, leading to confusion about who is the responsible party in decision making.

Nevertheless most GPs, particularly over the last decade, have given up their responsibilities for, and involvement in, intrapartum care. This decline reflects a shift in the place of confinement from home to hospital over the last 30 years, alongside a vast increase in technology which GPs now feel is best left to the specialist. Indeed, even for home delivery, few GPs are keen to get involved and Zander (1994) describes the midwife as the principal professional to practise what should only be the art of midwifery (not obstetrics) in the home environment. Zander (1994), goes on to explain that the GP's role should be complementary to that of the midwife, acting as her facilitator in the event of home delivery, thus recognizing the midwife's expertise and autonomy in this particular area of intrapartum care, particularly as skills such as perineal suturing and intravenous cannulation have now become part of the midwife's routine training and practice.

The midwife's autonomy is therefore often dependent on either the GP's indifference to being involved in maternity care, or on the establishment of a good relationship between GP and midwife which allows for mutual respect of each other's role and responsibilities and therefore promises equally the autonomy of both GP and the midwife.

The midwife and the obstetrician

When multidisciplinary team members hold differing views of care, interprofessional conflict may result (Siddiqui 1996). Also where one profession is deemed to have held professional supremacy over another during most of its history, a hierarchal structure that is deeply rooted and difficult to break down is inevitable. As midwifery, along with, for example, nursing, teaching and social work, may sometimes be described as a semi profession in contrast to the medical profession, who can boast all the sociological and historical hallmarks of a true profession (Symon 1996), then the struggle for midwives to assert their autonomy seems ever more difficult.

The medicalization of childbirth, with the shift from home to hospital birth and the conservative obstetric view that still upholds technological surveillance as the best means to achieve a successful outcome of pregnancy, has put the obstetrician rather than the midwife in control of the process of childbirth. Furthermore, as Symon (1996) comments, any group which has its standards of practice determined by another group forfeits its right to be autonomous. Midwives have in many instances been more than happy to be guided by their obstetric colleagues only to find that they are indeed accountable for their own practice. Calder (1994) states that in the past some obstetricians have even admitted to a tendency amongst their own profession to regard midwives as their handmaidens to do their bidding.

On a positive note, however, with the move to view childbirth as a normal event for the majority of women, there is optimism amongst midwives that their autonomy can at last be truly recognized. With the advent of midwife-led care and lead professional status, the satisfaction of professional autonomy is within the midwife's reach. The 1998 review of the statutory bodies for nursing, midwifery and health visiting (JM Consulting Ltd 1998) gave midwives a further opportunity to press for improved self-regulation. It is perhaps true that obstetricians, for a variety of reasons, are more ready than ever before in history to accept midwives as true colleagues, albeit in the care of women who present without complications. An example of this acceptance is described by Fraser (1997) in the area of education, where an academic division of midwifery education has become part of a new department of obstetrics, midwifery and gynaecology and is now working in collaboration both in the education of midwifery and medical students and in research, believing that such a partnership will have long term benefits for the childbearing woman. Calder (1994) addresses the medical profession's acceptance of midwives by putting forward a strategy which allows for interaction between midwives, GPs and obstetricians in planning care, taking into account the needs and safety of each mother involved, in addition to recognizing the lead professional status of all three health professionals that is dependent on each individual and their dynamic circumstances. Perhaps then real change in attitude is occurring amongst maternity care providers, both in the midwives' determination to be counted as autonomous practitioners and in their medical colleagues' decrease in resistance to allow them to practise autonomously.

Now undertake Activity 8.3.

 Activity 8.3

Jenny and Claire are midwives who work within the same Health Authority. Jenny has recently moved into a newly formed integrated midwifery team based in the community, whereas Claire is employed within the local hospital's maternity unit as a core member of the labour ward team.

1. Compare and contrast the extent of the autonomy that Jenny and Claire may have in these situations, on both a personal and a professional level.
2. Discuss the many factors that are likely to have an effect on the ability of Jenny and Claire to work as autonomous practitioners.

The midwife and the client

The relationship between the midwife and the mother has often evoked powerful and thought-provoking responses and discussion on the part both of the midwife and of the client population. According to Siddiqui (1996), this relationship has changed throughout time from the early part of the century, when the midwife was seen as a trusted and known supporter of women, helping the mother use her own powers to give birth naturally using a non-interventionalist approach. Arguably the midwife would much more easily be able to work autonomously at that time, when the midwifery skills were truly recognized and there was less recourse to the availability and subsequent dependence on technology. Therefore there was far less potential for conflict between mother, midwife and doctor. Siddiqui (1996) further describes how the situation has changed during the second half of the 20th century as potential for conflict became a reality. With the increase in technology the midwife often found herself in conflict balancing her own role as advocate to the mother against her loyalty to her obstetric colleagues.

In the early days of technological revolution, with the drive for 100% hospital births in the 1970s and 1980s, the midwife often sided with the obstetrician and bowed to what she considered their superior judgement. The midwife became a willing partner in promoting continuous fetal heart monitoring with the resultant immobility of the labouring woman. She undertook perineal shaves, enemas and routine episiotomies without questioning practice and searching for the evidence to support these practices, believing them to be in the woman's best interest. Therefore midwives were not always acting as the woman's advocate in such circumstances. It took the client to question the wisdom of these practices, and it was not until pressure from women gathered momentum that midwives remembered the meaning of their title and began themselves openly to question the changes. Siddiqui (1996) argues that there remains in some midwives a tendency to value maintaining a peaceful collaboration with the doctor rather than pursuing the principles of advocacy and autonomy for the client. Mander (1993) suggests that the midwife's autonomy has actually been reduced by the client's role and involvement in her own care. This, however, is a reduction which is supported and enjoys the collusion of the midwife.

Symon (1996) asserts that there may be tension between undertaking the responsibilities as a health care worker and at the same time enabling the client to achieve control over her care. McCrea (1993) also states that some clients have their own views on how they would like their midwifery care to be provided. She goes on to suggest that differences in perceptions may lead to conflict in the midwife–client relationship. This can be avoided if sufficient trust and respect for each other is present. McCrea (1993), in the conclusions of a research study looking at the relationship between midwives and clients, found that where midwives felt insecure or lacking in confidence in their role then the building of a positive relationship with the client was inhibited. She describes the blurring of both the public's perception of the midwife, as well as that of other health professionals, as being the result of the medicalization of childbirth. The questioning and doubt in people's mind as to midwives' authority to act on their own account brings into question their position as autonomous practitioners. Midwives therefore need to be confident, assertive practitioners who are able to exercise the authority that they do possess in order to inspire the confidence of the client group. This will then enable midwives to act as advocates for their clients in a mutually beneficial way which promotes the autonomy of the mother as well as that of the midwife.

Now undertake Activity 8.4.

Activity 8.4

Hilary is a 33-year-old woman who has had two previous caesarian sections because of failure to progress in labour. She is now 12 weeks' pregnant and meets Janet, the community midwife at the booking clinic. It is here she expresses her desire to have her third baby at home because of her past experiences of institutionalized births.

Hilary has already seen her GP, Dr Peters who, in view of her history, was unwilling to support her in her choice.

1. Discuss the conflict of interests between Hilary and the health professionals involved in this case.
2. Compare and contrast the autonomy of each individual, considering the professional, legal and ethical implications.
3. Suggest ways in which the situation may be resolved.

Summary

This chapter has attempted to examine the complex concept of autonomy as it affects health professionals and women in present day maternity services provision.

It has discussed the historical development of the role of the autonomous practitioner amidst the distribution of the balance of power between the midwife, doctor and childbearing woman.

It has also attempted to facilitate discussion and debate alongside self-examination of individual practice by the introduction of activities in the form of typical scenarios.

REFERENCES

American College of Obstetricians and Gynaecologists 1992 Ethical dimensions of informed consent. International Journal of Gynaecology and Obstetrics 39(4):346–355

Appelbaum P S, Lidz C W, Meizel J D 1987 Informed consent: legal theory and clinical practice. Oxford University Press, Oxford

Benjamin M, Curtis J 1986 Ethics in nursing, 2nd edn. Oxford University Press, Oxford

Bradshaw G, Bradshaw P 1997 The professionalisation of midwifery. Modern Midwife 7(12):23–25

Calder A 1994 Contributions of the professions. In: Chamberlain G, Patel N (eds) The future of the maternity services. RCOG Press, London, pp. 139–146

Campbell J M 1924 Reports of public health and medical subjects. HMSO, London

Cassidy J 1994 Indemnity costs puts the squeeze on go-it-alone midwives. Nursing Times 90(2):7

Committee on Nursing 1972 Report of the Committee on Nursing (Chairman: Asa Briggs). HMSO, London

Cronk M 1990 In-house debate: crisis in midwifery. Midwife, Health Visitor and Community Nurse (26): 280–287

DoH (Department of Health) 1982 Patients first. HMSO, London

DoH (Department of Health) 1990 The NHS and Community Care Act. HMSO, London

DoH (Department of Health) 1991 The patient's charter. HMSO, London

DoH (Department of Health) 1992 The health of the nation. HMSO, London

DoH (Department of Health) 1993 Changing childbirth part 1: report of the Expert Maternity Group. HMSO, London

DoH (Department of Health) 1994 The patient's charter: the maternity services. HMSO, London

DoH (Department of Health) 1997 The new NHS: modern–dependable. HMSO, London

Donnison J 1977 Midwives and medical men. Heinemann, London

ENB (English National Board for Nursing, Midwifery and Health Visiting) 1991 Guidelines for midwifery programmes of education, leading to entry to part 10 registered midwife) of the register. ENB, London

Feinberg J 1973 Social philosophy. Prentice Hall, New Jersey

Fraser D M 1997 Change for whose benefit?: The merger of midwifery and obstetrics in the University of Nottingham. MIDIRS Midwifery Digest 7(4):425–426

Fraser D M, Murphy R J L, Worth-Butler M 1997 An outcome evaluation of the effectiveness of pre-registration midwifery programmes of education. ENB, London

Garnett C A 1969 Conscience and conscientiousness. In: Feinberg J (ed) Moral concepts. Oxford University Press, Oxford, pp 80–92

Gillen J 1995 Can midwives practise autonomously? British Journal of Midwifery (editorial) 3(5):245–246

HMSO 1979 The Nurses, Midwives and Health Visitors Act. HMSO, London

Holden R J 1991 Responsibility and autonomous nursing practice. Journal of Advanced Nursing 16(4):398–403

House of Commons Health Committee 1992 Second report: maternity services (the Winterton Report). HMSO, London

Hunter B 1998 Independent midwifery: future inspiration or relic of the past? British Journal of Midwifery 6(2):85–87

J M Consulting 1998 The regulation of nurses, midwives and health visitors: invitation to comment on issues raised by a review of the Nurses, Midwives and Health Visitors Act 1997. J M Consulting, Bristol

Jackson K 1994 Preceptorship involves irreconcilable concepts. British Journal of Midwifery 2(4):174–175

Johns C 1990 Autonomy and primary nurses: the need to both facilitate and limit autonomy in practice. Journal of Advanced Nursing 15(8):886–894

Jones S R 1995 Ethics in midwifery. Mosby, London

Lee S 1986 Law and morals. Oxford University Press, Oxford, p 16

Lewis F M, Batey M V 1982 Clarifying autonomy and acountability in nursing service: part 1. Journal of Nursing Administration 12(9):13–18

Lewis P 1998 Boundaries to practice: when is a midwife not a midwife? RCM Midwives Journal 1(2):60–61

McCrea H 1993 Valuing the midwife's role in the midwife/ Client relationship. Journal of Clinical Nursing (2):47–52

McKay S 1997 The route to true autonomous practice for midwives. Nursing Times 93(46):61–62

Mander R 1993 Autonomy in midwifery and maternity care. Midwives Chronicle and Nursing Notes October:369–374

Maternity Advisory Committee 1970 Domiciliary and maternity bed needs (Sir John Peel, Chairman). HMSO, London

The Medical Act 1858: An Act to regulate the Qualification of Practioners in Medicine and Surgery. In: A Collection of Public General Statutes 1858. Eyre & Spottiswoode, London, Ch. 90 pp 297–307

The Medical Act 1886. In: The Law Reports: The Public General Statutes 1886–1888. Eyre & Spottiswoode, London Vol. XXII, Ch. 48, pp 121–133

The Midwives Act 1902: An Act to secure the better training of Midwives and to regulate their practice. In: The Law Reports: The Public General Statutes 1899–1902. Eyre & Spottiswoode, London, Vol. XL, Ch. 17, pp 19–25

The Midwives (Scotland) Act 1916: An Act to secure the better training of Midwives in Scotland and to regulate their practice. In: The Law Reports: The Public General Statutes 1915–1916. Eyre & Spottiswoode, London, Vol. LIII, Ch. 91, pp 325–335

Rogers J 1991 Practitioner in your own right?: myth or reality. Midwives Chronicle and Nursing Notes May:131–134

Rothman B 1984 Childbirth management and medical monopoly: midwifery as (almost) a profession. Journal of Nurse-Midwifery (29):300–306

RCM (Royal College of Midwives) 1992 A philosophy for midwifery. RCM, London

RCM (Royal College of Midwives) 1997 Debating mid-wifery: normality in midwifery. Davies Communications RCM Publication, London

Siddiqui J 1996 Midwifery values: part 1. British Journal of Midwifery 4(2):87–89

Silverton L 1998 The NHS White papers and the future of midwifery. RCM Midwives Journal (editorial) 1(2):40

Smith F B 1979 The peoples health. Croom Helm, London

Spencer J A D 1994 Working together. In: Chamberlain G, Patel N (eds) The future of the maternity services. RCOG, London, pp 159–165

Symon A 1996 Midwives and professional status. British Journal of Midwifery 4(10):543–550

Towler J, Bramall J 1986 Midwives in history and society. Croom Helm, London

Tyler S 1996 Independent midwives' insurance: the stance of the RCM. British Journal of Midwifery 4(3):151–152

UKCC 1992 Scope of professional practice. UKCC, London

UKCC 1998 Midwives rules and code of practice. UKCC, London

Walton I, Hamilton M 1995 Midwives and Changing childbirth. Books for Midwives, Hale

Zander L I 1994 The contribution of the general practitioner to maternity care. In: Chamberlain G, Patel N (eds) The future of the maternity services. RCOG, London, pp 147–158

9

Clinical risk management

Iris G Cooper

CHAPTER CONTENTS

This chapter aims to provide midwives with an understanding of how the process of risk management can assist with improving the quality of the service they provide and develop their skills and knowledge of the risk management system. Guidance describing the need for risk management was produced by the DoH in 1993 and this advised all trusts to set up a risk management process. Although most trusts now have a risk management process in place, the availability of literature describing their experiences is minimal and therefore many of the systems and examples described in this chapter use the author's personal experience gained after being involved in a risk management team since its inception in 1993. It is hoped that by portraying this experience others will benefit as they form and develop their own risk management systems.

INTRODUCTION

Risk management in obstetric and midwifery practice is a process which identifies and examines unforeseen outcomes happening during pregnancy and childbirth. The knowledge gained from this identification is then used in the prevention of similar occurrences. The decision to develop a risk management process in the NHS arose because in 1990 there was a sudden increase in the number of litigation claims being made against health authorities and trusts

(Vincent & Clements 1995). This rise, in part, was associated with the change in the eligibility for legal aid (Clements 1991) but there was also an increasing expertise in medical litigation amongst plaintiff solicitors and progress in paediatrics was increasing the chance of survival of more infants born prematurely, thereby increasing the expectations of parents. The majority of expensive claims are for cerebral palsy, and in spite of continuous improvements in obstetric care the incidence remains stable at 1 in 400 cases (Capstick 1994).

When risk management began to be implemented in the health service it sometimes caused anxiety amongst professionals as it was seen as threatening for a risk management team to be examining the clinical judgement of others. As, however, the development of risk management progressed the advantages of having such a system became clearer, and most hospital trusts have, or are developing, a system. Initial guidance was produced by the DoH (1993) to assist trusts with implementing risk management, and this publication covered potential risks in all aspects of the health service.

When considering the advantages of risk management it can be seen as a process which is based on being proactive and improving the quality of the service. Placing the emphasis on improving quality rather than reducing costs has a greater impact on the service, is more acceptable to the professionals, and the original aim of reducing litigation claims and costs is also aided.

Although risk management can be applied to any aspect of the health service it can be divided into two main areas: clinical risk and health and safety risk. This chapter will address only clinical risks relating to the obstetric service, midwives and obstetricians. The obstetric specialty has the highest number of claims and the highest costs in regard to settlements, therefore NHS trusts would probably initiate a risk management strategy in this specialty before devolving it to other areas within the trust. The reasons for the high number of claims in obstetrics is described by (Clements 1994) as being:

- there are two potential claimants
- emergencies are common

- the quantum of injury for a baby damaged for life is high.

When implementing risk management in obstetrics and midwifery it is important that all professionals are knowledgeable about the process, understand the need for early reporting where a risk factor is present and receive ongoing information about the effectiveness of the service and related statistical data. Without the cooperation of the senior clinicians (Marlock & Malitz 1991) the system would certainly falter and without the commitment of all the staff extreme difficulties would be experienced in making the system work.

FORMATION OF A RISK MANAGEMENT TEAM

The membership of a risk management group will differ from unit to unit according to local needs and circumstances but all maternity groups should have senior obstetricians and midwives as team members. There may be occasions when it is necessary to co-opt professionals from other specialties such as anaesthetics or pathology to obtain specialist advice.

A risk management team should include:

- consultant obstetricians
- lawyer or legal claims manager, or both
- midwifery manager
- paediatrician or neonatologist
- risk manager
- senior obstetric registrar
- supervisor of midwives.

Although the overall responsibility for managing risk lies with the chief executive of the trust, that person will mainly ensure that the appropriate teams are formed in the required specialties thereby delegating the day to day functioning to the experts within each team. The members of the team need to be those who have responsibility for managing the staff and the service, as implementation of the risk management process and acting upon findings is seen as their responsibility by the NHS Management Executive (DoH 1993).

Establishing such a team provides a focus for risk management and a forum for discussion and decision making. Meetings held monthly and of about 2 hours' duration will probably be sufficient for most units. There should be an agenda and minutes, although minutes which give only a brief outline of the meeting may be prudent as discussions of this nature should be regarded as highly confidential.

Cases brought for discussion will be judged on whether they are high or low risk. Once the level of risk is identified the appropriate action will be determined and this will be waiting for contact from the patient or client, or her solicitor, acceptance of liability or defence of the case. Those cases where liability is accepted or the case is to be defended will, from this point on, follow the claims management process, which will involve consulting with the trust's legal advisors. Once this decision has been made, and it may have taken a lengthy discussion to reach, then the next step is to consider why the events occurred and if any action is necessary to prevent similar instances in the future. Recommendations may be made and these could include the revision of a policy or procedure. If this is so then the chair of the risk management team should request a copy of any such revision. Some of the decisions are not straightforward and will require the contribution of all team members to bring their own expertise and breadth of experience to enable the analysis of the risk factors present or absent in each case. Participation in the discussion by all the team members means the cases are viewed broadly from all aspects. A cohesive team of mixed disciplines which gathers information and exchanges knowledge will progress towards achieving the ultimate aim of improving the quality of the service and reducing costs related to litigation.

THE ROLE OF THE RISK MANAGER

A risk manager should be appointed where an obstetric service is provided. The size of a unit is usually judged by the number of deliveries per annum and this would help to decide whether a full- or part-time post is required. For example, a unit with 4000 deliveries or more and where gynaecology is included in the directorate would probably need a full-time person.

The risk manager is notified by staff of all cases where a risk factor is present. Each notification is investigated by reviewing the case notes and talking with the staff involved in the care. This review may result in the case only being summarized and noted as not requiring further action. An example would be a third degree tear of the perineum where the mother makes a full recovery. Where, however, an obvious error has occurred, such as a swab being left in the abdomen at caesarean section, then the risk manager would undertake a full investigation of the facts and statements would be taken from those present at the operation. This latter case would be presented at the risk management meeting by the risk manager providing a clear summary of the facts and the action taken to date. Action taken should include the patient being seen by the consultant for her to receive an explanation and apology. Full explanatory details of the case would then be filed by the risk manager to be available if a solicitor's letter is received at some time in the future.

The overall role of the risk manager can be described as coordination of all the aspects of clinical risk in a maternity unit and forming of judgements in conjunction with the risk management team as to the necessary action to be taken to reduce future risk. It is important that the postholder, and in many instances to date this is an experienced midwife, has certain skills and qualities. It is suggested that these include:

- the ability to communicate with all levels of professionals
- the ability to provide support to staff particularly when they are being interviewed to ascertain the facts of a case
- the ability to be non-judgmental thereby encouraging staff to state the facts in an open and honest way
- possession of a professional qualification with sufficient experience and expertise to be clinically credible (and therefore not requiring input from another suitably qualified person).

An example of a job description can be seen in Box 9.1.

Box 9.1 **Job description for clinical risk manager**

Job summary
The postholder is responsible for identifying areas of clinical risk and for coordinating the process of risk management within the obstetric and midwifery service.

Job duties
These are:
- to define an up to date list of areas of clinical risk and ensure all rèlevant staff have ease of access to it
- to receive notifications of potential risk cases
- to take appropriate action when a clinical risk has been identified
- to interview all grades of staff involved in an identified case of clinical risk
- to ensure any member of staff involved in an incident is given advice, help and support with writing statements
- to ensure the case notes are appropriately completed when a clinical risk is identified
- to organize the monthly meetings of the risk management team and ensure the case notes and other relevant documents are available
- to liaise with the legal advisors and the solicitors employed to service the hospital and to attend case conferences and coroner's court hearings as required
- to work with the midwifery managers in order to action recommendations arising from the process of risk management and ensure that policies or procedures are changed as necessary
- to provide audit information of the risk management process and findings
- to review the risk management process and make change recommendations as required
- to secure confidentiality at all stages of the risk management process and ensure any electronically stored data meets with the conditions of the Data Protection Act
- by precept and example to ensure the rights and dignity of the patient are protected at all times
- to keep abreast of current research and developments in clinical practice thereby maintaining credibility.

MANAGEMENT OF RISK

All professionals need to recognize a risk situation confidently and take the appropriate action. A guidance list of risk situations should be readily available in all clinical areas of a maternity unit but with the proviso that it cannot be exhaustive. If there is some uncertainty as to whether a risk exists then it would be wiser to report it. The facts can then be reviewed by the risk manager and the risk management team and a decision made as to whether to proceed further.

Both management and staff need to work in partnership when implementing a risk management process. Managers have a responsibility to ensure a strategy is developed for safe care within available resources and staff have a responsibility to ensure they practise in a safe manner and report adverse outcomes or equipment failures.

Areas of management that will contribute towards having a safe environment include:

- maintaining adequate staffing levels
- continually providing training, supervision and support for staff
- providing equipment that is regularly serviced, updated and for which there is an organized scheme of training in its usage
- establishing an effective system of communication at all levels of staff
- encouraging staff to report instances of risk and near misses in an open and confident manner.

This last point in particular can be assisted by managers being seen to be supportive towards staff. A midwife involved in a serious adverse outcome can have her confidence in her ability severely affected unless this is recognized and the appropriate action taken. A midwife in this situation would benefit from contact with her supervisor of midwives (ENB 1997).

At trust level, management should be seen to be providing support for managers within the specialties, have a management of claims system in place which reduces costs and employ lawyers who are competently experienced in the specialty and have a good knowledge of the risk management system.

A management structure which accepts responsibility for providing the best possible working environment will be effective in reducing risks and enable those giving direct patient or client care to have confidence in the system. Providing a system with which the staff feel confident will help them to accept their role and responsibility in fulfilling the requirements of risk management. As the risk management process proceeds and develops the advantages to staff should become more apparent.

The responsibilities for staff include:

- constantly improving their professional knowledge and skills
- identifying their own training needs
- developing their record-keeping skills
- increasing their communication skills
- always acting in the best interest of the mother and baby (UKCC 1994).

Case scenario 9.1 illustrates most of these points.

In this case the outcome was good but it may have been different if the placental site had bled and an emergency caesarean section performed with subsequent wound infection which

Case scenario 9.1

A midwife is caring for a mother on the antenatal ward who has a grade 1 placenta praevia. Previously the midwife had cared only for mothers who had had an elective caesarean section for placenta praevia. She has therefore already added to her experience and further increases her knowledge by reading about placenta praevia outcomes. The midwife takes the time to read the mother's case notes thoroughly and discovers in the medical notes that 10 years previously she had an appendicectomy with peritonitis which had required a hospital stay of 3 weeks. The midwife discusses this with the mother and discovers that her memory of this surgery is one of pain, feeling unwell for a long time and having a wound that would not heal. She has a consequent dread of having a caesarean section. The midwife records this information in the notes and reassures the mother that as the placenta is lying anteriorly the risk of caesarean section is reduced, but should it be necessary she will ensure the medical staff are aware of the need for antibiotic cover and she will be closely observed for signs of infection. The mother had labour induced the next day and the midwife was able to care for her during a normal labour and delivery. The midwife had acted in the best interests of the mother and had displayed good communication and record-keeping skills (UKCC 1993).

required return to theatre for wound drainage. At this point a risk management form would need to be completed and a full explanation of the possible causes and necessary treatment given to the mother by senior medical staff. The notes would then be reviewed and a check made that details of all actions and explanations had been recorded. If the mother was unhappy with her condition or she felt there was a lack of explanation then a letter of complaint could be received and if she did not feel the reply was satisfactory a solicitor's letter could follow perhaps alleging poor treatment and unnecessary pain and suffering.

Risk assessment chart

Use of a risk assessment form may be useful to clarify, in general terms, whether the risk is high, medium or low or whether, at this point, a risk is not present (Table 9.1). Additional information or a change in circumstances may increase or decrease the risk score either at the time or many months later.

If, for instance, a mother who sustains a third degree tear at delivery is notified to the risk manager but on investigation is found to be recovering normally then the risk score of 1 (unexpected poor outcome) is low. However, suppose that when the mother returns for her postnatal check at 6 weeks she is found to need surgery to correct the damage caused by the tear and subsequent repair. This has caused her a loss of earnings and psychological trauma so a claim is received for compensation, via a solicitor's letter. At this point the risk has increased to 4.

On the other hand a reduction in score may occur and is illustrated by the following situation. A baby has an unexpected Apgar 4 score at birth. The case notes are checked by the risk manager and it is ascertained that all the required information is correctly recorded. Eighteen months later a solicitor's letter is received as the baby is apparently suffering from cerebral damage. The risk score of 1, unexpected poor outcome, rises to 6 with the addition of an indication of litigation and a solicitor's letter. The case notes are reviewed again, the

Table 9.1 Risk assessment chart				
Score	0	1	2	3
Clinical circumstances	Satisfactory standard of care	Unexpected poor outcome	Care lacking in some aspects	Injury due to suboptimal care
Patient circumstances	Happy with explanation	Written or verbal complaint	Hostile	Solicitor's letter
Other circumstances	Nil	Witness missing	Indication of litigation	Notes missing

Score indicator: 0 = no risk, 1–3 = some risk, 4 = potential risk, 5+ = high risk.

whereabouts of the staff involved are identified and contact is made with them to formulate statements. Some months later it is found that the cerebral condition of the baby has been diagnosed as being of genetic origin. The case against the trust is discontinued.

Using a risk assessment chart not only gives clarity to the risk being considered, particularly for those inexperienced in risk management, but collating the scores and eventual outcomes provides statistical information for future auditing purposes. Also where a high risk is identified an estimated figure for possible compensation can be prepared.

Reviewing complaints

One of the areas to be noted on the risk assessment chart is that of complaints; the range here is from a verbal complaint (Spinks 1995) where the matter is dealt with at the time and to the satisfaction of the complainant, to the continuation of dialogue between the complainant and the trust because satisfaction has not been achieved and a claim for compensation is received by the trust. If complaints are not dealt with satisfactorily risk scores can leap from 1 to 5 at any point.

Reviewing all the complaints received by the obstetric directorate is part of the responsibility of the risk management team and a system should be in place to collate the various aspects of complaints. This would involve noting the types of complaints, the personnel involved, how each complaint was initially handled,

whether this was effective or proceeded to receipt of a solicitor's letter and, importantly, whether action was needed to improve care for the future.

Some trusts are experiencing an increase in the number of letters from solicitors asking, on behalf of their client, for details of the treatment given or why the events occurred. The increase in these letters may be partly because solicitors are now advertising this service in the local press or because the woman or her relatives may feel the only way to receive an adequate explanation is to go via a solicitor. These letters are not seeking compensation, at this stage, but are merely stating dissatisfaction about the care given by the midwifery or medical staff and are seeking details of the situation. If the complaint proceeds and the woman obtains legal advice there is now a system called mediation which may be used. In these cases a mediator is appointed whose role is to act as a facilitator to settle the dispute and, although both parties may be legally represented, the case does not go to court (Hallett 1995) but is settled by discussion and agreement.

Letters of complaint should always be taken seriously. Providing an adequate explanation, apologizing where appropriate and, if the circumstances warrant it, offering the complainant a meeting between themselves and the senior midwifery or medical staff to explain the events should be seen as normal practice. When giving explanations honesty and openness are essential. Mistakes do occur and they should be admitted, a sincere apology given and an assurance that action has been taken to prevent similar occurrences.

Complainants who feel they have been told the truth and have had the events and actions clearly explained will often feel satisfied and the matter will end there. There have been many instances where families have proceeded with the litigation process because they are desperate to find the truth and financial compensation is only a side issue or not important (Simanowitz 1985).

Taking complaints seriously and answering them with care and concern is good practice as it ensures the quality of the service improves and litigation costs are lessened. The Wilson Report (1994) and subsequent government guidance was produced to provide nationwide standards to assist trusts when dealing with complaints from patients, and all trusts should be complying with the standards contained within the document.

Risk factors

Every unit where risk management is being practised should have guidance for staff of likely cases where a risk might exist. Lists of risk factors will vary from unit to unit according to local need and they should be formed in consultation with the staff using them. The practice at St Mary's Hospital, London is described by O'Connor & Beard (1996) and comprises lists based on episodes of high mortality or morbidity or having litigation potential, whereas Williams (1995) divides risks into categories of direct or indirect risk. Whichever method is used it is wise to review the contents of the lists at least yearly and make adjustments as necessary, taking into consideration the previous year's notifications.

An example list of both mother and infant risk conditions can be seen in Box 9.2.

Notifying cases for risk management

When a patient or client's care has a risk factor, such as those listed in Box 9.2, a standard form should be completed as well as when any

---

Box 9.2 **Example of mother and infant risk conditions**

Mothers
- Miscarriage following amniocentesis
- Complications of cervical cerclage
- Drug errors/adverse reaction
- Eclampsia
- Infection after prolonged membrane rupture
- Complications of the perineum after suturing
- Third degree tear
- Epidural anaesthetic problems
- Retained swabs/foreign bodies
- Injury to other organs during surgery
- Rectovaginal fistula
- Ruptured uterus
- Severe haemorrhage
- Retained products of conception
- Severe illness following delivery
- Faulty equipment causing a complication
- Breach of protocol.

Infants
- Apgar 4 or below
- Fracture due to trauma
- Nerve palsy due to trauma
- Severe bruising due to birth trauma
- Iatrogenic trauma after delivery
- Hypoxic ischaemic encephalopathy
- Major resuscitation at birth or subsequently
- Neonatal death
- Drug errors/reaction
- Faulty equipment complications
- Jehovah's Witness blood transfusion.

---

untoward outcome of care occurs. A list of suggested risk conditions (not exhaustive) should be kept with the supply of unused forms. A form such as that in Box 9.3 should be completed as soon as possible after the event. If the outcome is death or serious injury then reporting must be immediate. 'Near misses' should also be reported.

Assessment of risk

When a risk management form is received by the risk manager the details within it will be noted immediately and in most instances the case notes will be reviewed. This is necessary to understand all aspects of the events and to note any relevant background medical history of the mother in all cases where further action may be required. The case notes should be read from

---

Box 9.3 Notification of case for risk management

Date of incident _____ Time of incident _____ Ward/area _____
Consultant . _____ Named midwife _____

Patient identity label

Factual account of incident (without opinions)

Person(s) carrying out the procedure/operation present

Name	_____	Grade	_____	Was there any equipment failure? yes/no
Name	_____	Grade	_____	Was this incident a 'near miss'? yes/no
Name	_____	Grade	_____	Initial explanation given to patient yes/no
If yes by	_____	Grade	_____	
Form completed by:	_____	Name	_____	Grade	_____

Completed forms to be taken by hand to risk management office

---

cover to cover, not just the entries relevant to the current situation, as it is important to gain as much information as possible about the mother. Also, there may be some previous medical history which has a bearing on the current situation.

The records relating to the event should be in sufficient detail to provide a clear picture of all the actions taken and all dates, times and identifiable signatures present. The risk manager will check that the recorded times are those of the events and not of the time of writing. Also the midwifery and medical timings should agree as if, at a later date, there is a suggestion that an action was delayed then a difference in timings recorded between professionals is not helpful, particularly if the case is to be defended. If such discrepancies exist or clarification on a point is needed the risk manager may need to have a preliminary discussion with the staff involved. If the case is serious the details should be discussed with the midwifery manager as soon as possible so that the midwife can be given support and advice at this early stage; the same opportunity should be given for the consultant to address similar needs with junior medical staff (Ennis & Grudzinkas 1993).

The risk manager will then prepare a summary of the case for discussion at the risk management team meeting and if the team feel the risk is high they will request statements to be taken from all staff involved in the case. These statements should be taken as soon as possible whilst the details are still clearly remembered. An example of a high risk case that would require statements to be taken without delay is where a baby sustains a brachial plexus injury as the eventual outcome is not predictable in many cases of this type of injury (Birch 1995).

If a high risk case is thought likely to proceed then discussion with legal advisors would be appropriate at this point. The event may highlight that immediate action is necessary to prevent a recurrence. If for example there is equipment failure then action should be taken immediately, not only to prevent danger to further women or babies but because a second incident of a similar nature would be difficult to defend.

A percentage of forms received by the risk manager will not, after an initial investigation, require any action and these will be put on file for statistical purposes. They may include such forms as notifying third degree tears which heal normally or low Apgar scores where the baby recovers quickly and makes normal progress.

Witness statements

Statements should be taken as soon as the details of the case have been assessed and a judgement made that litigation is a fair possibility. This may be within days of the discovery if the case is considered serious, (e.g. a swab left in the vagina after suturing the perineum or suspected misreading of a cardiotocograph with a low Apgar score) or statements may be requested after the risk management team meeting where the risk was thought to be high. Formulating statements sooner rather than later is beneficial as the details will be recalled more easily and the staff will either still be in post or will have a known forwarding address.

The main aim of such statements is to preserve information that is not recorded in the case notes and is in a format that can be used as evidence. The actions recorded should be in as much detail as possible as this will help the claim to be defended or give clarity if liability is to be admitted. If sufficient information has not been recorded then it is very difficult to defend a case particularly if several years have passed or a key witness cannot be traced.

An experienced risk manager will assist staff to formulate their statements and ensure that only relevant facts are included, the information contained is pertinent for defending the issues and appropriate explanations are included.

When involved in such a process it is normal not only to feel stressful but to feel a sense of guilt (Firth-Cozens 1993). When the outcome is poor and the individuals examine their actions phrases such as 'I should have' or 'if only' are often used. This common occurrence of self-blame is mainly unjustified and mostly exaggerated, sometimes out of all proportion. It is also common for some staff to feel defensive of the actions they have taken and others will suggest the 'blame' lies with another. All these reactions need to be recognized as existing and talked through with sympathy and understanding before the final version of the statement is produced.

A guide to the preparation of witness statements is provided in Box 9.4. If the case proceeds these witness statements will be used in evidence and it is important that aspects such as timings agree with the case notes or an

---

Box 9.4   A guide to the preparation of witness statements

- Record full name, address, place of work and brief details of work experience to date.
- Thoroughly read the case notes including all medical, midwifery and paramedical entries.
- Write a narrative of the events recalled of actions taken or not taken, who was called or spoken to and when involvement in the care ceased. Explain why actions were or were not taken as appropriate.
- Clearly state the dates and times of each action and record them in chronological order.
- Include only factual information and not hearsay or opinion.
- Inaccuracies in the notes should be explained in the statement and an amendment prepared for the patient's notes which is signed, dated and witnessed.
- No other circumstances exist for adding, deleting or altering information contained in the notes.
- Typed statements are easier to read though this is not essential.
- All copies of the statement should be signed and dated at the foot of each page.
- A copy should be retained by the individual.
- Witness statements must not be stored in the case notes.

---

explanation included as to why they differ. The practice of recording the time of writing rather than the times of events should now be obsolete but some instances may be found in past case notes. Written statements clearly identifying the facts and produced at an early stage will be of great assistance to the individual if needed for use in court. Writing them should be regarded as advantageous as a valid record of the events will be available, even if not used for up to 25 years, and this record can be used if at the time of the court hearing a witness cannot be traced.

CLAIMS HANDLING

It is important that where there is a risk management process in place an identified series of steps is designed to ensure claims are dealt with efficiently and cost effectively. The NHS Management Executive (1996) gave guidance to claims handling and this states the responsibility of the chief executive to establish a framework for claims management. These include ensuring that:

1. the trust has a clear policy for handling claims of clinical negligence
2. there is a board member who has responsibility for clinical negligence issues
3. A claims manager is appointed.

The claims manager will be responsible for the process from this point onwards but will work closely with the risk manager, the risk management team and the trust's legal advisors.

Letter before action

This is a letter received from the plaintiff's solicitor giving a brief summary of the sequence of events and basic allegations of negligence with a request for a full copy of the case notes. A form of consent signed by the patient or client agreeing to this release should be enclosed. Before notes are released it is important to use a checklist including the following:

- check the claim has sufficient details to warrant voluntary disclosure of the case notes
- check the patient or client has given authority for release
- inform the consultant, senior midwife and risk manager (as applicable) of the potential claim
- request from the consultant or senior midwife:
  —a preliminary opinion of allegations
  —the identity of staff involved
  —an agreement to disclosure
- obtain the whereabouts of all staff involved
- obtain two sets of accurately photocopied medical and midwifery records and include all additional information such as CTG tracings, X-rays, scans and any complaints correspondence
- instruct trust solicitors
- ensure internal data collection and statement taking are in progress.

Disclosure

This is effected by the serving of a list of documents required. It will state: 'all documents which are or have been in your possession, custody or power'. The fact that any document may harm or help either party is irrelevant and all must be disclosed.

Action for disclosure

The following actions are necessary once a list of documents for disclosure has been served by the plaintiff's solicitor:

- arrange disclosure of records through the trust's solicitors
- recover photocopying costs from those requesting disclosure
- assess position on liability
- depending on the circumstances, trace any missing key witnesses
- obtain an outside expert witness who is willing to produce a written opinion on the events.

After disclosure of the medical and midwifery records the plaintiff may decide there is not sufficient grounds to continue or the limitation period may expire. In both instances the claim will be discontinued, staff should be informed and the file archived. If the claim proceeds then a writ and statement of claim will be received from the plaintiff's solicitors and the outcome is either to admit liability and negotiate a settlement or to deny liability. If liability is denied the case can still be discontinued at this late point if the plaintiff's evidence is weak. If the case continues then proceedings will be issued, the trust will continue to defend and preparations for trial will begin. The trust's legal advisors will hold conferences composed of lawyers and medical and midwifery expert witnesses, plus any key witnesses involved in the care, to discuss all the surrounding issues and formulate the defence. The trial will be held, the decision made and the file will be archived. The case can be discontinued for a variety of reasons at any point right up to the day before the trial; in spite of a large increase in the number of claims submitted most are not heard in court.

CLAIMS AUDIT

If the main aims of risk management are to improve the quality of the service and reduce the associated costs then undertaking an audit will provide valuable information about how successful the process is in progressing towards meeting these aims and in identifying any necessary changes. When a risk management team has been functioning for a few years a database of factual information will have been collected and this should be reviewed on a regular basis to detect the number of risks, their outcome and whether the same or similar risk situations are recurring (Ennis & Vincent 1990). It is apparent from studies already undertaken that there are a few conditions arising in obstetric practice where solicitors are consulted on a regular basis (Capstick & Edwards 1990). These are: failure to act appropriately on CTG recordings, meconium-stained liquor or delay in expediting delivery of the baby.

A claims audit should include analysis of all legal claims received and not just those that have progressed to formal proceedings. Each case will need at least the following information recorded, preferably using a computer program:

- classification by severity of the clinical details
- date of incident
- date of claim
- time period between incident and claim
- predicted or known cost
- possible year or period of payment
- final costs—subdivided into payments to plaintiffs and legal costs
- date case was archived.

If this information is recorded using an appropriate computer program then numbers of each classified case, frequency of occurrence, timespans from start to finish, outcomes and costs will be readily available (Capstick 1995). When sufficient data have been collected to be numerically valid then decisions can be made to change any identified aspect of the risk management process. If, for example, the maternal and infant notifiable risk lists have a condition which has not been notified in the last 3 years because it has always been linked with a more serious condition then it should be removed and the midwives' time saved in completing forms unnecessarily. A more major change may be that when legal costs are compared with other trusts they seem high; this could result in the trust changing its legal advisors.

Building up audit information over a period of time will enable comparisons to be made year by year for identification of trends or claims which may be peculiar to a particular area. If risk management audit information becomes available on a regional basis then comparisons between each will be possible and the reasons for any major differences examined. Although claims audit in risk management provides very necessary information, merely collecting activity data does little to change clinical practice unless action is taken on areas where change is agreed. Once change has been implemented its effectiveness should be evaluated by measuring it against future rises or falls of adverse outcomes (Beard & O'Connor 1995).

Collecting information on quality issues would probably require a more sophisticated computer program but details of changes to policies or procedures should be collected because the date a certain practice started or ceased could be useful in defending a case in the future (see Case study 9.3). A database of the reasons for complaints and their outcomes can be used for monitoring quality issues, and acting upon such information should be initiated by the risk management team.

Audit information collected in a unit should be shared with all staff, particularly when areas acted upon as a result of risk management show that an improvement in practice has occurred.

CASE STUDIES

The following cases (Case studies 9.1 to 9.6) are included to illustrate some of the aspects and actions taken from a risk management point of view. Most are based on incidents that have happened in various maternity units in Britain but the details have been sufficiently altered to comply with confidentiality.

Case study 9.1

Bacterial Meningitis

Pamela had progressed normally during her first pregnancy and labour started spontaneously at 39 weeks' gestation. On admission to the labour ward she was established in labour and the first stage of labour progressed well with all recordings and observations normal. During the second stage of labour a severe fetal bradycardia occurred and when the membranes were ruptured the liquor was stained with fresh meconium. A Ventouse extraction was performed and Peter was born with an Apgar score of 9 at 1 minute and 10 at 5 minutes. He was transferred to the postnatal ward at 2 hours of age.

The next day he was being held by Pamela who had fallen asleep and had not noticed that he was blue and lifeless. One midwife started resuscitation whilst another called the paediatric cardiac arrest team. By the time the medical team arrived Peter had a good heart rate but was not breathing spontaneously. He was intubated and transferred to the neonatal unit. Seizures were apparent within one hour of collapse. A lumbar puncture was performed and cerebral spinal fluid sent for culture, which did not grow any organisms but three doses of antibiotics had already been given. A presumed diagnosis of meningitis was made and Peter received a 2 week course of ampicillin and gentamicin.

A cranial ultrasound revealed changes compatible with hypoxia and also showed thrombosis of the superior sagittal sinus. Peter remained on artificial ventilation for 8 days. His seizures gradually settled and he was discharged home aged 16 days to be followed up in paediatric outpatients in 4 weeks' time. When Peter was 3 months old a solicitor's letter was received alleging that Peter had been allowed to contract bacterial meningitis and was suffering from consequential brain damage. The case notes were reviewed and the contents discussed by the risk management team who thought the possibility of this allegation proceeding to be of low risk. The case notes were disclosed to the plaintiff's solicitor. Eight months later the case was discontinued.

Comments on Case study 9.1

It was fairly obvious from the beginning of this case that the allegation was lacking in evidence. There is, however, little doubt that this baby was damaged and requires frequent follow-up support and care. If any lessons are to be learnt from this situation the question needs to asked as to why Pamela needed to consult a solicitor. Was sufficient information and support given to her in those first few months?

Case study 9.2

Laparoscopy in pregnancy

Ann was seen in the accident and emergency department when she was 26 weeks' pregnant suffering from severe abdominal pain. She was booked for confinement and had been receiving antenatal care at this same hospital. The general surgeons assessed her and decided she was suffering from appendicitis. She was taken to theatre for laparoscopy where it was found the appendix was normal. She was admitted to a surgical ward and discharged home 2 days later.

There had not been any communication between the surgeons and the obstetrician/gynaecologist and the first knowledge they had of this admission was when a solicitor's letter was received alleging unnecessary surgery during pregnancy. Ann was now nearly 36 weeks pregnant and due for her next visit to the hospital clinic. Ann had á normal delivery at 39 weeks' gestation.

Comments on Case study 9.2

In this case the surgeons had to answer the allegations, which were considered defendable. The allegations were withdrawn after Ann had a full discussion with the surgeon. The obstetrician/gynaecologist felt that contact should have been made with him so that he could have been present during the laparoscopy and gynaecological causes for the pain could have been diagnosed or discounted. The clinical director of obstetrics and gynaecology wrote to the clinical director of surgery requesting involvement of a gynaecologist when pregnant women are taken to theatre in the future, and the senior midwife made contact with the accident and emergency department and surgical sisters asking to be informed of any similar cases. This enabled an antenatal check to be made after surgery and the opportunity given to the mother to discuss any worries she may have had regarding her pregnancy.

Case study 9.3

Cerebral palsy

Carol booked for her second pregnancy in her local maternity hospital in January 1980. This unit undertook about 1500 deliveries per year and, although full obstetric cover was available, both the paediatrician and the anaesthetist were on call from the local district general hospital, 3 miles away.

Carol's antenatal period was normal and she was admitted in established labour at 40+weeks. On admission contractions were every 7 minutes, the os uteri was at 1.5 cm dilatation, the membranes were intact and all other findings were normal. Her labour progressed and 4 hours later when the membranes ruptured the liquor was noted to be slightly stained with meconium. Examination per vaginam showed the os uteri to have reached 5 cm dilatation. Owing to the presence of meconium, the relatively new procedure of fetal blood sampling to assess the acidity of the fetal blood was performed. The pH was 7.23. Two hours later another fetal blood sample showed a pH of 7.18. The os had now reached 9.5 cm dilatation and as the fetal heart rate was causing concern it was decided to deliver the baby by Ventouse extraction. This was applied but failed so Carol was taken to theatre for emergency caesarean section. The paediatrician was already present but the anaesthetist had to be called from the other hospital. Lucy was born half an hour later with Apgar scores of 2 at 1 minute, 3 at 5 minutes and 5 at 10 minutes. She was intubated and extubated 10 minutes later with a normal heart rate and respirations. Carol and Lucy were discharged home after 10 days in the postnatal ward. When Lucy was nearly 3 years of age she was diagnosed as having cerebral palsy. A solicitor's letter was received in 1994 claiming delay in undertaking a caesarean section and thereby causing cerebral damage due to hypoxia.

Comments on Case study 9.3

Attempts were made to trace the midwives who cared for Carol in labour but only one, who had only had minimal input, could be traced. The midwives notes were just sufficient to describe the actions they took and these were considered appropriate. The doctor, however, had recored only the results of the fetal blood samples, without any comment. The case went to court but the plaintiff lost as fetal blood sampling was only just starting to be used as a method of detecting fetal hypoxia. A doctor is not considered negligent if he has acted in accordance with accepted practice (Watts 1995).

Case study 9.4

Preterm labour and delayed transfer

Sylvia booked at 12 weeks' gestation for her second pregnancy. Her first pregnancy had been a miscarriage at 14 weeks when she had been living abroad. She was found to be Rhesus negative with antibodies and therefore most of her antenatal care was at the hospital antenatal clinic. At 28 weeks' gestation Sylvia was admitted for a raised antibody titre and an intrauterine transfusion was carried out. Sylvia returned to the antenatal ward for close observation and later that day uterine contractions were present but labour was not established. The hospital's neonatal unit did not have any intensive care cots and so it was decided to transfer Sylvia to an obstetric unit in the next county where an intensive care cot was available.

The senior houseman said he would arrange the transfer and spoke to the obstetric and paediatric registrars in the accepting hospital. Four hours later, by which time a shift change of midwives had occurred, Sylvia was still on the ward. Another hour passed and the senior midwife rang the ambulance service to ascertain the delay. The ambulance booking office did not have a record of such a request for transfer but were able to take Sylvia as an emergency.

Close monitoring of the fetal heart rate and the uterine contractions had been undertaken and, although the contractions were starting to increase in intensity, the fetal heart had not given cause for concern until the midwife went to tell Sylvia the ambulance crew were on their way to collect her. The fetal heart could not be heard and an ultrasound scan confirmed an intrauterine death.

Labour was induced the following day and Sylvia delivered a stillborn infant.

Comments on Case study 9.4

Statements were taken from all the staff involved in this case as it was regarded as a high risk case of the trust's liability. Sylvia and her husband were seen and spoken to at length and apologies were given for the delay in transfer due to poor communications. A solicitor's letter was received 9 months later alleging delay in transferring Sylvia to a unit which could have provided the required care, and this delay contributed to the loss of her baby.

The defence asked for the opinion of an expert witness as, in spite of the delay in transfer, the chance of this baby surviving was slim. The expert witness confirmed the liability of the trust. An agreed settlement of £14 000 was made to the parents. The delay occurred because the midwife thought that when the senior houseman said he would arrange the transfer this included arranging the ambulance. A similar occurrence would be prevented by ensuring clear guidelines are available stating the responsibility of midwives when arranging transfers of mothers and babies to other units.

The lack of intensive care cots also needed to be addressed and some units have decided that intrauterine transfers will not take place if labour has started but that delivery will be expedited as necessary and mother and baby transferred as appropriate.

Case study 9.5

Vaginal tampon

Joan was booked for her first pregnancy at the local hospital and had a normal antenatal period, labour and delivery. An episiotomy was necessary and this was sutured by the medical student who had delivered Joan under the supervision of the midwife. When the last suture was being put in, the midwife was asked to assist with a mother having a breech delivery in the next room. The midwife knew the medical student and his competency so left him to complete the task. The medical student had already asked the mother next door if he could observe her breech delivery and she had agreed. He therefore finished the suturing, made Joan comfortable and left.

Joan was transferred to receive care at home on her 4th postnatal day. During a home visit on the 7th postnatal day the midwife observed that Joan's lochia smelt very unpleasant. On further inspection the midwife removed a tampon from Joan's vagina. Joan denied using a tampon so it was assumed that it had not been removed after the suturing was completed. The Trust accepted liability and made a payment of £500 via Joan's solicitor.

Comments on Case study 9.5

This is a situation of accepted liability but with a low cost because Joan had not been harmed. Had, however, she suffered an intrauterine infection which had affected her fertility and this had been proven then the costs would have been much higher.

To ensure tampons are not left in situ in the future it would be necessary to revise the suturing procedure to include an instruction that states: 'if tampons are used during suturing of the perineum the string of the tampon must be attached with forceps to the sterile towel placed over the abdomen.' It might be wise to add that gauze swabs or cotton wool balls should never be inserted into the vagina during suturing.

Case study 9.6

Ventouse delivery

Annabel had married at age 29 and, although she eventually wanted children, developing her career in teaching had remained her priority until she discovered she was pregnant. Annabel began to read about pregnancy and became intensely interested in natural childbirth attending local classes on the subject and reading every available book or leaflet she could find. She became determined to have a natural birth and formulated a birth plan that clearly stated that the only form of pain relief she wished was to use the birthing pool. She did not want any drugs that stimulated uterine action, Syntometrine for the third stage, or her membranes ruptured artificially.

She began labour spontaneously at 41 weeks and was admitted to the labour suite at 22.00 hours. On admission her contractions were moderate in strength and were occurring about every 6 minutes. Examination per vaginam revealed the os uteri to be at 2 cm dilatation, the presentation was cephalic and the presenting part was at the level of the ischial spines. Annabel continued with moderate contractions throughout the night but she was quite relaxed and managed to sleep for an hour or so on several occasions.

The doctors round was at 08.00 hours and although they were informed of Annabel's labour and progress they did not see her as she was considered to be in normal labour and therefore under the care of a midwife. At 10.00 hours Annabel's contractions were stronger and every 4 to 5 minutes. She asked to go in the birthing pool for pain relief but another mother had just delivered in the pool room and it was not available until 12 midday.

Annabel was examined prior to entering the pool and the os uteri was then 6 cm, the position of the head was left occipitoposterior and still at the level of the ischial spines. She was relaxed and comfortable in the water and her recordings were normal until 14.30 hours when the fetal heart rate showed a late deceleration with slow recovery. The medical staff were informed and Annabel was told they would be coming to see her. She returned to her labour room and the

Case study 9.6 Continued

doctor examined her. The os uteri was 9 cm, the membranes were bulging and the doctor ruptured them revealing fresh meconium. A further late deceleration of the fetal heart occurred and the doctor decided to deliver Annabel by Ventouse extraction. A live baby boy was delivered at 15.15 hours with an Apgar score of 6 at 1 minute and 9 at 5 minute.

Another midwife had entered the room just before the birth and given Annabel Syntometrine with the birth of the anterior shoulder. Annabel and her son were transferred to the care of the community midwife on the 5th postnatal day.

Several months later a solicitor's letter was received by the hospital stating that at the time of her son's birth Annabel had not been informed of the reasons for a Ventouse delivery. This had not been discussed with her at the time and she had not given her consent to this type of delivery.

The hospital received the following allegations:

- Annabel's membranes had been ruptured without her consent.
- a Ventouse delivery had been performed without her consent.
- Syntometrine had been injected without her permission ignoring her request not to have it.

She was suing because she had suffered extreme psychological trauma as a result of the circumstances of her delivery and had been unable to return to work at the agreed time, which meant she was suffering a loss of earnings.

Activity 9.1

Give your judgement on the following:
1. If Annabel's case appears to be proceeding, detail the necessary actions to be taken by: the risk manager, the midwifery manager and the hospital legal advisor.
2. If the case does not proceed, what action needs to be taken to prevent a similar letter being received in the future?

Summary

Risk management should be seen as a tool to assist midwives to take a positive course of action when the clinical outcome is unexpectedly poor. Risk areas need to be identified without fear of recrimination, acted upon and if not eliminated at least reduced in occurrence and severity. Having an understanding and acceptance of risk management will both enhance midwifery practice and improve the quality of the service provided for mothers and babies.

The risk management team have a key role to play in ensuring staff are supported when involved in a case of risk and in keeping all staff informed of changes recommended as a consequence of risk management audit. Constant analysis of actions that could result in harm to a mother or her baby and implementing preventative measures as appropriate will not only reduce costs but will also result in the best possible outcomes for all concerned with the maternity service.

REFERENCES

Beard R W, O' Connor A 1995 Implementation of audit and risk management—a protocol. In: Vincent C (ed) Clinical risk management. BMJ Publications, London

Birch R 1995 Obstetrical brachial plexus palsy. Clinical risk 1:71–73

Capstick B 1994 Risk management in obstetrics. In: Clements R V (ed) Safe practice in obstetrics and gynaecology: a medico-legal handbook. Churchill Livingstone, New York, pp 405–416

Capstick B 1995 Incident reporting and claims analysis. Clinical risk, vol 1, Churchill Livingstone, New York, pp 165–167

Capstick B, Edwards P 1990 Trends in obstetric malpractice claims. Lancet Oct 13:931–932

Clements R V 1991 Litigation in obstetrics and gynaecology. British Journal of Obstetrics and Gynaecology 98:423–426

Clements R V 1994 (ed) Safe practice in obstetrics and gynaecology: a medico-legal handbook. Churchill Livingstone, New York, pp 1–4

DoH (Department of Health) NHS Management Executive 1993 Risk management in the NHS. HMSO, London, ch 24, pp 95–98

ENB (English National Board) 1997 Clinical risk management and the supervisor of midwives. Preparation of supervisors of midwives. Module 3, section 5. ENB, London, pp 45–50

Ennis M, Grudzinkas J G 1993 The effects of accidents and litigation on doctors. In: Vincent C, Ennis M, Audley R J (eds) Medical accidents. Oxford University Press, Oxford, pp 167–180

Ennis M, Vincent C A 1990 Obsteric accidents: a review of 64 cases. British Medical Journal 300:1365–1367

Firth-Cozens J 1993 Stress, psychological problems and clinical performance. In: Vincent C, Ennis M, Audley R J (eds) Medical accidents. Oxford University Press, Oxford, pp 131–149

Hallett D 1995 Mediation for clinical negligence cases. Health Care Risk Report, vol 2, issue 2. Eclipse Group, London, p 1

Marlock L, Malitz F E 1991 Do hospital risk management programs make a difference? Law and Contemporary Problems 54:1

NHS Management Executive 1996 EL (96)11 Guidance notes on clinical negligence and personal injury litigation. NHS Management Executive, Leeds

O'Connor A, Beard R W 1996 Risk management—what is it and how does it work? MIDIRS Midwifery Digest Mar. 6(1):61–64

Simanowitz A 1985 Standards, attitudes and accountability in the medical profession. Lancet 11:546–547

Spinks M 1995 First line of defence. Nursing Times 91 (16):53

UKCC 1993 Midwives rules. 42, UKCC, London, pp 21–22

UKCC 1994 Midwife's code of practice, 40, UKCC, London, pp 8–9

Vincent C A, Clements R V 1995 Clinical risk management— why do we need it? Clinical Risk 1(1):1–4

Watt J 1995 Bolam v Friern Hospital Management Committee. Clinical Risk 1(1):84–85

Williams J 1995 A midwife's view. Clinical Risk 1(5):175–177

Wilson Report 1994 Acting on complaints. EL(95) 37, EL (95)121, EL (96) 19. NHS Management Executive, Leeds

10

Supervisors and managers

Colleen Drury   Margaret Staples

CHAPTER CONTENTS

The aims of this chapter are to: enable
practitioners to develop a greater
understanding of the supervision of midwives;
explore the tensions and potential conflicts of
the dual roles of midwifery manager and
supervisor of midwives, and consider the role
of the supervisor of midwives in the current
climate of changing midwifery practices.

Supervision is what makes us strong, helps us to
develop our practice, provides support and distinguishes us as a profession.   (Davis 1994, p 304)

INTRODUCTION

The continuation of the debate for and against
the supervision of midwives requires a re-ex-
amination of its many different perspectives—
for example, the statutory framework, the tensions
of the dual role and the different perspectives
of supervision of midwives held by midwives,
supervisors and childbearing women. The knowledge base of both newly qualified and practising
midwives in relation to supervision of midwives
is often criticized even though there is a plethora
of literature now available. However, midwives
may in some areas lack access to some of this
information, for example the Preparation of
supervisors of midwives distance learning pack
(ENB 1997a–d), which would enable a greater
understanding of the role. In addition, and this
chapter is no different, whilst the role of manager and that of supervisor of midwives are

often linked in the literature to help develop understanding, it is possible that this could add to the lack of clarity between the roles.

THE HISTORICAL PERSPECTIVE OF THE SUPERVISION OF MIDWIVES

Statutory control—from the Central Midwives Board to the United Kingdom Central Council

The role of the supervisor of midwives has been a part of the statutory law controlling midwives' practice since the 1902 Midwives Act (HMSO 1902), although Donnison (1988) suggests that as long ago as 1512 Henry VIII made formal arrangements for the control of midwives. This arose as a result of concerns about infant and maternal mortality and from the need to protect the public from the unsafe practices of unqualified birth attendants.

As a result of the 1902 Midwives Act the CMB was formed and it was able to register midwives and establish and maintain a roll of practising midwives. The CMB also defined and limited the midwife's sphere of practice by formulating midwives rules. Those midwives who disobeyed or ignored the rules or were guilty of negligence, malpractice or misconduct were to be disciplined. This controlling of midwives was from a medical dominance, as midwives were not allowed to be members of the CMB until 1920 and even then were statutorily forbidden to form a majority.

The LSAs were established as a result of the 1902 Act and the CMB delegated the supervision and monitoring of midwives to these bodies. The LSAs were in fact county councils and their main function was to exercise general supervision of midwives who practised in their area. The LSAs' duties included investigating charges of misconduct, negligence or malpractice, suspension of midwives who were likely to be a source of infection and ensuring that midwives notified their intention to practise. All of these activities were reported to the CMB. The LSAs performed the supervision of midwives through a midwifery committee, which included the medical officer of health who was mainly responsible for general supervision. The medical officer had the power to delegate the task to a non-medical supervisor, this person often being a lady, usually a non-midwife or sometimes a health visitor (RCM 1991). The supervisors at this time were called inspectors of midwives and the Institute of Inspectors of Midwives was thus formed in 1910.

It was not until the 1936 Midwives Act (HMSO 1936) that the CMB was empowered to make rules relating to the qualifications of non-medical and medical supervisors who until this time had been known as inspectors of midwives. This Act therefore allowed for the appointment of midwives to the role of non-medical supervisor although they still had to work under the direction of the medical officer of health.

The Ministry of Health letter of 1937 (see Appendix p. 175), was of great significance in stating the function and qualifications of the supervisors of midwives. Section 3 of the letter acknowledged the ill effects of inspection of midwives and therefore the title was changed to 'supervisor'. The supervisor was required to have 'adequate' experience in midwifery although it was not explicit that the supervisor should be currently practising as a midwife. Section 4 also required that she should be regarded as a 'counsellor and friend to midwives, rather than a relentless critic' and have 'sympathy and tact'. However, the structure in which the 'new' supervisors worked did not change. The Institute of Supervisors of Midwives became the Association of Supervisors in 1937.

The 1936 Act and section 7 of the Ministry of Health letter highlights the role of the supervisor of midwives as a separate function to that of managing midwives as a salaried midwifery service became mandatory at this time (Association of Supervisors of Midwives 1992). As the LSAs were local government authorities this only applied to community midwives.

The LSAs continued to provide the service of supervision of midwives until the 1974 National Health (Reorganization) Act (HMSO 1974) when existing LSAs were abolished and the service was delegated to regional health authorities as the new LSAs. These new LSAs further delegated some duties of supervision of midwives to district health authority level. Supervisors of midwives were thus nominated in each health district and approved by the LSA. It was not until 1977 that the role of the medical supervisor was eradicated and the words 'non-medical' removed from the title of 'supervisor of midwives' (The Midwives [Qualifications of Supervisors] Regulations 1977 no. 1850). As health authorities had responsibility for both hospital and community health services this opened the way for midwifery managers to become supervisors of midwives. This situation has over the years led to a lack of clarity between the distinct roles of midwifery manager and supervisor of midwives.

The 1979 Nurses, Midwives and Health Visitors Act (HMSO 1979) abolished previous statutory bodies and created the UKCC and the national boards. The function of supervision was then divided between the boards, having been retained in Section 15 and Section 16 of the Act.

DEVELOPMENT OF LOCAL SUPERVISING AUTHORITIES AND THEIR FUNCTION

In the Health Authorities Act 1995 (HMSO 1995), health authorities took over the functions of the LSAs from the regional health authorities, which were dissolved. This arrangement was introduced in England in 1996. Technically under these new arrangements the eight NHS executives and the 119 health authorities were to provide the LSA function. However, to achieve a consistent approach the health authorities combined to form consortia for the LSA function. This resulted in 12 LSA consortia and, for the first time, all LSA officers were practising midwives. This new system, according to the ENB (1998), is effective.

The functions of the LSA

The functions of the LSAs are stated in Midwives rule 45 (UKCC 1998). The Nurses, Midwives and Health Visitors Act 1997 states:

Each local supervising authority shall—exercise general supervision, in accordance with the rules under section 14, over all midwives practising within its area; report any prima facie case of misconduct on the part of a midwife which arises in its area to the Council; have power in accordance with the Council's rules to suspend a midwife from practice.

(Nurses, Midwives and Health Visitors Act 1997, section 15(2) p. 10)

In addition, this Act (section 15(4) p. 10) requires the national boards to provide the LSAs with advice and guidance in respect of exercising their functions in relation to the supervision of midwives.

The LSA is therefore responsible for ensuring that statutory supervision of midwives is undertaken to a satisfactory standard within its geographical location. This applies to all midwives working within its geographical area whether employed in the NHS, the private sector, in higher education, prisons, in independent practice or employed by general practitioners.

The UKCC may prescribe in the formulation of rules the qualifications of persons to be appointed by an LSA to exercise supervision of midwives within its area. A person who is not qualified in accordance with the rules cannot be appointed (UKCC 1994). The person appointed to undertake the duties of the LSA in accordance with the statutory requirements is known as the LSA responsible officer. Where LSAs have formed a consortia to undertake the discharge of the statutory function of supervision of midwives the lead authority appoints the responsible officer. However, each health authority is required to identify a named supervisor of midwives to ensure effective communication with the LSA responsible officer (ENB 1996). This named supervisor is known as the link supervisor.

Activities of the LSA responsible officer

The activities of the LSA responsible officer are wide ranging and likely to expand as the responsibility for the LSA function transfers to the purchasers. The officer's role is described by Duerden (1996) as:

- advising purchasers of contract specifications
- contributing to trust policies

- providing expert advice to outside agencies
- acting as a catalyst for change.

Further responsibilities of the LSA responsible officer can be found in ENB (1996) Supervision of midwives.

As management structures in the NHS change, and with many senior midwifery posts being axed, the involvement of midwives at this high level is seen as a crucial development (Henderson 1997). This relocation of the statutory role of the LSA can only benefit midwifery by ensuring close links are maintained with health authorities, there are more opportunities for involvement in commissioning and expert midwifery advice is provided by midwives. This brings the LSA much closer to midwifery practice and better able to relate to local situations. The importance of supervision of midwives is beginning to be recognized by trust boards and district health authorities in terms of its potential role in risk management initiatives, clinical audit, quality assurance and primary care initiatives (Mayes 1996). In the long term this should additionally facilitate the move towards a woman-centred service placing midwifery firmly on the political agenda.

In addition to the activities stated, the LSA officers play an important role in the delivery of courses for the preparation of supervisors of midwives and the ongoing education of existing supervisors. This provides an opportunity for LSA officers to influence and support supervisors of midwives and facilitate a more cohesive and consistent approach to supervision (Sauter 1997).

PREPARATION OF SUPERVISORS OF MIDWIVES

The role of the supervisor of midwives is, according to Mayes (1995), very complex, therefore the individual who undertakes this role must be credible in making professional judgements, approachable and acceptable to the midwives who will be supported in practice.

Since 1974, it has been common practice to appoint managers as supervisors of midwives, the combination of which has been extensively debated (Lansdell 1989, Magill-Cuerden 1994). Issues also highlighted in the literature relate to the lack of a common understanding of the responsibilities and authority of supervisors of midwives as well as inconsistencies in the approach to supervision (Isherwood 1988). The national boards recognized these problems and the need for development of the supervision of midwives in terms of enabling supervisors to acquire knowledge of the role and the skills to empower midwives in the rapidly changing maternity services. As a result the ENB developed an open-learning course for the preparation of supervisors of midwives (ENB 1992). These courses require a minimum of diploma level study with some now encouraging degree level study. At the end of 1995, 480 midwives had undertaken this new preparation for the role (Thomas & Mayes 1996).

The formal preparation of supervisors of midwives initially began as a result of the 1977 Regulations with the CMB introducing courses of instruction in 1978. The Nurses, Midwives and Health Visitors Act 1979 (HMSO 1979) and the amendments to the Act in 1992 (HMSO 1992) passed the responsibility for setting standards for supervision of midwives to the UKCC. The UKCC therefore sets the standards, qualifications, appointment and preparation of supervisors of midwives in addition to the duties of the LSAs. The responsibility for ensuring these standards are met is delegated to the national boards. The national boards are also responsible for providing advice and guidance to the LSA with regard to their function.

Rule 44 of the Midwives rules (UKCC 1998) requires midwives nominated for the role to complete a national board approved course successfully prior to appointment as a supervisor of midwives. The UKCC's Midwifery Committee has also identified the preparation of supervisors of midwives as an issue that requires even further consideration. Steene (1996) highlights the recommendation for a set of learning outcomes for the preparation of supervisors to be included in legislation, which would be broad enough to allow flexibility in the courses offered throughout the UK. The ultimate aim of this standardization would be to achieve a more consistent approach in the exercise of supervision of midwives. A further proposal for changes to the rules is that the national boards should provide guidance to LSAs in relation to the process of selection and appointment of supervisors of midwives (Steene 1996). Again this is an attempt to achieve consistency in the approach to the function of supervision of midwives. Future developments relating to selection, preparation and appointment to the role of supervisor of midwives have been incorporated into the Midwives rules published in 1998 (UKCC).

The changes in the NHS have resulted in a reduction of the number of midwifery managers and hence a reduction in experienced midwifery supervisors (Thomas & Mayes 1996). This reorganization of management structures has opened the way for new supervisors of midwives to be selected from a range of grades enabling the separation of management from supervision of midwives. However, for supervision to be effective it must impact at all levels within trust structures. This influence is required in policy development, total quality management, risk management and to provide the essential professional leadership in the maternity services (Thomas & Mayes 1996).

Mayes (1996) identifies the areas of practice of the 480 midwives who completed the supervisors of midwives programme by the end of 1995 as follows:

- clinical practice   54%
- management   34%
- education   3.5%
- unknown   3%
- other (research, practice development)   5%.

The majority of these supervisors are clinical-based midwives, a situation that has changed from one where supervision of midwives was mainly seen as management dominated. Johnson (1996) argues for a team approach to the supervision of midwives similar to that adopted by general management, as described by Kakabadse, Ludlow & Vinnicomke (1988). The team approach developed at Southmead (Johnson 1996) recognizes that supervisors cannot realistically

maintain consistent competency in every area of midwifery practice and, therefore, aims to offer midwives a broad range of support in practice. The range of expertise and background from which supervisors develop serves to raise the profile of supervision and the range of complementary support for midwives. The strengths and opportunities this creates can enable a more innovative and proactive perspective of supervision to be achieved, benefiting both midwives and childbearing women. It is, therefore, the function of supervision of midwives, rather than any continuing debate of who should or should not be a supervisor, which requires further consideration (Mayes 1997).

The ENB (1996) advise that LSAs establish a policy for the selection and appointment of supervisors of midwives. The requirement is that any such policy should address local needs and meet the UKCC's standards. A 'person specification' is recommended, identifying essential and desirable criteria (ENB 1996 p. 15, RCM 1996 no. 6) which include:

- experience
- knowledge and academic ability
- effective communication
- assertiveness with leadership skills
- approachability
- political awareness
- ability to use evidence and research to underpin practice
- commitment to own personal and professional development.

However, Johnson (1996) suggests that if a team approach is to be achieved a generic person specification will no longer be required as the team's requirements will need to be reflected. If a team approach to managing midwifery practice is seen to be endorsed then a team approach to supervision would appear to complement this style of practice. Supervisors may then utilize skills and knowledge for team building (Belbin 1981) to enable effective supervision of midwives and in their facilitation of midwives participating in team-working practices.

Mayes (1996) suggests that, in some maternity units, midwives are encouraged to nominate colleagues whom they consider to be suitable for appointment as supervisors of midwives. This stance may enable midwives and supervisors to work together in achieving the common aim of providing optimum care for mothers and babies. In addition, it would enable the supervisor to fulfil the requirement to act as a colleague, counsellor and advisor and offer support to the midwife, thereby promoting a positive working relationship to improve standards of care (UKCC 1994).

It is suggested by Mayes (1995) that the majority of midwives are linked to a named supervisor of midwives but have open access to other supervisors within the locality. The literature also reveals an increasing trend towards midwives choosing their own supervisor of midwives. This is highlighted as a key issue by Stapleton, Duerden & Kirkham (1998) suggesting that, whilst this stance would facilitate a more empowering approach for midwives, the case load of the supervisor must also represent a balance of the supervisors' choice.

An important development in the supervision of midwives is that of deselection. The ENB (1996 p. 14) consider one of the responsibilities of a supervisor of midwives is: 'identifying when peer supervisors are not undertaking the role to a satisfactory standard, and taking appropriate action'.

It is further recommended by the ENB (1996) that the LSA establishes a policy for deselecting identifying the reasons and evidence for such an event. The policy for deselecting supervisors of midwives provides not only a quality assurance mechanism but also a clear move away from the historical perspective of supervision being seen as restrictive, punitive and intimidating. Indeed, Stapleton, Duerden & Kirkham (1998) further suggest that a mechanism of appeal against supervisory decisions should also be in place to enhance the process of supervision.

The role of the supervisor of midwives

The UKCC's Midwifery Committee identified that there is a lack of understanding of both the purpose of supervision of midwives and the role of the supervisor (Steene 1996). A clarification of the definition of a supervisor of midwives is contained within the Midwives rules 1998 (UKCC 1998), which will enable a greater understanding of the role and function of supervision. Spend a few minutes considering the questions contained within Activity 10.1 before continuing this chapter.

 Activity 10.1

The role of the supervisor of midwives
Consider the following questions:

• What do supervisors of midwives do?
• What makes a good supervisor of midwives?

According to the ENB (1996 p. 13), the purpose of supervision of midwives is 'to safeguard and enhance the quality of care for the child-bearing mother and her family'.

The specific duties of a supervisor of midwives are identified as:

• safeguarding the public by:
  —monitoring standards of midwifery practice
  —monitoring the integrity of the service
  —investigating critical incidents
  —reporting to the LSA serious incidents involving professional conduct
  —contributing to activities such as risk management and clinical audit
• giving professional advice, guidance and support by:
  —ensuring midwives notify their intention to practise
  —ensuring midwives have access to statutory rules, guidance and local policies
  —providing support to enable midwives to discuss their practice
  —meeting individual midwives at least once annually to help evaluate their practice
  —providing guidance on maintenance of registration
  —providing professional leadership
  (ENB 1996, 1997a).

Safeguarding the public

As previously mentioned, the supervisor's role in terms of safeguarding the public stems from the existence of the practice of untrained birth attendants (Williams & Hunt 1996). Today, midwives in Europe are educated and trained to take full responsibility for the care of child-bearing women and practice as accountable practitioners supported by legislation. Therefore, protecting the public today involves actively ensuring a safe standard of midwifery practice measured against the Midwives rules and code of practice (UKCC 1998). Winship (1996) argues that supervision is about quality, about caring and preventing poor practice through a supportive process seeking excellence in midwifery care. It most certainly is about facilitating midwives to practise competently, demonstrating confidence, in an appropriately resourced environment.

Supervision of midwives is seen as significant in supporting the changes in the provision of maternity services as highlighted in The Patient's Charter (DoH 1992a), The Named Midwife (DoH 1992b), the Second Report, Maternity Services (House of Commons 1992) and the Government's response (DoH 1992c). If supervision is as significant as the above documentation would suggest then why, questions Lewison (1996), are women not more adequately informed of the role of the supervisor of midwives? She highlights the low profile of supervision of midwives and the various documents available to women that could contain this information but rather tend to suggest it merely as a complaint mechanism, if at all. If the purpose of supervision is to protect the public then the role of supervisors of midwives needs to be better understood by women and in addition how these supervisors may be accessed.

According to Page (1995), when supervision works well it is invisible to the general public. Indeed, Beech & Robinson (1992) consider that the public are safeguarded against incompetent midwives because they can be immediately suspended from duty by their supervisor of midwives. This statement clearly highlights the lack of clarity regarding the power and authority of a supervisor of midwives. If the supervisor of midwives is also a midwifery manager then the decision to suspend a midwife from duty may be actioned from the authority of the managerial position. However, a supervisor of midwives not in this dual role would have to make a recommendation to the midwifery manager for a midwife's suspension from duty. Beech & Robinson (1992) also believe that midwives are subject to a more effective and swifter disciplinary proceedings than are doctors, dangerous practitioners being dealt with more easily. In addition, they state that women are safer in midwives' hands because midwives are subject to an 'ethically superior and more consumer oriented code of conduct than doctors' (Beech & Robinson 1992 p. 27).

If midwifery care is to be effective it has to be acceptable to the woman, outcomes being more favourable if the woman has control. As women are becoming more assertive and more actively involved in their care then there is a need for the balance of power to move from medical staff and midwives to the women themselves. If midwives feel supported and confident in practice then they are in a pivotal position to support women. If, however, the woman rejects the advice of the midwife then the supervisor involvement becomes necessary in upholding the safety of the woman and providing support for the midwife. A commonly cited example of such a scenario is when a woman insists on home care against medical advice. Lewison (1996) points out that in such cases the supervisor may not be protecting the woman but rather the GP who is unwilling to agree to women's requests for home births.

Beech (1993) also expresses concerns on behalf of AIMS of the requirement on many trusts for the midwife to inform the supervisor of midwives of planned home births. She further questions this practice arguing that women booked for hospital confinements are not visited at home by supervisors of midwives to discuss the risks and dangers of their decision (Beech 1995). This issue needs to be considered from a professional perspective rather than just a managerial one. The Midwife's code of practice (UKCC 1998 para. 12 p. 28) states that, 'it is the duty of the supervisor of midwives to ensure that agreed local policies are easily available to all practising midwives within their jurisdiction'. Furthermore, paragraph 36 refers directly to home births and may be interpreted by midwives that the supervisor should be informed of any home births and provide advice and support as necessary depending on the individual case. Therefore, the supervisor acting as a support for midwives and safeguarding the mother and baby is able to ensure appropriate arrangements are in place prior to the event. This situation also raises the issues of accountability and risk management. Consider all of these issues in relation to the Case scenario 10.1.

Case Scenario 10.1

Maria is a 32-year old woman, gravida 12 para 10. She has gestational diabetes and her obstetric history reveals a number of previous problems including a previous postpartum haemorrhage. She is well known to the community midwives as she presents late in each pregnancy and does not always attend for antenatal care. On this occasion she is requesting a home confinement; she is already 36 weeks pregnant.

Whilst recognizing the dilemmas in practice and promoting choice for childbearing women it must not be forgotten that the primary role of the supervisor of midwives is to: 'uphold the balance between safety for the mother and support for the midwife' (Mayes 1993 p. 141). In addition, Kirkham (1994) believes supervision to be beneficial for mothers, babies and midwives, and states that: 'There are two reasons why we need supervision ... so that we can practice from a secure basis in the face of vulnerability, change and uncertainty ... and to guide, support and inspire us in improving our practice' (Kirkham 1994 p. 27).

Supporting professional conduct

As it is the primary responsibility of the supervisor of midwives to ensure the safety of childbearing women it is necessary that if a midwife's competence is in question that the supervisor conducts an investigation into misconduct. Although incidences of alleged professional misconduct in midwifery are fairly uncommon (ENB 1997d), it is necessary for both the midwife and the supervisor of midwives to understand the process of dealing with such issues.

The Nurses, Midwives and Health Visitors Act 1997 (HMSO 1997) states that each LSA shall: 'report any prima facie case of misconduct on the part of a midwife which arises in its area to the Council' (section 15(2)(b)).

The LSA must be certain that there is a case to answer before it is reported to the UKCC. The key questions that must be considered are:

- Have the mother and baby been placed at risk by the midwife?
- Have the UKCC standards, i.e. the Midwives rules and code of practice, failed to be adhered to by the midwife?

The ENB (1997d p. 13) state that 'as a general rule, a case of alleged misconduct relates to a failure to maintain the standards in these documents'. Examples of situations where the mother and baby may be placed at risk are:

- drug errors
- not referring to a doctor in a case of emergency or deviation from normal
- failing to write records of care.

Case scenario 10.2 is an example of an incident investigated by a supervisor of midwives. The supervisor of midwives must undertake an investigation of the incident.

Case Scenario 10.2

A mother wrote a letter of complaint to the supervisor of midwives regarding the care she received during the birth of her son, 10 months previously. Her son had been diagnosed as having early signs of cerebral palsy. The mother implied that a midwife had failed to recognize fetal distress and she believed this to be the cause of her son's condition.

The ENB (1997d) list the principles that should govern an investigation as:

- inform the midwife
- provide an opportunity for the midwife to give her explanation of events
- recognize and clarify similarities with witnesses
- do not make a final judgement until all the evidence is available
- maintain records of all interviews
- always ask for a second person to witness the interviews e.g. another supervisor of midwives.

During the investigation the midwife should be provided with support from another supervisor of midwives. This is in preference to the same supervisor who conducts the investigation as the role will conflict with that of a supportive colleague, friend and counsellor.

After completing the investigation the supervisor of midwives determines whether there have been any extenuating circumstances that may have influenced the midwife's actions. These are taken into account when deciding on any action to be taken. The following options are then considered:

- No further action is required.
- Local action only is taken.
- The case is formally reported to the LSA.

If the case is forwarded to the LSA then it becomes the responsibility of the LSA to determine whether it is reported to the UKCC. It is worth noting that a case of alleged misconduct can be reported to the UKCC by the woman, her partner, or one of her relatives (e.g. a parent).

Further details of the process on managing professional conduct can be found in ENB (1997d) Preparation of supervisors of midwives, module 4.

Giving professional advice, guidance and support

The supervisor of midwives must ensure that midwives in her area of practice notify their intention to practise on an annual basis (UKCC 1998 p. 27). This enables the supervisor to verify that the statutory requirements for practice have been fulfilled. These forms are forwarded to the LSA and then to the UKCC for correlation with the register. The focus for giving professional support will be discussed in relation to encouraging accountability in practice and individual professional development, which is needed to ensure quality midwifery care. (See Ch. 6 for a comprehensive discussion on acountability in practice.)

To achieve quality of midwifery care, midwives and supervisors of midwives need to work in partnership. The code of practice (UKCC 1998) puts more emphasis on partnership with midwives: 'Your supervisor of midwives should give you support as a colleague, counsellor and advisor. This should be developed in order to promote a positive working relationship which is conducive to maintaining and improving standards of practice and care' (UKCC 1998 para. 34).

For safe care to be ensured for women, midwives must, according to Caldwell (1996), have professional support from their supervisor of midwives which includes enabling midwives to reflect on their practice and identify professional development needs. This support needs to have a commitment from both parties and, although a degree of formality is required, openness and availability are vital components.

The ENB endorse the view that supervision is about supporting midwives in maintaining professional competence and enabling development (ENB 1992, 1997c). However, midwives' views on supervision vary widely, from it being seen as a 'valuable asset' (Williams, unpublished work, 1994) to causing considerable tension for the independent midwife (Demilew 1996).

One issue raised in the literature by midwives is that some supervisors do not share the same philosophy of care. This, according to Seaman (1995), can have damaging consequences in terms of balancing the monitoring and supporting aspects of supervision. Caldwell (1996) describes a programme called 'care for the carers' which was devised to complement the more formal stance of supervision. The philosophy underpinning the scheme acknowledges the problems midwives experience in their professional and personal lives whilst striving to provide the level of care expected of them. If supervision alone cannot ensure confidentiality, an individually focused approach to professional development and a non-threatening environment for discussion then it must be considered how the midwife will receive the desired support in practice.

There is a minority view emerging from within the profession that questions whether supervision of midwives is still relevant on the premise that a mature profession has no need for this control. The paradox is that nurses and health visitors are using midwifery supervision as a model and are examining ways in which a similar system might be implemented (Kargar 1993). For example, the NHS Management Executive (DoH 1993a p. 15) defines clinical supervision as:

A term used to describe a formal process of professional support and learning which enables individual practitioners to develop knowledge and competence, assume responsibility for their own practice and enhance consumer protection and the safety of care in complex clinical situations. It is central to the process of learning and to the expansion of the scope of practice and should be seen as a means of encouraging self assessment and analytical and reflective skills.

From this definition there are a number of comparable features between clinical supervision and statutory supervision of midwives. Refer to Activity 10.2 and try to identify both the

Activity 10.2

Clinical supervision and supervision of midwives

Consider the definition of clinical supervision (DoH l993a) and compare this to that defined by the ENB (1996 p. 3), which states:

The supervision of midwives and midwifery practice is a statutory responsibility and provides a mechanism for support and guidance to every midwife practising in the United Kingdom. The aim of supervision is to ensure competent practice so that the needs of mothers and their families can be met through appropriate midwifery care. When executed effectively supervision develops professional leadership, which creates a practice environment to support innovation and where midwives develop new roles to practise autonomously and contribute to cost effective ways of achieving woman-centred care.

Identify the similarities and the differences.

comparable features and those which clearly differentiate the practices.

It is worth noting that Faugier & Butterworth (1993) and Kohner (1994) have reported the value of clinical supervision in nursing, and models of supervision in the different professions are being explored. Comparisons can also be made with supervision in the field of counselling and social work. Stewart (1992) recognizes that the components of supervision are those of support and encouragement, a tutoring role which enables the integration of theoretical knowledge and practice, an ongoing assessment in the maintenance of standards and the opportunity to transmit professional values and ethics. These components within supervision may similarly be translated into supervision of midwives highlighting the various dimensions of the role, which include the expert practitioner, the researcher, the educationalist, the manager and the supervisor (ENB 1997a p. 12). A full discussion of clinical supervision is not within the scope of this chapter but is well worth further reading.

The studies conducted with midwives overall firmly suggest that supervision should be maintained and improved in the interests of midwives and midwifery as well as of childbearing women (Demilew 1996, Duerden 1996, Williams, unpublished work, 1994). It is further argued by Mayes (1993) that supervision has developed over the past decade from a restrictive and punitive control towards a positive, enabling process capable of being audited. The underpinning standard has been to improve the quality of midwifery care through proactive supervision. Supervisors of midwives need to work proactively with midwives and ensure they are clear about the statutory requirements which govern midwifery practice. The midwife herself must recognize that it is her own responsibility to ensure she has the required UKCC documentation and is familiar with the contents. Opportunities must be created to promote a greater awareness of the statutory legislation and the supervisor of midwives is ideally placed to assist in this process. The annual supervisory review is one such opportunity.

The annual review

This meeting between the midwife and her supervisor of midwives provides the forum for the midwife to reflect on her practice and identify professional development needs. The annual review is similar to the management tool of appraisal but it should not be confused with the employment review. It is not surprising that midwives are confused when both reviews are conducted simultaneously by the manager/ supervisor of midwives. Now consider Case scenario 10.3

Case Scenario 10.3

Cathryn has been a practising midwife for 10 years. For the past 6 years she has practised in the community setting providing antenatal and postnatal care. Mary has been appointed as manager/supervisor of midwives to the community where Cathryn practices. At a recent meeting between Mary and Cathryn it is apparent that all women in Cathryn's case load are referred to the local consultant unit for intrapartum care. Cathryn does not offer a choice of place of confinement for the women and states she is unwilling to participate in intrapartum care.

Consider how Mary might respond to this situation:

- In her role as manager of the area,
- in her role as supervisor of midwives

The manager has a responsibility to ensure that the organization provides a framework that allows individual development of staff thereby contributing to the service offered. The supervisor of midwives is responsible for enabling midwives to evaluate their practice, identify areas for development and agree the means in which this can be achieved. The focus quite clearly is on the midwife's clinical competence (ENB 1997c). The standards monitored in the case of supervision relate to the Midwives rules and code of practice (UKCC 1998) whereas the manager relates to the midwife's job description and organizational goals. In the authors' experience it is suggested that both reviews are successful when conducted separately. The management tool of appraisal and the annual supervisory review both have links to quality assurance processes as an individual's performance has to be directly linked to the quality of care provided to women and their families. The important role for supervisors is to assist and support the midwife in her self-reflection without making judgements. It is clear in relation to professional development that there is an overlap of roles of the manager and supervisor of midwives. The supervisor in enabling midwives to acquire new skills and knowledge to meet the statutory requirements must also acknowledge the changing requirements of a dynamic, progressive service.

The supervisor of midwives is required to maintain records of supervisory activities. It is not clear what form these records take as it is not defined by the ENB but may be locally determined by the LSA. The supervisory review record should be kept by both the midwife and the supervisor of midwives, an example of which is offered in the 'Preparation of supervisors of midwives' module 3 (ENB 1997c).

Providing guidance on maintenance of registration

The supervisor of midwives has a responsibility to promote a climate which encourages questioning and innovative approaches to midwifery care, and to identify the development needs of midwives (ENB 1994 p. 8). It is also stated that she should be the: 'focal point for the discussion of information to midwives ... matters of professional practice ... 'assist midwives to identify their own educational and training needs and advise the approved midwife teacher of these requirements' (ENB 1994 p. 9).

The supervisor therefore has an important role to play in facilitating and supporting midwives to develop their practice. The ENB (1997c) consider that the supervisor of midwives can enable midwives in developing their practice by motivating, enabling reflection and counselling. Kirkham (1994) emphasizes the need for the supervisor to be skilled in counselling: 'We must be able to discuss those aspects of our practice which we want to improve, without feeling that our present practice will be judged as "substandard"' (Kirkham 1994 p. 27).

The annual review meeting is an ideal opportunity for the professional development needs of midwives and allowing refresher course requirements (UKCC 1998) and post-registration education and practice requirements to be discussed. Furthermore, the compilation of a professional portfolio will, according to Price (1994), help midwives to identify their career aspirations and reflect on their practice. Supervisors in this instance can be described as facilitators of growth (ENB 1997c).

THE ROLE OF THE MIDWIFERY MANAGER

The concepts of management and supervision of midwives are often considered together partly because the roles have been undertaken by one person. To combine the role of the midwifery manager with that of supervisor of midwives may either enhance or impinge on the effectiveness of supervision of midwives.

A definition of management

Although there is no generally agreed definition of management in the literature management can be described as: 'the art of getting work done through people' (Vaughan & Pillmore 1989). Management is therefore not an activity that exists in isolation but is a variety of activities carried out by individuals within an organization whose role is that of manager.

A manager may be considered to be someone in the organization who has a position of authority with formal responsibility for the work carried out by other workers. The activities of a manager are generally grouped together in the literature and are described under the auspices of a process of management (Gillies 1982, Marquis & Huston 1987). The activities related to this process are:

- planning
- organizing
- directing
- controlling.

It is important that the process of management is understood as its components impact on decision making in the organization. The term 'process' implies a series of movement or actions which, rather than having a start and end point, needs to be viewed as a cyclical structure which never ends. This can be compared to the nursing and midwifery process and the decision-making process. The process is generally considered to start at the planning stage, which in management spheres includes assessment, and ends at the controlling or evaluation stage. However, because the process is viewed as a cycle, many different stages may be occurring at the same time. For example, the midwifery manager may be determining how her budget is to be managed during the year; this involves the planning stage; she may also be meeting with staff to reorganize the teams to meet Changing Childbirth (DoH 1993b) indicators of success, operating in the organizing stage; for the directing stage the manager may be liaising with the multidisciplinary team in devising protocols to guide practitioners; finally in controlling midwives the manager may be conducting individual performance appraisals. Each of these aspects has an influence on decision making as the manager begins with her plan, implements it and then evaluates the outcomes.

It is argued by Cole (1990) that managers utilizing this process of management are operating from a leader-centred approach. This approach to managing staff does not take account of the additional key roles of resource allocator, coordinator, negotiator and conflict handler as described by Mintzberg (1991).

Midwifery managers must have well-developed personal ethics which they consistently enact and the ability to inspire organizational colleagues to realize the goals of the organization. Within the decision-making process, decisions made at one level of the hierarchy may have profound implications for those who are expected to implement such decisions. This is a situation which Drucker (1966 p. 52) argues that 'management without values, commitment, and convictions can only do harm'. Decision making by managers is set in a more client-centred and consumer-oriented service where choice is made according to standards set and acknowledgement of the implications of the choices made. The rules or ethics of behaviour in the work environment require, therefore, a constant re-evaluation in the light of continually changing practice. To solve really difficult ethical dilemmas managers must be ready to act on both their life values and their professional values. A full discussion of ethical decision making can be found in Ch. 5.

The main objective for the midwifery manager is to 'achieve a high quality service, which meets contractual obligations' (Brears 1995 p. 45). Therefore, in attaining this objective managers need to be able to determine the goals to ensure organizational outcomes are achieved. The supervisor of midwives, on the other hand, ensures the statutory requirements for practice are maintained by monitoring the professional standards. The individual undertaking the dual role of midwifery manager and supervisor of midwives should, if she is to be effective, recognize and endeavour to overcome any constraints.

Professional leadership

Managers are not necessarily leaders but, according to the ENB (1997a), a responsibility of a supervisor of midwives is to provide professional leadership. Magill-Cuerden (1992) argues that supervisors need to be leaders who are politically aware at all levels of management in the NHS. If the head of midwifery services in each unit is not a supervisor how will midwives be represented at unit or district level?

The management structures in the NHS have, over the years, been changed from hierarchies to a more flattened organizational structure. As a result a manager's sphere of management has expanded and their responsibilities in terms of staff numbers has increased. This has inevitably led to an increase in the ratio of midwives: supervisors of midwives, which meant that, supervisors did not 'know' the midwives they managed.

The ratio of midwives: supervisors of midwives has been an issue addressed by the ENB (1992) to offset this position. The recommended standard for effective supervision (UKCC 1998 para. 33) is no more than 40 midwives: 1 supervisor. According to Mayes (1996) there were approximately 930 supervisors of midwives practising in England which facilitated the achievement of a ratio of approximately 30 : 1, which more than met the requirements of the standard specified by the UKCC (1998). The midwives: supervisors of midwives ratio continues to reduce, as demonstrated in Table 10.1, and is reported by the UKCC (1997) as being 21 : 1. Therefore, as previously highlighted, a midwife today may not now necessarily be supervised by her line manager but by a supervisor from a clinical, educational or other background (ENB 1997b).

Characteristics of leaders

The literature reveals many studies of leadership traits and, although it is not clear which traits are essential to acquire or maintain leadership, examples of such values are:

- adaptable
- brave
- clever
- decisive
- enthusiastic
- friendly
- loyal
- organized
- reliable
- stable
- versatile
- well informed.

Table 10.1 An analysis of the number of midwives per supervisor shown in England and the UK

Year	England	UK
1988	46	51
1990	39	44
1992	37	41
1994	33	36
1996	32	34
1998	21	22

Adapted from statistical analysis of the UKCC's professional register 1 April 1997 to 31 March 1998, UKCC July 1998.

Leadership is often thought of as being undertaken by 'special' individuals who may be described as 'born leaders' when they are seen to be making useful contributions to a group activities (Abraham & Shanley 1992). This implies that leadership is related to personality but the literature fails to prove this and refers rather to leadership behaviours and situations that enable leadership behaviour to emerge. However, Crainer (1988) argues that effective leaders do demonstrate six characteristics:

• mastery
• assertiveness skills
• a belief in self
• goal orientation
• a need for recognition
• an acceptance of the need for
  self-development.

If supervisors of midwives are to fulfil their role as professional leaders then these characteristics, when considered in relation to the criteria for selection of supervisors of midwives, may provide a useful starting point for appointment to the role.

It must be considered that leadership theories tend to relate to either traits, which are based on personal characteristics of the leader, or on leadership styles, based on leader behaviours including contingency or adaptive leader behaviours in differing situations (Cole 1990). The focus on leadership functions enables common leadership skills to emerge.

Leaders need to be able to understand group functioning, be able to communicate with group members and demonstrate specific knowledge and expertise relevant to the group's activities. This will enable leaders to influence commitment, whereas a manager's position would rather take care of positional responsibilities and exercise authority. An important concept is that a person can be a manager without being a leader or be a leader without managing.

Hersey & Blanchard (1982) believe there is an essential difference between management and leadership. They define leadership as 'the process of influencing the activities of an individual or a group in efforts towards goal achievement in a given situation' (p. 83). These goals may not be organizationally focused. In contrast, a manager may further be described as someone who brings things about, who accomplishes, who has responsibility, who conducts (Cross 1996). Management requires a particular style of leadership where organizational goals must be achieved—the difference being the organization, the commonality between the two roles being the achievement of goals.

A leader, alternatively, is one who influences and guides direction, opinion and course of action to follow. Leaders create rather than master routines. Leadership is needed to assist organizations to develop visions, then to mobilize the workers towards achieving the vision. Management and leadership are therefore, complementary; without management leadership could become overwhelming and volatile, but without leadership management can be bureaucratic and less creative.

The strategy for nursing (DoH 1989), formulated to assist practitioners to meet the changes in healthcare, considered leadership and management as one of five main issues for action. It advocated that the way to achieve change in the NHS was to develop clinical and professional leadership, a stance reiterated in A vision for the future (DoH 1993). The latest consultation document on A strategy for nursing, midwifery and health visiting (DoH 1998) highlights the need to re-examine A vision for the future to determine which elements are of continuing relevance. Continuing changes in practice create opportunities for midwives to demonstrate clinical skills and managerial and leadership capabilities, which will enable the profession to deliver high quality care. Furthermore, leaders in midwifery will have the opportunity to influence developments as well as ensure effective care continues to be provided. The development of clinical and professional leadership therefore, must remain one of the essential elements in any government strategy if it is to achieve a quality health service.

Now that supervisors of midwives are from varied backgrounds and not just managerial positions a more dynamic professional leadership may impact on the delivery of midwifery care. The preparation for the role and ongoing education of supervisors of midwives must also be geared to the development of leadership skills rather than just a knowledge of the role itself, a stance supported by Mayes (1996) and reiterated by Stapleton, Duerden & Kirkham (1998).

Styles of management

It may be assumed that styles of management are determined by the personality of the manager. Some common approaches to management are known as 'bottom up' and 'top down', which may be considered to relate to both strategies for change (Bennis et al 1976) and leadership styles (Cole 1990). In addition, Scammell (1990 p. 3) adds 'within certain boundaries' and 'according to outcomes of managers work'. The bottom-up approach to management relates to the individual manager's style which may be influenced by other managers within the organization and the actual role functions of the manager. The top-down approach considers the influences from society in general as well as local and national policies. Role boundaries need to be taken into account as these will determine the sphere of authority of the manager, their accountability and responsibility. Finally, the manager's ability to motivate and control the workforce will ultimately relate to the achieved management outcomes.

Johnston (1990) identifies four ways in which influence may be exerted:

- by offering rewards or applying pressures
- by building cooperation and trust
- by appealing to a common vision
- by logical argument.

In relation to the supervisor of midwives this role does not provide the power or authority to suspend a midwife from practice but rather a recommendation to management to suspend the midwife from duty and then refer the case to the LSA. The manager, on the other hand, does have the authority to suspend from duty.

In the scenario of a midwife requiring supervised practice or updating, the supervisor of midwives cannot force a midwife to follow this course of action. She would need to negotiate with the midwife and encourage her to recognize her own personal and professional developmental needs. If an agreement cannot be reached then the case would need referral to the LSA. However, the midwifery manager has the power and authority to compel midwives to follow a course of action, such as updating or supervised practice, as their employment terms would make this a requirement.

Box 10.1 demonstrates the difference between the role of supervisor of midwives and that of the midwifery manager.

Box 10.1	**A differentiation of the role of supervisor of midwives and that of the midwifery manager**

Supervisor of Midwives	*Midwifery Manager*
Appointed by the LSA Accountable to the LSA and the UKCC	Trust employee Accountable to the trust
Must fulfil the statutory duties and responsibilities of the supervisor of midwives	Must fulfil the job description of employment in terms of duties and responsibilities
Undertakes a statutory course of preparation for the role prior to appointment to the role of supervisor of midwives	May or may not have been provided with management training
Ensures agreed policies are available to all practising midwives within their supervisory jurisdiction	Must be conversant with trust policies
Ensures midwives have access to statutory rules and professional codes of practice/guidance documents.	Issues protocols/ procedures/guidelines for employment
Receives notification of intention to practise forms from midwives	Checks UKCC registration is current to on appointment to post and then 3 yearly
Non-budget holder	Manages a budget
Carries out supervisory reviews with midwives annually	Undertakes staff appraisal and individual performance reviews
Investigates incidents in practice to determine professional misconduct and reports to the LSA if appropriate	Implements disciplinary policy as required

Box 10.1 (*Continued*)

Recommends suspension from practice to LSA	May suspend a midwife from duty
Protects and maintains professional standards consistent with the Midwives rules and codes	Sets organizational goals and standards and ensures they are met
Facilitates development of competency in new skills to meet statutory professional practice	Facilitates development of competency in new skills to meet organizational developments and changes

Management of change

If managers and supervisors of midwives are to facilitate change within the maternity services then knowledge of the process of change is imperative. The literature highlights the pressures for change, taking into account internal and external forces, the most commonly cited influence being the Changing Childbirth report (DoH 1993b). This report recommends a service that provides women-centred care facilitating choice, continuity and control. It firmly places midwives as the lead professional working in partnership with women, which enables midwives to practise their full range of skills. This provides midwives with the opportunity to develop their role and meet the needs of childbearing women. If midwives are truly to be given this opportunity then the role of management and the supervisor of midwives must be considered.

It is not uncommon for change to be met by resistance, a situation which is highlighted in the literature (Cross 1996, Vaughan & Pillmore 1989). If Changing Childbirth is offering midwives a great opportunity to strengthen their role then the issues in relation to resistance must be considered if partnership with women is to be achieved. It is understandable that change brings with it uncertainty and a fear of the unknown but it also brings possibilities for innovation and achievement of a shared vision for the future of the midwifery profession. Rowan & Steele (1995) argue that no one really wants to change as the status quo offers a predictable and

safe situation. Some of the reasons they cite for the resistance to change are:

- lack of trust or confidence in managers or change agents
- a dislike of how the change is being implemented
- not feeling involved or lack control in the proposed change
- a previous bad experience of change.

Each of these issues has implications for both the manager and the supervisor of midwives. If midwives do not receive the support and guidance they require from their manager then they are free to consult a supervisor of midwives. However, midwives must have a clear understanding of supervision and how this process can support practice.

If change is to be successful then the process of change needs to be determined. Change processes have been described for example by Lewin (1951) and Wright (1989). Lewin identifies change as a series of three stages:

1. *Unfreezing*—this is where the change agent unfreezes the forces which maintain the status quo and people become dissatisfied and aware of the need to change
2. *Changing or moving*—the change agent assesses, plans and implements the change strategy
3. *Refreezing*—the new change is integrated into the system creating a status quo.

Alternatively, Wright (1989) likens the change process to a cycle similar to the nursing or midwifery process, the stages being:

- assessment
- planning
- implementation
- evaluation.

First, the situation is assessed for the need to change. This may be determined by utilizing a management tool such as a SWOT analysis or a force field analysis (Broome 1990). The latter will enable the identification of the resisting forces, which need to be overcome, as well as the forces driving for the change. The next step is careful planning, which is crucial for the change to be a success. This stage involves identifying issues such as who will be the change agent, the strategy for change, midwives' training needs, formulation of protocols, etc. The implementation stage requires effective communication and support for midwives, recognizing stress and dealing with any conflict. The final stage involves evaluation of the change in terms of how successful has it been, which will lead to the whole cycle starting again enabling further change and developments.

Throughout the change process the manager or supervisor of midwives must display effective leadership skills ranging from directive leadership to non-directive counselling. Operating in each of these opposing actions the leader prescribes what is best for midwives in one situation but then enables reflection with midwives without offering judgement in another. Influencing change also requires enthusiasm and commitment, which can enable midwives to release creativity and thereby move the organization to the desired state. Facilitating change in this way requires a person who can positively help midwives to help themselves and then fade into the background (Cole 1990, Mayes 1995). The supervisor of midwives is ideally placed to do exactly that.

Summary

It is recognized that there is some lack of clarity and understanding regarding the role of the supervisor of midwives and the purpose of supervision of midwives. By examining the role of the supervisor of midwives and the role of the manager separately a greater understanding of each should be achieved. The areas of potential tension have been highlighted and exploration enabled through the case scenarios posed. The supervision of midwives needs to be reflected upon continuously, particularly in times of change to ensure it adapts to meet the needs of the midwife and the profession. It is envisaged that supervision of midwives will continue to strengthen the midwifery profession and promote excellence in practice.

APPENDIX: MINISTRY OF HEALTH LETTER

I am directed by the Minister of Health to enclose for the information of the Council copies of the Regulations which he has made under Section 9(2) of the Midwives Act 1936, prescribing the qualifications of persons appointed by Local Supervising Authorities under section 8 of the Midwives Act 1902, to exercise supervision over midwives practising in their areas. The Regulations, which have been made after consultation with the Central Midwives Board and the Association of Local Authorities concerned, will come into operation on the 1st June next.

It will be observed that the Regulations apply to persons appointed as Supervisors of Midwives on or after that date, but in view of the importance of entrusting this work to persons with the necessary qualifications and experience, the Minister suggests that each Authority should review their arrangements for the supervision of midwives and should take the earliest opportunity for effecting any changes which may be desirable having regard to the qualifications prescribed by the Regulations. This is of particular importance at the present time when the new service of salaried midwives under the Act of 1936 is about to be established throughout the country.

The Departmental Committee on midwives, which reported in 1929, pointed out that the inspection of midwives by a person without experience of practical midwifery has a bad psychological effect upon the midwife and reacts unfavourably on her methods of practice, as she is deprived of the opportunity for guidance on professional matters affecting the well-being of her patients which she would receive from a properly qualified inspector. In particular, the Committee strongly deprecated the employment as inspectors of midwives of health visitors with little or no practical experience of midwifery. The Minister endorses these views and it will be seen that the Regulations require the persons appointed in future to supervise midwives shall have an adequate experience in the practice of midwifery.

The Departmental Committee also drew attention to the fact that an inspector of midwives should be regarded as a counsellor and friend of the midwives, rather than a relentless critic and should be one who is ready to instruct the midwives in the various points of difficulty which arise from time to time in connection with their work and make them feel that there is always someone to whom they can look for sympathetic understanding of the laborious nature of their profession. The Minister feels that it is scarcely necessary for him to emphasize the importance of appointing persons who do not only possess the necessary professional qualifications, but who also have the essential qualities of sympathy and tact, and he thinks it is desirable that the title of 'Inspector of Midwives' should be superseded by that of 'Supervisor of Midwives' which is used in the Regulations.

The Regulations prescribe qualifications for a Medical Supervisor, and a non-Medical Supervisor, respectively, and it is within the discretion of each Authority to appoint either one or the other, or both. But in large areas it appears to the Minister that the most desirable arrangement would generally be to appoint a Medical Supervisor, acting under direction of the Medical Officer of Health, to exercise general supervision over the midwives practising in the area, and non-Medical Supervisors to work under the instructions of the Medical Supervisor and perform routine duties of supervision.

The Minister appreciates that at the outset it may be difficult in some cases to secure Medical Supervisors who possess all the qualifications prescribed in Article 3 of the Regulations, and if necessary he will be prepared to consider the question of using dispensing power which is contained in Article 5. He thinks it desirable, however, to point out that the words 'some branch of obstetric work' in Article 3 have a wide range, and include the conduct of antenatal clinics, the duties of administrative officers in a maternity department, the investigation or treatment of puerperal fever, obstetric research, etc.

In conclusion, the Minister wished to emphasize the fact that the duties of a Supervisor of Midwives extend to all midwives practising in the area of the Authority and that a distinction should be drawn between an officer holding this post and one who is appointed as a Superintendent or Senior Midwife to control the work of the salaried midwives appointed by the Authority. The Minister is advised that it is not desirable for a Supervisor of Midwives to be engaged in the actual practice of midwifery.

A copy of this circular has been sent to the Medical Officer of Health. I am, Sir, Your obedient Servant, Assistant Secretary.

REFERENCES

Abraham C, Shanley E 1992 Social psychology for nurses. Edward Arnold, London

Association of Supervisors of Midwives 1992 Supervision the whys and where-forces ASM, Great Yarmouth

Beech B L, Robinson J, 1992 Hard labour. Health Service Journal 102(5286):26–27

Beech B L 1993 Supervision of midwives. AIMS Journal 5(2):1–3

Beech B L 1995 The consumer view. In: ARM (ed) Super-Vision Consensus conference proceedings. Books for Midwives, Hale, pp 51–60

Belbin R M 1981 Management teams—why they succeed or fail. Butterworth Heinemann, London

Bennis G W, Benne K D, Chin R, Corey K E 1976 The planning of change. Holt, Rinehart & Winston, London

Brears D 1995 Towards a model of midwifery management. In: ARM (ed) Super-vision. Consensus conference proceedings. Books for Midwives, Hale, pp 45–50

Broome A 1990 Managing change. Macmillan, London.

Caldwell K 1996 Care for the carers in Exeter. In: Kirkham M (ed) Supervision of Midwives. Books for Midwives, Hale, ch 6, p 84

Cole G A 1990 Management: theory and practice. DP publications, London

Crainer S 1988 Making boss-power positive. The Sunday Times. 9th October

Cross R E 1996 Midwives and management. A handbook. Books for Midwives, Hale

Davis K C 1994 Is statutory supervision central to our professional identity? British Journal of Midwifery 2(7):304–305

Demilew J 1996 Independent midwives' views of supervision. In: Kirkham M (ed) Supervision of midwives. Books for Midwives, Hale, pp 183–201

DoH (Department of Health) 1989 A strategy for nursing: report of the Steering Committee. HMSO, London

DoH (Department Health) 1992a The patient's charter. HMSO, London

DoH (Department of Health) 1992b The named midwife. HMSO, London

DoH (Department of Health) 1992c Maternity services: Government response to the second paper from the Health Committee, session 1991–1992. HMSO, London

DoH (Department of Health) 1993a A vision for the future. The nursing, midwifery and health visiting contribution to health care. DoH, London

DoH (Department of Health) 1993b Changing childbirth: the report of the Expert Maternity Group. HMSO, London

DoH (Department of Health) 1998 A consultation on strategy for nursing, midwifery and health visiting. DoH, London

Donnison J 1988 Midwives and medical men: a history of the struggle for the control of childbirth, 2nd edn. Historical Publications, London

Drucker P 1966 The practice of management. Heinemann, London

Duerden J 1994 Audit of supervision of midwives in the North West Regional Health Authority. British Journal of Midwifery 4(1):26–28

Duerden, J 1996 Supervision of midwives is alive and well in the northwest. British Journal of Midwifery. 4(1):26–28

ENB (English National Board) for Nursing, Midwifery and Health Visiting 1992 Preparation of supervisors of midwives. Modules 1–4. ENB, London

ENB (English National Board) for Nursing, Midwifery and Health Visiting 1994 Supervision midwives. The English National Boards advice and guidance to local supervising authorities and supervisors of midwives. ENB, London

ENB (English National Board) for Nursing, Midwifery and Health Visiting 1996 Supervision of midwives—the English National Board's advice and guidance to local supervising authorities and supervisors of midwives. ENB, London

ENB (English National Board) for Nursing, Midwifery and Health Visiting 1997a Preparation of supervisors of midwives—supervision and you: what is your role? Module 1. ENB, London

ENB (English National Board) for Nursing, Midwifery and Health Visiting 1997b Preparation of supervisors of midwives—your statutory role and organisational models for supervision. Module 2. ENB, London

ENB (English National Board) for Nursing, Midwifery and Health Visiting 1997c Preparation of supervisors of midwives—supporting good midwifery practice and professional development. Module 3. ENB, London

ENB (English National Board) for Nursing, Midwifery and Health Visiting 1997d Preparation of supervisors of midwives—managing professional conduct. Module 4. ENB, London

ENB (English National Board) for Nursing, Midwifery and Health Visiting 1998 Report of the LSA function in England. DCL/09/GM. April. ENB, London

Faugier J, Butterworth 1993 Clinical supervision. A position paper. School of Nursing Studies, University of Manchester, Manchester

Gillies D A 1982 Nursing management—a systems approach. W.B. Saunders, Philadelphia

Henderson C 1997 Changing childbirth and the west midlands 1995–6. Report of changing childbirth RCM/DoH scholar. RCM, London

Hersey P, Blanchard K 1982 Organizational behaviour: utilizing human resources. Prentice-Hall, New Jersey

HMSO 1902 Midwives Act. HMSO, London

HMSO 1936 Midwives Act. HMSO, London

HMSO 1974 National Health (Reorganization) Act. HMSO, London

HMSO 1979 Nurses, Midwives and Health Visitors Act. HMSO, London

HMSO 1992 Nurses, Midwives and Health Visitors Act. HMSO, London

HMSO 1995 Health Authorities Act. HMSO, London

HMSO 1997 Nurses, Midwives and Health Visitors Act. HMSO, London

House of Commons Health Committee 1992 Second report, maternity services. HMSO, London

Isherwood K 1988 Friend or watchdog? Nursing Times 84(24):65

Johnston R 1990 Leadership. In: Marson S, Hartlebury M, Johnston R, Scammell B (eds) Managing people. Macmillan, London, pp 20–28

Johnson R 1996 Enabling midwives to practice better. In: Kirkham M (ed) Supervision of midwives. Books for Midwives, Hale, ch 7, p 90

Kakabadse A, Ludlow R, Vinnicombe S 1988 Working in organisations. Penguin, Harmondsworth

Kargar I 1993 Whither supervision? Nursing Times 89(40):22

Kirkham M 1994 First draft proposal for the future of midwifery supervision. Midwifery Matters 60(Spring): 26–27

Kohner N 1994 Clinical supervision in practice. Kings Fund Centre, London

Lansdell M 1989 Friend and counsellor. Nursing Times 85(28):76

Lewin K 1951 Field theory in social science. Harper & Row, New Yory

Lewison H 1996 Supervision as a public service. In: Kirkham M (ed) Supervision of midwives. Books for Midwives, Hale, ch 5, p 72

Magill-Cuerden J 1992 Are supervisors of midwives necessary? Modern Midwife March/April:4–5

Magill-Cuerden J 1994 The silent haemorrhage. Modern Midwife 4(2):4–5

Marquis B, Huston C 1987 Management decision making for nurses. Lippincott, Philadelphia

Mayes G 1993 Quality through supervision. British Journal of Midwifery 1(3):138–141

Mayes G 1995 Supervisors of midwives. How can we facilitate change. In: ENB The challenge of Changing childbirth. Midwifery educational resource pack. Section 5(5.4)

Mayes G 1996 The changing face of supervision of midwives. British Journal of Midwifery 4(1):23–25

Mayes G 1997 Supervisors of midwives. How can we facilitate change. In: ENB preparation of supervisors of midwives. ENB, London, Module 3

Mintzberg H 1991 The effective organisation, forces and forms. Sloan Management Review Winter:54–67

NHS Executive 1997 (add ref)

Page L 1995 Effective group practice in midwifery. Blackwell, Oxford

Price A 1994 Midwifery portfolios: supporting the midwife. Modern Midwife 4(11):23–26

Rowan M, Steele R 1995 Effective change through vision, attitude, reflection and innovation. In: ENB the challenge of Changing childbirth. Midwifery educational resource pack. ENB, London, 5, 5.1

RCM (Royal College of Midwives) 1991 Report of the Royal College of Midwives commission or legislation relating to midwives. RCM, London

RCM (Royal College of Midwives) 1996 Supervision of midwives the strength of the midwifery profession. Position Paper 6. RCM, London

Sauter S 1997 Supervision from a LSA office's perspective. British Journal of Midwifery 5(11):697–699

Scammell B 1990 The science and function of management. In: Marson S, Hartlebury M, Johnston R, Scammell B (eds) Managing people. Macmillan, London, ch 1, p 1

Seaman B 1995 Where supervision goes wrong. In: ARM super-vision: consensus conference proceedings. Books for Midwives, Hale pp 75–82

Stapleton H, Duerden J, Kirkham M 1998 Evaluation of the impact of the supervision of midwives on professional practice and the quality of midwifery care. ENB, London

Steene J 1996 UKCC strengthens statutory supervision of midwives. British Journal of Midwifery 4(1):32–33

Stewart W 1992 An A–Z of counselling theory and practice. Chapman Hall, London

Thomas M, Mayes G 1996 The ENB perspective: preparation of supervisors of midwives for their role. In: Kirkham M (ed) Supervision of midwives. Books for Midwives, Hale, ch 4, p 58

UKCC 1997 Statistical analysis of the UKCC's professional register 1 April 1996 to 31 March 1997. UKCC, London

UKCC 1998 Midwives rules and code of practice. UKCC, London

Vaughan B, Pillmore M 1989 Managing nursing work. Scutari Press, London

Williams E, Hunt S 1996 Supervision in midwifery practice: the debate and some evidence. British Journal of Midwifery 4(1):28–31

Winship J 1996 The UKCC perspective: the statutory basis for the supervision of midwives today. In: Kirkham M (ed) Supervision of midwives. Books for Midwives, Hale, ch 3, p 38

Wright S G 1989 Changing nursing practice. Edward Arnold, London

11 Delivering quality in midwifery practice and education

E Rosemary Buckley   Nicola J Dunn

With the emergence of clinical governance, it is more important than ever that midwives not only give effective, evidence-based quality care, but that they are able to demonstrate they are doing so. This chapter aims to show how quality in clinical practice is implemented, based on the quality cycle model through standards, audit and implementation of change and demonstrate the importance of 'quality assured' midwifery education both before and after qualification.

INTRODUCTION: A HISTORICAL OVERVIEW OF QUALITY IN MIDWIFERY

Midwives have been in existence almost as long as humanity itself. For centuries midwives have supported and helped mothers in childbirth and there is evidence that, even as far back as the time of Moses around 2000BC, midwives sought to give quality care. In one instance, even though Pharaoh had decreed that all baby boys should be killed at birth, the Hebrew midwives refused to do so, risking their lives for what they felt was a spiritual and ethical issue (Holy Bible 1982).

In the United Kingdom, midwifery was practised for centuries by lay women. In 1616 a group of midwives mounted a campaign for a system of instruction and regulation, asking the King for a charter. Their petition was opposed by the physicians and their campaign was unsuccessful (Baly 1986 p. 65).

Florence Nightingale addressed the issue over two centuries later, endeavouring to get recognition for midwives as a profession. Her concern was the high maternal mortality rates at that time and the lack of availability of trained midwives, and she used audit results to make her point:

But with all their defects, midwifery statistics point to one truth; namely that there is a large amount of preventable mortality in midwifery practice, and that, as a general rule, the mortality is far, far greater in lying-in hospitals than among the lying-in at home ... One feels disposed to ask whether it can be true that, in the hands of educated accoucheur, the inevitable fate of women undergoing, not a diseased but an entirely natural condition, at home, is that 1 out of every 128 must die? (Nightingale 1871)

It was not until 10 years later, in 1881, that the Midwives Institute (now the Royal College of Midwives) was established to unite midwives and provide pressure for a Midwives Act. The aim of the organization was: 'to encourage the training of midwives so as to lead to a better standard of care for mothers and babies' (Cowell & Wainwright 1981).

Midwifery was formally recognized as a profession 21 years later. The Midwives Act of 1902 (HMSO 1902) legalized and restricted the practice of midwifery to those who had been educated, its purpose 'to secure the better training of midwives and to regulate their practice' (Baly 1986 p. 80).

Hence, the newly born midwifery profession was built on the aim of upholding standards of care for mothers and babies. Throughout the century since the Midwives Act of 1902, midwives have strived to give good quality care to mothers and babies. However, in common with the other health disciplines relatively little had been done to formally audit care.

It was only when the Government produced its white paper 'Working for Patients' (DoH 1989) that quality and audit issues came formally onto the agenda of the health professions. In this paper, far-reaching changes to the NHS were set out, among them 'improving the quality of service' and 'bringing all parts of the Health Service up to the very high standard of the best' (DoH 1989). Medical audit was the subject of Working Paper no. 6, defining it as: 'the systematic, critical analysis of the quality of medical care, including the procedures used for diagnosis and treatment, the use of resources, and the resulting outcome and quality of life for the patient' (DoH 1989).

Nothing was mentioned about audit in nursing, midwifery or the therapies. This medical bias, to the apparent exclusion of nursing, midwifery and the therapies, was corrected in 1993 when the concept of multidisciplinary *clinical audit* was introduced along with the recognition that, although health professionals had made critical analyses of the quality of care, it had not been systematic. In the booklet 'Clinical Audit-meeting and improving clinical standards in health care', clinical audit was defined as: 'looking at the procedures used for diagnosis, care and treatment, examining how associated resources are used and investigating the effect care has on the outcome and quality of life for the patient' (DoH 1993a).

In 'Targeting practice: the contribution of nurses, midwives and health visitors', the concept of audit as a way of demonstrating clinical effectiveness was put forward: 'Nothing shall be called good practice until there is evidence that it achieved and continues to achieve the desired outcome. This evidence has therefore to be in the form of a routine audit of outcome against predetermined objectives/targets/standards' (DoH 1993b).

This introduction of quality issues also affected education. In the past, midwifery education had been regulated by the relevant national board which inspected premises where midwifery was taught and practised. Approval for training establishments was given or withheld depending on whether the institution attained various standards. Midwifery teaching establishments have now increasingly become integrated with the university system and education audit is now carried out by higher education (HE), the relevant national board and the education consortia. The English National Board (ENB) for Nursing, Midwifery and Health Visiting Report of midwifery practice audit (ENB 1997a) is an example.

DEFINITIONS

Quality is one of those concepts which is easy to understand but is difficult to define. Pirsig (1974) famously defined quality as 'what you like'. Crosby (1979) emphasized the objective aspect of quality when he described it as 'conformance with requirements'. Donabedian (1966), the guru of quality in health care, captured the essence of quality when he said 'quality may be almost what anyone wants it to be, although it is ordinarily, a reflection of values and goals current in the medical health care system and in the larger society of which it is a part'. Fundamental to quality is the concept that a standard is set and measured against, by individuals, groups or society itself. How far actual practice conforms with the standard is the measure of quality achieved.

Quality assurance 'is the measurement of the actual level of the service plus the efforts to modify, when necessary, the provision of those services in the light of the results of measurement' (Williamson 1978). A *quality service* 'gives people what they need as well as what they want at lowest cost' (Ovretveit 1992).

Quality can be analysed into component parts. Maxwell (1984) outlined six constituents of quality in a famous article in the British Medical Journal. These are: access to services, relevance to need, effectiveness, equity, social acceptability and efficiency. However, a service may have all these characteristics and not be ethical. This characteristic is therefore included (Box 11.1).

Box 11.1 **Dimensions of a quality service**
• Accessible • Acceptable • Appropriate • Equitable • Efficient • Effective • Ethical.

THE QUALITY CYCLE

Quality is not just a set of static characteristics however. It is a process. The process of quality can

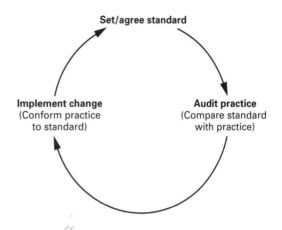

Figure 11.1 The quality cycle.

be demonstrated by the 'quality cycle' first described by Lang in 1976. It has also been represented as a 'spiral' (Bucknall et al 1992) indicating that quality is a dynamic, ongoing process. Figure 11.1 shows a simplified version of the quality cycle.

The process of quality assurance is simple, whether applied to clinical or educational practice or, indeed, any service. It starts with a *standard*, an expectation, something to measure against. This standard is *audited* to see how far actual practice conforms with the standard. *Change* is implemented in order to conform practice to the standard. The standard is then reviewed again. And so the process continues in a continuous spiral of improvement. Quality in clinical practice and education in this chapter will be based on this model.

QUALITY IN CLINICAL PRACTICE
Setting standards

Standards are the starting point in implementing a quality service. A standard has been defined as 'a measure or specification to which others (should) conform or against which others are judged; required degree of excellence' (Little Oxford Dictionary 1980). In relation to clinical practice, standards have been defined as 'professionally agreed levels of performance appropriate to the population addressed which are achievable, observable and measurable' (Sale 1991) and 'a representation of care which all patients should receive' (Bednar 1993), either as 'a minimum level of acceptable performance or results or excellent performance or results' (Grimshaw & Russell 1993). Wilson (1987) coined the acronym 'RUMBA' to summarize the ideal standard statement as Relevant, Understandable, Measurable, Behavioural and Achievable.

How do standards relate to clinical practice? Midwives' practice is regulated by statute. Their day to day practice is required to conform to the standards of the UKCC namely the Midwives rules and code of practice (UKCC 1998a), Standards for the administration of medicines, (UKCC 1992) and Guidelines for records and record keeping (UKCC 1998b) among others. These documents enshrine broad standards for midwifery practice.

Parliament also produces standards which have a bearing on midwifery practice, for example: The Patient's Charter (DoH 1991), Maternity Charter (DoH 1994), Changing Childbirth (DoH 1993c) and Health of the Nation (DoH 1992).

Other standards are set locally by purchasing authorities or by hospital or community unit management or directorates. In recent years, the setting of standards has also taken place in local health care settings. Quality circles, consisting of clinicians and sometimes known as standard setting groups, have been established to set standards for clinical practice at a local level. Standards produced are either initiated and developed for use at a local level, or taken from existing professional or government standards and adapted to the local situation. Box 11.2 gives examples of different professional standards.

One method used for setting standards is based on Donabedian's (1966) 'structure, process, outcome' model, which is defined as 'a statement which outlines an objective with guidance for its achievement given in the form of criteria sets which specify required resources, activities and predicted outcomes' (RCN 1990). In this method, the groups aim to set standards which are acceptable to their peers through feedback and discussion and which therefore are more likely to be 'owned' and implemented.

Box 11.2 Examples of professional, national and local standards

- 'A practising midwife shall keep as contemporaneously as is reasonable detailed records of observations, care given and medicine or other forms of pain relief administered by her to all mothers and babies' (UKCC 1998)
- 'The Charter Standard is that you will be given a specific appointment time and be seen within 30 minutes of that time.' (DoH 1991)
- 'All mothers will be aware of the measures to be taken to reduce the risk of cot death, in the light of recent research' (Maternity Ward Standard Setting Group, Nottingham City Hospital (NHS trust) maternity unit 1992).

Whether standard setting and audit should be unidisciplinary or multidisciplinary has been a matter of debate. The DoH publication Clinical audit (DoH 1993a) recognized that there is a place for both types. Midwifery and obstetrics overlap in major areas and for many topics standard setting and audit should be multidisciplinary. Other areas, for example, supporting mothers with breast feeding, involve both midwives and support workers, and it is obviously more appropriate that they set and implement standards in this area. What is important is that the most relevant people are involved, be they midwives, obstetricians, paediatricians, anaesthetists, medical records clerks, estates personnel or lay people, to take account of different perspectives, skills and experience. Establishing quality groups to set maternity and audit standards is addressed in Buckley (1997 pp. 33–61).

Audit

Audit is the next stage in the cycle of quality. The definition of audit in the clinical field has changed over recent years. The word derives from the Latin 'audire' which means 'to hear' and refers to the hearing of oral accounts of financial records as a way of assessing whether accounts literally 'added up' and giving auditors a chance to judge. Audit in its narrowest definition refers to the process of measurement with the implicit meaning of 'systematic measurement with a view to evaluation' (Buckley 1997 p. 11).

Audit as related to clinical audit has been broadened to include the whole process of quality in clinical practice and, indeed, the term is often used synonymously with quality. 'Nursing audit is part of the cycle of quality assurance. It incorporates the systematic and critical analyses by nurses, midwives and health visitors, in conjunction with other staff of the planning, delivery and evaluation of nursing and midwifery care ... and introduces appropriate change in response to that analysis' (DoH 1993b).

All aspects of practice need to be audited (DoH 1993b) and they should be audited against existing standards. This may involve measuring a practice directly against the standard statement itself, outcomes or some aspect of structure or process. There are many ways of carrying out audit. A detailed discussion is beyond the scope of this chapter; however Table 11.1 gives a brief outline of the various methods with their respective strengths and weaknesses. Audit methods fall into three main categories: surveys (interviews, questionnaires) observing practice, and examination of records.

Examples of audit projects using different methods are given in Box 11.3. Audit should be systematic, regular and part of an overall strategy. 'One-off' audits are of little value in improving

Table 11.1 Audit methods

Method	Advantages	Disadvantages

Questionnaires	Cheap
	Easy to administer
	
	Suitable for large
	  numbers
		Low response rate
		Unsuitable for those
		  unable to read or write
		Unsuitable for those who
		  cannot understand English
		Questions may be
		  missed or understood
		Susceptible to bias as
		  less motivated people
		  less likely to complete

Interview schedules	High response rate
	Suitable for those
	  unable to read or write
	Extra comments can
	  be noted
		Time consuming
		Inter-interviewer variation

Observation	Direct view of what is
	  actually happening
	Qualitative information
	  gained
		'Hawthorne effect'
		
		Possible observer
		  bias/difficulty with
		  interpretation of data
		Time consuming
		Not suitable for large
		  scale studies

Examination of
records: manual
	Direct record of care
	
	Analysis of original
	  records
	Contemporaneous data
		Possible incomplete
		  records
		May be difficult to interpret
		
		Time consuming

Examination of
records: computer
	Easy
	
	Quick
	Confidential
		Depends on those with
		  computer programming
		  skills
		Missing or inaccurate data
		Training of personnel to
		  access data
		Expensive equipment
		  required

> **Box 11.3** **Examples of audit methods in midwifery practice**
>
> - Questionnaires: Patient charter standard no. 6 waiting times in antenatal clinics
> - Interview schedules: audit of information given to mother about vitamin K
> - Observation: audit of information given to mothers at booking
> - Examining manual records: manual case notes, audit of signatures, times, dates, storage, CTGs, advice about smoking
> - Examining computer records: postnatal haemoglobins, breast-feeding rates, low risk care in labour, waiting times for induction, waiting times for suturing, antibiotics at caesarean section, application of pneumatic boots at caesarean section, advice about smoking.

quality. Carrying out audits can be time consuming and expensive in terms of time and resources and this needs to be planned and resourced accordingly. Increasingly, maternity units are employing a midwife to work full or part time on quality and audit issues.

There is no such thing as an ideal audit method, even with all the money, time and personnel available. The method which is chosen will usually be a trade-off between the optimum and the practical. Further, audit is constrained by midwives with clinical workloads, limited time and resources. For example, it would probably be ideal to audit a mother's views of the support she received with breast feeding, after she had been discharged from hospital and by a person (maybe a lay person) not involved with her care. It could (rightly) be argued that her answers may be biased if she is asked for her views in hospital, by clinicians. She may not want to make negative comments to the staff concerned for fear of consequences. It has been shown that patients may be reluctant to complain about their treatment in hospital because of possible repercussions (Zimkin 1985) or resentment from staff (Kaye & MacManus 1990). However, practicalities need to be considered. To carry out an audit of the mother's views at home would be possible but there would be the organizational problems of communicating to community midwives, getting surveys to them, giving instruction about completing the forms,

answering queries, collection and coordination of the audit. The time and resources needed would be considerable. A compromise solution would be to interview mothers on the day of discharge, or give out anonymous questionnaires to complete. Questionnaires (as opposed to interviews) may encourage more 'honest' comments, but at the cost of a lower overall response rate.

Implementing change

Implementing change is the third step in the quality cycle. It refers to the process of taking steps to conform practice to the standard. Implementing change has already been referred to in the DoH's (1993a) definition of nursing and midwifery audit. It is a vital part of the quality cycle for, without it, standards remain aspirations and audit data is 'orphaned' (Shaw 1980). Once changes have been made, the standard is reviewed (a local standard may be amended in the light of audit), and the process of audit and implementing change continues.

Achieving change which actually improves care is perhaps the greatest challenge of all. It is relatively easy to set standards, given the resources. It is fairly easy to audit them. The real challenge however is to interpret the results, evaluate them against the standard, decide what needs to be done and implement change which conforms practice to the standard. Relatively few people may actually be involved in setting standards and carrying out audit, and it is usually over a short period of time. The sustained effort of implementing change which works, makes a difference to care and can actually be demonstrated to do so, takes a great deal of planning, effort and people management.

Bringing about change in clinical practice is easier said than done. Just because something *ought* to be done does not mean that people will do it. Putting posters up or sending out edicts as the sole approach will not work. People think up all kinds of excuses about why the change does not apply to them, at that time or in that particular situation. Much change is dependent on what others do and how they are influenced and it should be recognized that people take on change in different ways and at different rates.

Rogers (1983) has done extensive studies on how people accommodate change and found that innovations are typically taken on in an 'S'-shaped curve. It is taken on slowly at first by *innovators*, about 2.5% of the population. These are venturesome individuals who play a key role in launching new ideas and methods. As they make up only a small percentage of the organization, it is vital that they persuade the *early adopters* to take on the change, otherwise the initiative will fail. Early adopters are open to ideas and enthusiastic in carrying them out. Their role is key. They account for about 13.5% of the workforce and are influential in the organization. They tend to be opinion leaders who are respected and are in positions of relative seniority. They are able to influence the next group of people, the *early majority* to take on the proposed changes. The early majority account for around 34% of the workforce and, once they are persuaded, the momentum is created for the *late majority*, also about 34%, to implement the change. The late majority tend to be sceptical and cautious and are reliant on the proposed change being well embedded and on peer pressure before they take it on. Once the late majority have taken on the change, it is at this stage that the change is embedded and established. Only the *laggards* remain to take on the change. They make up about 16% of the organization, tend to be traditional in outlook and adopt change very late and some do not do so at all.

Effective communication is the most important factor in effective change. This involves considering both people and the way they take on change, and the methods used to communicate the change. Some will work better than others depending on the situation.

Clinical effectiveness, clinical guidelines and clinical governance

How can successful change in clinical practice be ensured? Practice in midwifery has traditionally been handed down through education, learned from midwifery and obstetric colleagues and sometimes influenced by research findings. In the past, obstetric practice has been accused of being the speciality 'least likely to be supported by clinical evidence' (Cochrane 1979). Midwifery, as a close relation to obstetrics, is no doubt implicated in the charge. Since midwives have been required to demonstrate the efficacy of their practice they, along with other health professionals, have started to question the basis of their practice and are attempting to place their practice on a more rational footing to demonstrate that their care is effective. In recent years, several important concepts have emerged which have a direct bearing on quality in clinical practice. They are *clinical effectiveness, clinical guidelines* and *clinical governance*.

Clinical effectiveness

Clinical effectiveness has been defined as 'the extent to which specific clinical interventions when deployed in the field for a particular patient or population do what they are intended to do, i.e. maintain and improve health and secure the greatest possible health gain from the available resources' (DoH 1996a). In other words 'doing the right thing in the right way for the right patient at the right time' (RCN 1996). Clinical effectiveness cannot be demonstrated until it has been measured (DoH 1996b). It is important that all aspects of midwifery practice are evaluated and shown to be effective or otherwise discontinued.

Clinical guidelines

It is increasingly being recognized by health professionals that to achieve clinical effectiveness they need to use clinical guidelines. Clinical guidelines (sometimes known as practice guidelines or protocols (Conroy & Shannon 1995)) have been defined as 'systematically developed statements to assist practitioner and patient decisions about appropriate health care for specific circumstances' (Institute of Medicine 1992). They are used to achieve standards and have been found to produce improvements in the quality of health care by reducing inappropriate practice (Conroy & Shannon 1995, Grimshaw et al 1995).

Clinical guidelines may be developed and produced at a national or local level (Duff et al 1996). As a rule those developed nationally tend to be broad statements and are produced by professional colleges. They are standards of good practice and are usually based on research findings. Those developed locally tend to be more detailed, often, though not always, based on national standards and adapted to the local situation. Guidelines may be based on formal meta-analyses, systematic reviews of the literature, or expert opinion and professional consensus, where no research is available. There are large resource implications in producing guidelines which are based on the best available evidence. Not every practice or procedure is amenable to a randomized controlled trial.

Guidelines have been described as 'one person's opinion sent round in the mail to be uniformly ignored' (Wright 1997). Certainly if that is how guidelines are perceived at local level, they will be doomed to failure and the waste bin. So will those which appear to be emanating from external or remote sources (Conroy & Shannon 1995) or are imposed without discussion and agreement. Locally agreed guidelines which are 'owned' by the health professionals involved (Renvoize et al 1997, Wray & Maresh 1997), have the support and input of senior staff and 'opinion leaders' (Conroy & Shannon 1995), are well disseminated using reminders and incentives and audited regularly with the opportunity for feedback are the most effective way of making change work (Duff et al 1996).

Clinical governance

Clinical governance was introduced in the Government's white papers, 'The New NHS: modern–dependable' (DoH 1997) and 'A First Class Service' (DoH 1998). They describe new arrangements to 'put quality at the core of individual NHS organizations and individual NHS professionals'. This is to be reflected in:

- a new statutory duty for ensuring quality of care
- ultimate responsibility for this resting with the chief executive

- a trust board subcommittee chaired by a senior clinical professional with responsibility for ensuring that systems for clinical governance are in place
- regular reports to the NHS boards on quality.

The concept of clinical governance requires every health institution to create a direct link from the 'shop floor' of clinical practice to the very top of the organization, increasing accountability and prompting health professionals to look ever more critically at their practice. Risk management and clinical audit are central. National standards will be set and monitored by new Government agencies. Midwives may be concerned that clinical governance and the trend towards adopting clinical guidelines to regulate large areas of clinical practice may limit their clinical freedom. This misses the point. The aim is not to regulate every single step of clinical practice but to provide parameters and guideposts along the way which enable safe, confident practice and allow flexibility, client choice and preferences. Clinical guidelines, properly produced, and based on best available evidence, not only protect the mother and her baby, but the midwife also.

'A subjective judgement about the quality of care is no longer tenable' (Duff et al 1996). For clinical practice at least, interventions need increasingly to be justified on rational, scientific grounds. That is not necessarily to reduce clinical freedom, although it may do in some cases. Reducing variability in practice is not to be feared. There is good evidence that clinical guidelines which are produced well, applied and implemented in the right way will improve clinical effectiveness.

Examples of quality in clinical midwifery practice

The two examples of quality and audit initiatives which follow were carried out in the Nottingham City Hospital maternity unit. The first one is a simple standard set in 1991, which has been audited regularly with change implemented and improved care as a result. The second example addresses an increasingly important and topical aspect of midwifery and obstetric practice and includes an example of clinical guidelines which have been developed and implemented locally and used effectively. Both are examples of the quality cycle in action.

Reducing waiting times for perineal suturing

It is generally acknowledged that there is morbidity subsequent to episiotomy or genital lacerations. Among these are bleeding (Sleep, Roberts & Chalmers 1989), pain (Howie 1995) and infection (Bennett & Brown 1989). Though prompt suturing secures haemostasis (Bennett & Brown 1989), promotes healing (Bobak & Jensen 1989), decreases infection (Bobak & Jensen 1989) and is kinder to the mother (Bennett & Brown 1989), little research has been carried out on the optimum time to suture after delivery.

In the Nottingham City Hospital, suturing delays were the cause of written complaints. After carrying out an audit of suturing times after normal delivery, the Labour Suite Standard Setting Group decided to reduce the waiting time for suturing and set a standard stating that: 'Every mother requiring suturing will be attended to within an hour of normal delivery, unless there are maternal or neonatal complications or maternal request to delay suturing'.

To implement the standard, more midwives were trained in perineal suturing and midwives were encouraged to make suturing a priority after delivery rather than, for example, writing up case notes. The standard was audited regularly by analysing the delivery–suturing interval times from the computer and by a short questionnaire completed by the midwife, which appeared on computer if suturing was delayed for more than an hour. This asked for the reasons for delay. Results of the audits are shown in Fig. 11.2.

There has been an overall reduction of 90.5% between 1991 and 1997 in the percentage of mothers delayed for more than an hour or 'avoidably delayed'. There has been a 53.7% increase of midwives involved in suturing over the same period of time. Since the standard was

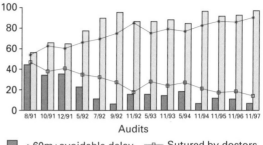

Figure 11.2 Reducing normal delivery–suturing times.

implemented, there have been no written complaints about suturing delays.

Improving CTG interpretation

Although CTGs have been part of midwifery and obstetric practice since the 1960s, interpretation of CTGs remains difficult and at times controversial. Research has found that there is considerable intra- and interobserver variability in interpreting fetal heart traces (Beaulieu et al 1982, Neilson et al 1987). Added to this is the finding that poor interpretation and response to abnormal CTGs have been implicated in avoidable fetal and neonatal deaths in the Confidential Enquiry into Stillbirths and Deaths in Infancy (CESDI) (Maternal and Child Health Consortium 1997) and in obstetric litigation (Capstick 1994).

At Nottingham City Hospital, we decided to address this issue and a multidisciplinary group was established to look at standardizing practice in this area. A standard was set: 'All midwives and obstetric staff will be able to recognise normal and abnormal CTGs and take appropriate clinical action in accordance with Unit policy' (Buckley 1997 p. 127).

Guidelines were produced by the group based on Federation Internationale de Gynaecologie et d'Obstetrique (FIGO 1987) guidelines, research findings and consensus, for antepartum, intrapartum first and second stages. These are colour coded for easy reference and include guidelines on consent, assessment, action, documentation, storage and definitions of terms. 'Credit card' size copies have been made which are sold to clinicians and students for a small charge. There is a rolling programme of education for all midwives, senior house officers and registrars.

The guidelines are reviewed, updated and monitored on a regular basis. A high degree of compliance has been found. Where midwives or doctors have not complied with the standard, steps are taken to ask the clinician involved to review the CTG along with the relevant guideline and to ascertain the need for further education.

Hence the quality cycle continues, with the aim of demonstrating improvements in the standard of CTG interpretation with the ultimate objective of giving better care to mothers and reducing perinatal mortality and morbidity.

QUALITY IN MIDWIFERY EDUCATION

Introduction

Quality in midwifery education has always been vitally important in securing high standards for both students of midwifery and midwives seeking additional qualifications. Assessment of quality in midwifery education has dramatically changed following integration with HE institutions. Education is now assessed both internally and externally using the same criteria as any other university department or faculty, and is required to meet all the demands expected of it, regardless of previous experience and background. It is important for students, midwives and midwife practitioners to understand the present demands and expectations. The emphasis is on quality, in both educational matters and student output.

Prior to midwifery education entering HE, the national boards for England, Wales, Scotland and Northern Ireland assumed full responsibility for approval of programmes and providers of midwifery education, and continued to do so in conjunction with individual HE institutions, once affiliation and subsequent integration took place. In 1995, the ENB agreed to change their guidelines for approval into standards for approval of institutions and programmes in the context of the rapidly developing quality assurance in HE. These standards were to be measurable, and their criteria were developed by the Professional Education Standards Group, which was established in April 1996 to be implemented in October 1998 (ENB 1997b).

Within the university quality system, there are three components of quality assurance: quality control, quality audit and quality assessment.

- *Quality control*—this is the process within institutions whereby mechanisms are put in place for maintaining and enhancing the quality of their provision.
- *Quality audit*—this allows external scrutiny to provide guarantees that institutions have proper quality control mechanisms in place. Until recently, this was undertaken by the Higher Education Quality Council (HEQC 1996).
- *Quality assessment*—this is the external review and judgement on the quality of teaching and learning in institutions. Until recently this was undertaken by the Higher Education Funding Council for Education (HEFCE 1996). Assessment by HEFCE is crucial in terms of monetary reward, and is the linchpin upon which quality recruitment and prestigious research projects can become achievable.

A Quality Assurance Agency (QAA) for HE has been formed in view of the overlap between audit and assessment. This agency coordinates both activities. Each institution will have an audit review on a 5 year cycle, and each subject area (e.g. nursing and midwifery) will have a review visit on a 5 year cycle. Institutional participation in the process is requisite.

Midwifery education will now be assessed using the university quality assurance mechanism. Its first assessment was between 1998 and 2000. Midwife educationalists were required to prepare for the assessment, having had no prior exposure to this system.

To illustrate how the university quality system works in practice, the quality cycle used in clinical practice and described earlier in the chapter will be adopted to illustrate how quality is implemented in education.

Standard setting in education

To initiate the process, each midwifery education provider completes a self-assessment document which is an evaluation of the quality of the student learning experience and student achievement (QAA 1997). This is measured against the aims and objectives that the midwifery education provider sets for the education of its students. This self-assessment addresses the following areas:

- aims and objectives of the educational provision
- factual profile of students, staff and learning resources
- an evaluation of the quality of midwifery education in six areas:
  - —curriculum design, content and organization
  - —teaching, learning and assessment
  - —student progression and achievement
  - —student support and guidance
  - —learning resources
  - —quality management and enhancement.

This self-assessment must be supported by evidence, and should discuss both strengths and weaknesses in the midwifery education provision. Where weaknesses are acknowledged, the education provider will be encouraged to discuss the issues and the steps necessary to improve the quality.

The set aims and objectives which are included in the self-assessment document provide a framework for the subsequent external assessment. The aims express the midwifery education provider's broad purposes in presenting each programme of study in midwifery. They focus on the level of the midwifery provision, the midwifery students and the midwifery programme being studied. Discrete aims for each programme should be specified, and the aims at different levels of study made explicit, for example level 2 (diploma) or 3 (degree).

An example of midwifery aims would be:

The broad aims of the midwifery department, as part of the school of nursing, faculty of health and in line with the University of Hull's (1995) mission statement are:

—to teach undergraduates of midwifery the role and responsibilities of a midwife as set out in the Midwives code of practice (UKCC 1998)
—to inculcate analytical skills in current areas of midwifery practice
—to produce midwifery graduates who can claim advanced knowledge in midwifery theory, research and practice which is detailed, critical and reflective
—to provide the midwifery service with graduate midwives who will be well placed in an increasingly demanding, selective and internationalized market.

The objectives set out the intended student learning outcomes and student achievements that demonstrate successful completion of a programme of study. The statement of objectives should communicate specific intentions of the student learning experience and learning outcomes. It should also articulate the relationship between the specific intentions (objectives) and broad purposes (aims) (University of Hull 1995).

An example of midwifery education objectives would be:

The midwifery department seeks to achieve its aims through an innovative and flexible programme in which a range of teaching and assessment methods are employed. The objectives of this modular programme are to enable students to:

1. achieve and maintain clinical competence in the specified activities of clinical midwifery practice as laid down in the European Community Midwives directives 80/155/EEC article 4 and Midwives code of practice (UKCC 1994)
2. demonstrate clear communication skills that are articulate, accurate and effective in meeting the needs of the service
3. critically analyse with confidence and academic rigour and apply as appropriate the findings of current research to clinical midwifery practice.

It is obviously in the midwifery education provider's best interests that the self-assessment document accurately reflects what their real aims and objectives are. It should not be too ambitious as the self-assessment sets the standard from which it is to be measured.

The HE sector is diverse, with variations in size of institutions, departments, subject provision, history and statement of purpose. This quality assessment method is designed to take as full account as possible of this diversity, and advises caution when making comparisons with different subject providers (e.g. department of mathematics with midwifery education) based solely on the quality assessment outcomes. Comparisons between subject providers with substantively different aims and objectives would have very little validity.

Auditing educational standards

Audit in education is fundamentally concerned with processes and outcomes. It considers the management systems currently in place, not individuals, and tends to underemphasize the contribution of the organizational processes generally. This basic principle underpins the quality assessment system in higher education.

Following submission of the self-assessment document, the department will have an assessment visit. Here, it is envisaged that the department will be peer reviewed by a team of subject specialist reviewers led by a review chair. The specialist reviewers are academic and professional peers in midwifery and nursing, with the majority being staff in other United Kingdom HE institutions. Others will be drawn from clinical practice, professional bodies, or both. All subject specialist reviewers are trained by the QAA, in collaboration with the Universities and Colleges Staff Development Agency, before the first visit.

The purpose of the review process is to gather, consider and verify the evidence of the quality of education, in the light of the midwifery education provider's aims and objectives. In reaching judgements on the quality of the provision, the subject specialist reviewers evaluate the extent to which the student learning experience and the student achievement contribute to meeting the aims and objectives set by the education provider. Quality assessment examines the wide range of influences that shape the learning experience and achievements of students. This range is captured within a core set of six aspects of provision, detailed on p. 189, each of which is graded on a fourpoint assessment scale (1–4, 4 being the highest).

The subject specialist reviewers establish a graded profile and an overall judgement on the quality of that provision. The tests to be applied to each core aspect of provision are:

1. to what extent do the student learning experience and student achievement, within this aspect of provision, contribute to meeting the objectives set by the midwifery education provider?
2. do the objectives set, and the level of attainment of those objectives allow the aims set by the education provider to be met?

The criteria for the achievement between 1 to 4 is for all subject areas within the university system and is illustrated in Box 11.4 (QAA 1997):

Box 11.4   Grade descriptors for subject review

1. The aims and/or objectives set by the subject provider are not met; there are major shortcomings that must be rectified.
2. This aspect makes on acceptable contribution to the attainment of the stated objectives, but significant improvements could be made. The aims set by the subject provider are broadly met.
3. This aspect makes a substantial contribution to the attainment of the stated objectives; however, there is scope for improvement. The aims set by the subject provider are met.
4. This aspect makes a full contribution to the attainment of the stated objectives. The aims set by the subject provider are met.

Source: QAA 1997, p. 51.

A grade of 1 means that either the aspect of provision makes an inadequate contribution to the attainment of the objectives, or that the objectives do not provide students with the experiences and achievements that would support a judgement that the aims were being met. A grade of 2 or more in an aspect of provision means that the particular aspect of provision (e.g. curriculum design, content and organization) makes at least an acceptable contribution to the attainment of the stated objectives and that the aims are at least broadly met.

The overall summative judgement is derived from the profile of the six core aspects of provision. All the aspects are treated as of equal weight. If all aspects are graded 2 or above, the department will be reported as 'quality approved'. A profile that has one or more aspects of provision graded 1 will be subject to a further review within a year and the following procedures are likely to apply:

1. A subject review report containing the decision of the first assessment will take place within 12 months. During this period of reassessment, normal HEFCE funding arrangements continue to apply.

2. If after reassessment within 12 months, the profile still contains one or more aspects of provision graded 1, the education provider will be recorded as being of unsatisfactory quality. In these cases funding issues are as yet undecided. There is concern that funding may be withdrawn or, more optimistically, it could be provided to allow improvements to be made.

The judgements are given as oral feedback from the review team to the institution at the end of the review visit. A review report is published after each visit and is the main documented outcome of the quality assessment process. The subject review report is very detailed. One component of the assessment visit is assessment of the teaching, learning and assessment aspect of provision. The subject specialist subject reviewers observe teaching and learning sessions, and tutorials with a sample of the teaching staff across the range of programmes of study offered by that education provider. For many lecturers this is likely to be the first time they have been observed since being a student teacher. The report will then detail the overall number of sessions observed and the overall grade given. It is unlikely, therefore that one individual would adversely affect the score, but it could potentially reduce the average sufficiently to warrant investigation. In the light of this, many institutions are now advocating systematic peer review of teaching and hence quality improvement before the QAA subject review.

Implementing change

The QAA report recommends where improvements could be made by raising certain issues.

Providing the subject provider attains a grade of 2 or more, education is 'quality approved'. For those who achieve grade 1 in one or more core aspects of provision they have a relatively short space of time of just 12 months to gain approval or risk having funds withdrawn by HEFCE. The recommendations will need to be actioned in order to achieve a grade 2 or more. This could cause problems if resourcing is an issue. The report also goes on the World Wide Web site, with thousands of 'hits' on those pages, especially during the applications period. This potentially has a knock-on effect for recruitment of quality staff and students.

To place the quality cycle in context, an example is demonstrated in Fig. 11.3.

Research assessment exercise

As a further way of ensuring quality within HE Institutions, the research assessment exercise (RAE) is undertaken periodically (Nyatanga 1995). HEFCE determines the frequency, which is approximately every 3–5 years and is a national exercise. It requires heads of departments or deans of schools to disclose the activities of its research-appointed staff.

The research activities are scored 1 to 5 (with an additional score of 5*, which is a grade similar to distinction) and carries significant potential monetary value for the department concerned and prestige for the university. All staff are categorized either as 'research active' or 'non-research active'. The proportion of research-active to non-research-active staff is taken into account in the assessment. To be termed 'research active' implies that a member of staff is appointed on the academic scale or is applying to be, has published their work in credible journals or recognized publishers on a regular basis and is currently engaged in research activity.

The score to the department is dependent upon the number of research-active members of staff put forward for assessment, the quality of their research to date, the number of publications and where they are published. In addition the number of research grants awarded and from whom, and the amount of current research

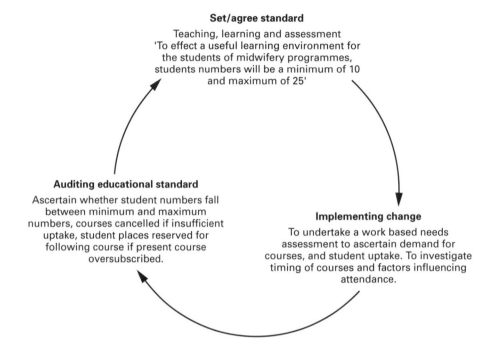

Set/agree standard

Teaching, learning and assessment
'To effect a useful learning environment for
the students of midwifery programmes,
students numbers will be a minimum of 10
and maximum of 25'

Auditing educational standard

Ascertain whether student numbers fall
between minimum and maximum
numbers, courses cancelled if insufficient
uptake, student places reserved for
following course if present course
oversubscribed.

Implementing change

To undertake a work based needs
assessment to ascertain demand for
courses, and student uptake. To investigate
timing of courses and factors influencing
attendance.

Figure 11.3   The quality cycle in context.

projects presently ongoing all count towards gaining a higher score.

A score of 5* is the maximum that can be awarded and attracts a substantial monetary contribution per active research member of staff. Conversely a low score or 1 or 2 seriously affects the income into that department per research active member of staff. This produces a chicken and egg scenario: more money is poured into areas already seen as centres of excellence and rich in terms of prestigious research grants and quality staff, yet other departments attempting to launch themselves into the research market can be penalized. This is the scenario currently facing most midwifery education departments today. The well-established fields and centres attract the majority of the funding, leaving the poorer-resourced areas struggling to compete.

Fortunately in July 1997 a report 'Higher education in the learning society' by the National Committee of Enquiry into Higher Education chaired by Sir Ron Dearing was released. This was commissioned to: 'make recommendations on how the purposes, shape, structure, size and funding of higher education, including support for students, should develop to meet the needs of the United Kingdom over the next 20 years, recognising that higher education embraces teaching, learning, scholarship and research' (National Committee of Enquiry into Higher Education, 1997).

There was much debate before midwifery entered HE, with concerns being raised that academia would sidestep the practical nature of the profession. The Dearing Report (1997) above outlines a new agreement for higher education with the following benefits:

To the employer:

- more highly educated people in the workforce
- clearer understanding of what HE is offering
- more opportunities for collaborative working with HE

- better accessibility to HE resources for small and medium enterprises
- outcomes of research activities.

To the staff:

- greater recognition to the value of their work, not just research activity
- proper recognition of their profession
- access to training and development opportunities
- fair pay.

To the students:

- more chances to participate in a large system
- better information and guidance to inform choices
- a high quality learning experience
- a clear statement of learning outcomes
- rigorously assured awards which have standing across the UK and overseas
- better support for part-time study
- larger access funds.

These benefits are dependent upon a contribution from employers, students and staff, which largely include:

1. commitment to excellence, and a willingness to seek and adopt new ways of doing things by the staff
2. for employers, to invest more in the training of employees, to increase their contribution to the infrastructure of research, and to provide more work opportunities for students, and greater support for employees serving the institutions' governing bodies
3. students will have a greater financial contribution to tuition costs, and will have to input more time and effort applied to learning.

The Dearing Report also acknowledges that, despite widespread support for the expansion of HE, current arrangements for quality assurance may not be sufficient to ensure comparability of standards in an enlarged sector. In addition, and more importantly to midwifery, it also acknowledges that current funding arrangements, as previously highlighted, reward high quality research and divert attention from the delivery of high quality teaching. The Dearing Report proposes a radical change in attitudes to teaching, and recommends that the representative bodies in consultation with the funding bodies immediately establish a professional institute for learning and teaching in HE, which would enable accreditation of professional achievement in the management of learning and teaching. Additionally, it recommends commissioning research and development work into teaching and learning practices, and stimulating innovation and coordination of the development of learning materials. This vision aims to put students at the centre of teaching and learning.

The Report proposes a qualification framework that would permit, for example, a fast track higher degree for midwives. This would produce 'high flyers' at a younger age, and encourage midwifery researchers earlier in their career. In other words, after undertaking a pre-registration midwifery programme, opportunities will exist for certain students to follow straight on with further studies at a higher level (i.e. master's or doctorate).

A further recommendation is that the QAA and funding bodies maintain this qualification framework, and participation by professional bodies in establishing the standards appropriate to their discipline. It is also considered necessary that funding policies currently supporting research should promote and fund high quality teaching. The need for high quality departments is recognized, but there is also a need for funding to support the research and scholarship which underpin teaching in those departments, such as midwifery, which do not aspire at this stage to be at the leading edge in research.

Leading on from this it is recommended that, at the next RAE, institutions are to be encouraged to make strategic decisions about whether to enter departments for the exercise, or whether to seek a lower level of non-competitive funding to support research and scholarship which underpins teaching.

Higher education and the national boards

Within midwifery education, all staff possess or are working towards a teaching qualification. Within many academic institutions this is not a requirement for full-time academic staff. It is reasonable to presume, therefore, that if the focus for funding is shifted from research to high quality teaching, this might just be the springboard midwifery education needs to create a strong presence within the HE structure.

There is a potential for education and practice to drift further apart following the move of midwifery education into institutions of higher education which are distanced from the NHS practice areas. The national boards still have statutory responsibility for education and training approval, which has created a situation in which responsibilities are being taken by two governing bodies: HE and the national boards. Therefore, agreement had to be reached to accommodate both parties in order for education and training in theory and practice to be consistent, unified and appropriate.

The change from regulations and guidelines, preintegration with HE, to standards and criteria should enable the professional standards of the UKCC and the European Union to be achieved within the QAA subject review. HE institutions are required to demonstrate how they meet the ENB's standards (ENB 1997b) through a process of annual monitoring and review of their midwifery educational programmes. Under this new system, approval of programmes is not subject to a fixed period, as has previously been the case, with midwifery education providers needing to request reapproval once the fixed term had been reached. This systematic annual monitoring and review should serve to ensure a continuing quality programme that is consistently striving to maintain approval, without the potential peaks and troughs between approval submissions.

Additionally course evaluations can be actioned quickly in view of the regular monitoring process.

Quality accreditation by national boards

Before HE institutions can offer midwifery programmes leading to registration or recordable qualifications, they need to gain national board approval. An essential requirement is that the institution works collaboratively with the designated education officer and provides an institutional self-assessment report demonstrating the institution's capacity and capability to achieve the board's standards. The timescale for approval is mutually agreed by both parties.

Once approved, an official correspondent is identified for all formal communication with the board. As the national boards will continue to span both the education providers and the clinical practitioners, the 18 ENB standards (ENB 1997b) have incorporated components of the previous educational audit of the practice placement. Following the review of the statutory bodies, although the composition of these professional bodies is likely to change, assessment of the quality of midwifery education programmes by the profession will almost certainly continue.

The ENB 18 standards address the whole spectrum of practice experience, staff resource and development, research, assessment, assessors of practice and curriculum design. Each standard has criteria which demonstrate to what extent the standards can be met. The standards mirror those contained in the report Improving the effectiveness of quality assurance systems in non-medical health care education and training (HEQC & NHSE 1996). This is useful as it spells out to HE institutions exactly what is expected, and safeguards appropriate midwifery input and supervision, placing its statutory obligations at the forefront.

Midwifery education has 'come of age' and entered the university system. It is required to meet all the quality requirements expected of any department within a HE institution. It is important that both students of midwifery and midwives in clinical practice understand the changes which have taken place. The focus is on quality, both in educational matters and student output. This needs to be followed through by quality in clinical midwifery practice.

THE WAY FORWARD

In a way, systematically auditing standards and implementing change on the basis of audit results is so obvious that it seems strange that no-one had thought of it long before. Yet it is only comparatively recently that the concepts of quality and audit were introduced to health professionals in the NHS. Since that time it has gone from being an almost unknown and often misunderstood concept, practised only by enthusiasts, to become a major issue underpinning clinical practice and education. It is a pity that its introduction, certainly in clinical practice, was prompted as much by the desire to save money as to give effective care.

Why should quality be so important to midwives and to midwifery? Midwifery, certainly in the UK, has travelled a long and tortuous path. For much of its history under medical domination and control, it has emerged to find its own identity, separate and distinct from other disciplines. These gains should not be lost. The way forward is through midwifery practice and education which is based on evidence-based, consensus standards which are produced by midwives in cooperation with other health professionals and, where appropriate, the consumer. These standards should be critically evaluated on a regular basis. Change then needs to be implemented using clinical guidelines where appropriate. Maintaining and continuously reviewing and improving the standard of education and clinical practice by means of audit is vital for the midwifery profession, its practitioners and consumers.

The present emphasis on quality and demonstrating clinical effectiveness provides the perfect opportunity for midwives to base their practice on a more rational, scientific footing, whilst at the same time giving individualized care which places the mother, her baby and family at its centre.

Quality and audit in midwifery have until recently been rather piecemeal as midwives have sought to find direction in evaluating and improving the service they give. The way forward is to focus on a few key areas of practice and education, statutory standards, standards produced by professional bodies and government and those adapted for local use. Quality and audit issues overlap with risk management as areas of high risk and this should inform planning. Midwifery supervision also is increasingly involved with ensuring that quality is maintained in midwifery (ENB 1996). One example of a key area is CTG interpretation, illustrated earlier in the chapter. In this particular area, it is likely that improving CTG interpretation is an area where perinatal mortality and morbidity can be reduced and, with it, litigation costs.

Although the achievement of progress should not be underestimated, it needs to be acknowledged that continuously improving the quality and outcomes of midwifery care is no easy task. Lack of support and commitment, conflicts between staff, willingness to participate and change practice are just some of the potential difficulties encountered when maintaining and improving the quality of service and care (Robinson 1996). However, down the years, midwives have demonstrated their ability to overcome problems and produce high standards of care.

The challenge for midwives and midwifery in the future is fourfold: balancing 'one to one' midwifery care with the wider realities of maternity care which involve interdependence with other health professionals; developing standardized clinical guidelines which reduce variability but allow for individualized care and consumer choice; rigorously and critically auditing their practice and acting on the findings; and not allowing concern with consumer choice to conflict with the responsibility to give confident, competent research-based direction when needed.

Quality issues are not an optional 'add-on' but, especially in the light of 'A First Class Service' (DoH 1998) a foundation stone of clinical practice and education. Of utmost importance and the 'raison d'etre' for every midwife, manager, teacher and researcher is that mothers, babies and their families get the highest quality care. Ensuring that their practice is 'quality assured' is the best possible guarantee.

Summary

Improving the quality of midwifery education and practice is of central importance in midwifery.

The first step is to set achievable, measurable standards for practice and education. The next step is to audit the standards regularly and disseminate the findings. The final step to 'close the audit loop' is to implement change to conform practice to the standard.

Midwifery clinicians, teachers, managers and researchers all have a part to play to achieve quality in midwifery

REFERENCES

Baly M E 1986 Florence Nightingale and the nursing legacy. Croonhelm, London

Beaulieu M D et al 1982 The reproducibility of intrapartum cardiotocogram assessments. Journal of the Canadian Medical Association 127:214–216

Bednar B 1993 Developing clinical practice guidelines: an interview with Ada Jacox. American Nephrology Nurses Association Journal 20(2):121–126

Bennett V, Brown L 1989 Myles textbook for midwives, 11th edn. Churchill Livingstone, Edinburgh, p 205

Bobak I, Jensen M 1989 Maternity and gynaecologic care. Mosby, St Louis p 441

Buckley E R 1997 Delivering quality in midwifery Baillière Tindall, London, pp 33–61

Bucknall C, Robertson C, Moran F, Stevenson R 1992 Improving management of asthma: closing the loop or progressing along the audit spiral? Health Care 1:15

Capstick B 1994 Risk limitation in obstetrics. In: Chamberlain G, Patel N (eds) The future of the maternity services. RCOG Press, London, p 83

Cochrane A 1979 1931–1971: a critical review with particular reference to the medical profession. In: Medicine for the year 2000. Office of Health Economics, London, pp 2–11

Conroy M, Shannon M 1995 Clinical guidelines: their implementation in general practice. British Journal of General Practice July:371–375

Cowell B, Wainwright D 1981 Behind the blue door. Baillière Tindall, London p 99

Crosby P 1979 Quality is free: the art of making quality certain. McGraw-Hill, New York, p 17

DoH (Department of Health) 1989 Working for patients. HMSO, London

DoH (Department of Health) 1991 The patient's charter. HMSO, London

DoH (Department of Health) 1992 Health of the nation. HMSO, London, p 18

DoH (Department of Health) 1993a Clinical audit. Meeting and improving clinical standards in health care. HMSO, London, p 15

DoH (Department of Health) 1993b Targeting practice: the contribution of nurses, midwives and health visitors. The health of the nation. HMSO, London, p 100

DoH (Department of Health) 1993c Changing childbirth. Report of the Expert Maternity Group, part 1. HMSO, London

DoH (Department of Health) 1994 The patient's charter. Maternity services DoH, London

DoH (Department of Health) 1996a Promoting clinical effectiveness a framework for action in and through the NHS. HMSO, London

DoH (Department of Health) 1996b Clinical audit in the NHS HMSO, London, p 2

DoH (Department of Health) 1997 The new NHS: Modern—Dependable. DoH, London, p 14

DoH (Department of Health) 1998 A first class service: quality in the new NHS. DoH, London

Donabedian A 1966 Evaluating the quality of medical care. Millbank Memorial Fund Quarterly 44:166–203

Duff L A, Kitson A L, Seers K, Humphris D 1996 Clinical guidelines: an introduction to their development and implementation. Journal of Advanced Nursing, 23:887–895

ENB (English National Board) 1996 Supervision of midwives: the English National Board's advice and guidance to local supervising authorities and supervisors of midwives. ENB, London, p 13

ENB (English National Board) for Nursing, Midwifery and Health Visiting 1997a Report of midwifery practice audit 1996–1997. ENB, London

ENB (English National Board) 1997b Standards for approval of higher education institutions and programmes. ENB, London

FIGO (Federation International de Gynaecologie et d'Obstetrique) 1987 Guidelines for the use of fetal monitoring. International Journal of Gynaecology and Obstetrics 25:159–167

Grimshaw J, Freemantle N, Wallace S, Hurwitz B, Watt I et al 1995 Developing and implementing clinical practice guidelines. Quality in Health Journal 4:361–364

Grimshaw J M, Russell I T 1993 Achieving health gain through clinical guidelines. I: Developing scientifically valid guidelines. Quality in Health Care 2:243–248

HEFCE (Higher Education Funding Council for Education) 1996 Assessors handbook October 1996–September 1998. HEFCE, Bristol

HEQC (Higher Education Quality Council) 1996 Quality standards and professional accreditation. HEQC, London

HEQC & NHSE 1996 (Higher Education Quality Council & National Health Service Executive) Improving the effectiveness of quality assurance in non-medical health care education and training, September. HEQC, London

HMSO 1902 Midwes Act. HMSO, London

Holy Bible (New International Version) 1982 Exodus i: 15–19, 6th edn Hodder and Stoughton, London

Howie P 1995 The physiology of the puerperium and lactation. In: Chamberlain G (ed) Turnbull's obstetrics, 2nd Churchill Livingstone, New York p 756

Institute of Medicine 1992 (eds Field M J, Kohr K N) Guidelines for clinical practice: from development to use. National Academy Press, Washington DC

Kaye C, MacManus T 1990 Understanding complaints. Health Service Journal 100(5215):1254–1255

Lang N 1976 Quality assurance—the idea and its development in the United States. In: Willis M, Linwood M (eds) Measuring the quality of care. Churchill Livingstone, Edinburgh

Little Oxford Dictionary 1980. Oxford University Press, Oxford

Maternal and Child Health Consortium 1997 Confidential enquiry into stillbirths and deaths in infancy (CESDI) 4th annual report 1 January–31 December 1995. Maternity and Child Health Consortium, London, pp 38, 39

Maxwell R J 1984 Quality assessment in health. British Medical Journal 288:1470–1472

National Committee of Enquiry into Higher Education 1997 Higher education in the learning society, summary report (the Dearing Report) July. Department of Education and Employment, London

Neilsen P V, Stigsby B, Nichelsen C, Nim J 1987 Intra- and inter-observer variability in the assessment of intrapartum cardiotocograms. Acta Obstret vicia et Gynaecologica Scandinavica: 66:421–424

Nightingale F 1871 Notes on lying-in institutions. Loughmans, Green. London. In: Baly M E 1986 Florence Nightingale and the Nursing legacy. Croonhelm London, p 65

Nyatanga L 1995 The research assessment exercise (RAE): criteria and issues. Nurse Education Today 15:395–396

Ovretveit J (1992) Health service quality. An introduction to quality methods for health services. Blackwell Scientific, Oxford, p 1

Pirsig R 1974 Zen and the art of motorcycle maintenance. Corgi, London

QAA (Quality Assurance Agency) for Higher Education 1997 Subject review handbook October 1998 to September 2000. QAA, Bristol

Renvoize E B Hampshaw S M, Pinder J M, Ayres P 1997 What are hospitals doing about clinical guidelines? Quality in Health Care 6:187–191

Robinson S 1996 Audit in the therapy professions: some constraints on progress. Quality in Health Care 5:206–214

Rogers E M 1983 Diffusion of innovations, 3rd edn. Free Press, New York pp 246–251

RCN (Royal College of Nursing) 1990 Quality patient care. The dynamic standard setting system. Scutari, Harrow, Middlesex

RCN (Royal College of Nursing) 1996 Clinical effectiveness. A Royal College of Nursing guide. RCN, London, p 3

Sale D 1991 Quality assurance Macmillan, London, p 54

Shaw C 1980 Acceptability of audit. British Medical Journal 14 June: 1443–1446

Sleep J, Roberts J, Chalmers I 1989 Care during the second stage of Labour. Effective care in pregnancy. Oxford University Press, Oxford, p 1136

UKCC (United Kingdom Central Council) for Nursing, Midwifery and Health Visiting 1992 Standards for the administration of medicines. UKCC, London

UKCC (United Kingdom Central Council) for Nursing, Midwifery and Health Visiting 1998a Midwives rules and code of practice. UKCC, London

UKCC (United Kingdom Central Council) for Nursing, Midwifery and Health Visiting 1998b Guidelines for records and record keeping. UKCC, London

University of Hull 1995 HEFCE quality assessment division: assessment of the quality of education—French. University of Hull, Hull

Williamson J W 1978 Formulating priorities for quality assurance activity: description of a method and its application. Journal of the American Medical Association 239:631–637

Wilson C R M 1987 Hospital-wide quality assurance. W.B. Saunders, Philadelphia, p 8

Wray J, Maresh M 1997 Multiprofressional guidelines: can we move beyond tribal boundaries? Quality in Health Care 6:57–58

Wright J 1997 Guidelines and clinical effectiveness conference notes. Meeting of Obstetric and Gynaecology Audit Networking Group, Hosted on behalf of the RCOG Clinical Audit Unit 3 October at Bradford Royal Infirmary 1997.

Zimkin T 1985 Do they mean us? New Age 28, 23. In: Webb B 1995 A study of complaints by patients of different age groups in an NHS trust. Nursing Standard 9(42):34–37 July 12–18

Lifelong learning

12

Ransolina Morgan

The dynamic nature of contemporary society requires practitioners who can respond positively to change in a creative and flexible manner. Learning should not cease at the point of registration; in fact, registration should be seen as the beginning of more meaningful learning when things learnt in the pre-registration period fall into place. Learning opportunities can be found everyday and in many situations, some of which are more obvious than others.

This chapter explores the concept of lifelong learning and its benefits not only to the individual, but also to the profession, as a means of protecting the general public. Maternity care expectations are changing; with better education women are more aware of their needs and rights and are articulate and assertive enough to rightly demand high standards of care. The Changing childbirth report (DoH 1993) advocates woman-centred care and challenges practitioners to provide sound information to enable women to make informed choices. To meet these demands, midwives have to be not only competent but also confident to work in a multidisciplinary team to deliver high quality care.

Post-registration educational requirements of midwives will be explored with suggestions of how these can be achieved and maintained. The value of learning from experience will be discussed, and how this can be used to gain academic credit.

THE LIFELONG LEARNER

The concept of lifelong learning is not new. Javis (1983) believes that people have an insatiable appetite for knowledge, which is necessary in order to relate to the society as a whole. This basic need to learn, he believes, is satisfied by adequate provision of learning opportunities. Knapper & Cropley (1985) who state that the individual continues to improve his knowledge, skills and attitude throughout life to meet the demands of a changing society, support this. Every experience offers a learning opportunity, which shapes our outlook on life. Learning is therefore a continuous process (Kolb 1984), which is added to by life's experience.

The acquisition of new knowledge may be from a variety of sources, both formal and informal, and learning may be intentional or unintentional. To make use of every learning opportunity, motivation and the ability to identify and utilize the opportunity are imperative.

To be a lifelong learner entails acceptance of learning as an integral part of life with necessary adjustment of one's life pattern to accommodate this. It should be an enjoyable experience with the learner taking full responsibility by:

- identifying one's own learning needs
- setting achievable goals
- exploring and utilizing relevant learning resources
- taking steps to achieve goals
- evaluating one's own learning.

Pre-registration education should lay the foundation for self-directed and lifelong learning; educationists therefore have the responsibility to equip potential midwives with the foundation and motivation to be independent learners, foster critical thinking and challenging attitudes. The ENB (1994) stressed that the curriculum must prepare midwives to be lifelong learners. This they hope will encourage them to accept learning as ongoing throughout their professional lives recognizing that each day presents opportunities for learning. Unfortunately, these opportunities are not always taken advantage of, as they are not always recognized for what they are.

Characteristics of a lifelong learner

The ENB (1994) identified lifelong learners as those who are:

- innovative in their practice
- flexible to changing demand
- resourceful in their methods of working
- able to work as change agents
- able to share good practice and knowledge
- adaptable to changing health care needs
- challenging and creative in their practice
- self-reliant in their way of working
- responsible and accountable for their work.

The Changing Childbirth report (DoH 1993) expects midwives to be flexible, and to evaluate their practices and respond effectively to the changing needs of the women that they care for. To be flexible, one has to be confident in practice. This can be achieved by engaging in continuous professional development.

Continuing education is not new in midwifery as it has been a statutory requirement since the Midwives Act of 1936 (HMSO 1936) for midwives to attend a minimum of 5 consecutive days residential refresher course, and midwives are often engaged in a variety of continuing education activities. There are now a variety of options open to midwives to meet this statutory requirement. National-board-approved courses such as the 'teaching and assessing in clinical practice', 'two week theoretical and practical refresher course' and the 'special and intensive care of the newborn' can be undertaken. The attendance of 7 national-board-approved study days within a 5 year period can also count as a refresher course. With the approval of the supervisor of midwives, a midwife can choose to use a non-national-board-approved course as a form of refreshment provided it can be justified as relevant to midwifery practice. Midwifery as a profession has progressed from the days when midwives were uneducated women whose only credential was personal experience of childbirth. From a 3 month training offered by the London Obstetrical Society, midwives now attain a high level of education at either diploma or degree level, preparing them academically and professionally to meet the demands of the community and fulfil the requirement of employers who expect highly skilled and knowledgeable employees (ENB 1998).

A practice-based profession such as midwifery necessitates continuous updating to keep abreast of knowledge that is evidence based to inform practice and enable midwives to meet not only the physical but also the sociological and psychological needs of women and their families. They also have to be equipped to work in both low and high technology areas and learn about new methods of managing different aspects of care.

The UKCC recognized the importance of supporting practitioners in the immediate post-registration period in order to consolidate what had been learnt and build the necessary confidence required to practise autonomously. This period of preceptorship is beneficial to the new practitioners who will be better prepared to take full responsibility of personal practice and work more effectively within the multidisciplinary team. Fulfilling this role will also enhance the preceptor's supervision and assessing skills. Supporting a new practitioner in the socialization process is a challenge and will provide the preceptor with the opportunity for reflection and self-evaluation. Being a preceptor to newly registered practitioners or supervisor/assessor to students and contributing to the education and development of others can be a means of professional development if the opportunities that these roles present are recognized and utilized appropriately.

How we learn

Many authors agree that we learn from experience (Boud, Keogh & Walker 1985, Javis 1983, Kolb 1984). Midwifery provides ample experiences from which one can learn; however, these opportunities are not always made good use of for a variety of reasons. Experience cannot be gained in isolation; for learning to take place links will have to be made with past and predicted future experience, as our past and current experiences will influence our future practice

and relationships in either a positive or a negative way. Learning from experience can therefore be seen as a 'magnetic cycle' that attracts new learning on its travels.

What is done with the experience gained is just as important, if not more important than simply gaining the experience. Each experience whether good or bad can be utilized in a positive way to promote growth and development; Boud, Keogh & Walker (1985) argued, however, that if the experience is stifled then learning will not take place.

Learning from experience will be addressed later in the chapter.

Adults as learners

Knowles (1980) used the term 'andragogy' to describe the theory of adult learning. This he explains, is the art and science of adult education where the learner is in control of the learning, assisted by the educator. Javis (1983) states that an adult learner takes an active part and directs the learning by seeking the relevant information. In contrast to this student-centred approach, 'pedagogy' (the way children are taught) can lead to frustration among adult learners as the teacher takes control of the learning in a non-negotiating way which may not fulfil the needs of the adult learner. Those whose past experience of learning was based on the pedagogical approach may find the shift to self-directed learning difficult if not daunting. This may be compounded if their work environment is hierarchical and they feel powerless and not part of the decision-making process, which is controlled by others. Directing one's own practice as an autonomous practitioner will foster confidence in directing one's own learning and professional development.

Knowles (1980) identified four features of andragogy:

1. *change in self-concept*—for learning to be self-directed a high self-esteem and self-confidence is important
2. *experience*—experience gained must be used as an important learning resource

3. *readiness to learn*—this will be stimulated by the relevance of the learning event
4. *orientation towards learning*—a problem-solving approach makes learning more meaningful.

To be in the position to empower women, midwives must feel empowered themselves. This will stem from self-confidence and self-esteem, which increase with sound knowledge, competence and confidence. Empowered practitioners are able to defend their practice and give correct and unbiased information to the women for whom they care. Confidence is gained when the competence gained at the point of registration becomes strengthened in an environment that is conducive to learning.

Although midwives are exposed to a variety of experiences every working day, these are not always recognized as learning resources and many valuable opportunities may be missed; some help may be required from more experienced midwives to help the less experienced ones to identify and effectively utilize learning opportunities. One's values and beliefs affect learning and may lead to inappropriate selection of available resources.

Attempting to deal with the complexities and uncertainty of midwifery often leads to misinterpretation of the selected material. It is understandable for people to respond to uncertainty by drawing on past experience and making predictions about the effect of possible actions.

Adults do not learn for the sake of learning; whatever they learn has got to be meaningful and relevant. Learners must not only want to learn but must also believe that learning is possible. They learn when they are motivated and are able to exercise choice and control over what they learn. The quality of their learning improves when they can pace their learning to meet their particular needs (Gibbs 1992). Accumulating knowledge for the sake of it is not attractive to adults; they regard learning as a tool to help them solve problems.

Learning styles

People adopt learning styles that they find beneficial to them. The end result may be the same though the route by which the outcomes are achieved may vary. Honey & Mumford (1986) suggest that each individual has a preferred or dominant learning style and agree with Brookfield (1986) that adults make use of a variety of learning styles in order to get the most out of the available experience. Being aware of what one's preferred learning style is will facilitate learning.

The four styles identified by Honey & Mumford (1986) are as follows:

- *Activists*—these are people who are willing to try new experiences without bias. They thrive on challenge and find excitement in activity.
- *Reflectors*—these like to take time to think about the situation before committing themselves. They stand back to ponder over experiences, and observe them from different perspectives before coming to any conclusions.
- *Theorists*—these try to make connections and relate one situation to another. They are analytical and objective and tend to be perfectionists.
- *Pragmatists*—these look for ways of applying theory to practice, searching for new ideas and taking the first opportunity to put it into operation.

No one style is superior to another; making use of one's own preferred learning style is likely to produce better results, but it can be helpful to develop different learning styles (Laurillard 1979, 1994, Miller, Tomlinson & Jones 1994) according to context or goal.

Following research and clinical observation, Kolb (1984) also described four basic learning styles, as follows:

- *Accommodators*—these thrive best in situations where they are involved in new experiences. They solve problems in a trial and error manner, relying on information gathered by other people.
- *Convergers*—these operate by problem solving and practical application. For them, there is only one answer to a problem. They relate better to technical problems than to social or interpersonal issues.

- *Divergers*—their strength lies in concrete experience and reflective observation and they view situations from different perspectives before arriving at a decision. They perform better in situations where alternative ideas and implications are generated.
- *Assimilators*—these are more concerned with ideas and abstract concepts. Their ability to create theoretical models and convert them into explanations is one of their strengths.

A flexible adult learner can utilize the learning style which suits the appropriate event in order to get the best out of the situation. Although Honey & Mumford's terminology are different from those used by Kolb to describe the different learning styles, it can be seen that the descriptions are similar; for example, activists and accommodators both enjoy the challenge of new experiences.

Learning from experience

Many authors agree that experiential learning is the most meaningful method of learning for adults and that it is a continuous process, going through various steps and arriving back at the concrete experience (Boud & Walker 1991, Javis 1985, Kolb 1984). It results from active participation in an event rather being told about it. This is supported by Brennan & Little (1996) who argue that learning is not confined to educational institutions but can and does take place in a variety of settings. Valuable as it is, it is often taken for granted and many find it difficult to articulate what they have learnt from a given experience (Clarke & Warr 1997). Taking full advantage of learning in the clinical setting promotes continuous professional development and learning becomes recognized and accepted as a lifelong event. How the learner perceives and responds to events, and the awareness of the factors which influence such behaviour, are all involved in the experience. Kolb (1984) describes his model of experiential learning in four stages:

1. *Concrete experience*—this is the actual involvement of the learner in the learning event.

2. *Reflective observation*—this is engagement in deep thought in an attempt to make sense of the experience, by asking difficult questions and challenging perceptions.

3. *Abstract conceptualization*—this is critical analysis of the event and examining alternatives, results in conclusions being formed and justification of concepts

4. *Active experimentation*—what is learnt is now put into practice in a variety of settings. The modified experience will be tested to foster continuation of the learning process and improvement of practice.

Kolb (1984) agrees that experiential learning can be quite complex, making it difficult to understand. Although this type of learning is in harmony with a practice-based profession such as midwifery, a lot of thought and planning is necessary if full benefit is to be achieved (Evans 1994). The ability to reflect is an important quality required by the practitioner, and should be done in a structured way.

REFLECTION

The terms 'reflection' and 'reflective practice' are now commonly used in midwifery and nursing practice but interpretations of what these terms mean and the result of reflection can be varied. Stuart (1997) agrees that the desired effect is not always achieved, as the process is influenced by the interval between the event and the reflective process. Reflection is a skill that develops over time. While some find it relatively easy, many people have to work hard to achieve effective reflection which enhances learning. Chapter 2 addresses reflection in more detail but the following definitions might also be helpful. According to Boud, Keogh & Walker (1985), reflection is 'those intellectual and affective activities in which individuals engage to explore their experiences in order to lead to new understandings and appreciations' (p. 19). Mezirow (1991) defines it as 'the intentional reassessment of prior learning to re-establish its validity by identifying and correcting distortions on its content, process or premises' (p. 15).

Broadly speaking, reflection encompasses returning to the experience, identifying the positive and negative aspects, giving meaning to them and making a decision as to how to improve on that experience. A change in one's knowledge, skills and attitude indicate that learning has taken place. Because reflection is often associated with critical incidents, the less experienced may misinterpret 'critical' to mean 'dramatic' and therefore may fail to reflect on events that, though subtle, can be a good learning experience. An incident that is critical to one practitioner may not be critical to another. Reflection may reveal uncomfortable truths about oneself, which have to be confronted if progress is to be made. Many midwives already engage in reflection in an informal way either alone or collectively with colleagues at meal breaks. A structured and more formal approach is necessary for a better result to be achieved. Reflection therefore has to be deliberate, conscious and exploratory. Kirkham (1997) points out how uncomfortable it can be to see oneself through the eyes of others, whether they are students or clients. The ability to justify one's actions will lead to evaluation of practice, which will enhance learning. Steele (1998) advocates honesty in self-examination to establish the effect of the incident on the person and vice versa. Learning results from reflection when the experience has been fully explored, taking into account not only actions but feelings of and thoughts about the situation. This will give a clearer insight and better understanding, which will inform future practice. Utilizing what has been learnt from experience to effect change will prevent mistakes being made over and over again.

Individuals attach different meaning and importance to any given event. The individual experiencing the event is as relevant as the event itself, which is of little significance unless it is put in context. The experience, motivation and personality of the observer will determine the interpretation of the event, which can be influenced by a variety of factors including mental or physical alertness, stress, attitude, beliefs and expectation.

Much has been written about reflection by educational theorists (Boud, Keogh & Walker 1985, Mezirow 1981, Schön 1991). They are all in agreement that reflection is a continuum which starts with an experience, has an analysis and evaluation stage, and then goes back to the experience to recommence the cycle. Schön (1991), however, places the emphasis on awareness of the situation, while Mezirow (1991) believes that self-awareness is more important.

Schön (1991) makes a distinction between reflection in action and reflection on action. With reflection in action, the experience and the reflection occur simultaneously. The practitioner identifies a new situation, thinks about it and makes a decision on how to respond to it. Experience and confidence are necessary prerequisites for this type of reflection to take place.

Reflection on action occurs after the event when the practitioner is able to devote time to critical analysis and evaluation.

Aids to reflection

The meaning given to an experience is personal and is influenced by one's perception of the event. A woman's decision to stop breast feeding may seem insignificant to someone who may regard it as her choice. However, much can be learnt about the preparation for and support of breast-feeding mothers if the event is recognized as a learning experience. In order to aid accuracy, the facts of the event should be recorded, as it happened, as soon as possible after the event. The steps outlined in Activity 12.1 may be helpful. Those who are not familiar with reflection may wish to start by focusing on the events of the last shift, being aware of any particular feelings such as happiness, satisfaction, elation or disappointment. Self-awareness and probing questions may reveal the reasons for such a feeling.

Not every day will provide opportunity for new learning; indeed learning is not synonymous with new information, and the opportunity to consolidate previous learning should not

Activity 12.1

Aids to reflection

You may wish to ask yourself a number of questions to aid reflection. The following suggestions might be helpful:

- What events occurred during the last shift?
- Which of the events were significant?
- What made it/them significant?
- Who else was involved?
- Am I pleased with the part I played?
- Why?
- What went particularly well?
- Was I unhappy about anything?
- Why?
- What have I learnt from the experience?
- What effect has it had on me, including emotional and psychological?
- How will this change my practice?

be missed. Two tools are necessary to aid reflection. These are:

- reflective log—a factual record of events
- reflective diary—interpretation and reaction to the event—physical, emotional and psychological; these may be subjective.

Deciding what is relevant to be included in a reflective log comes with experience, and develops over time. It is better to record more than is necessary until the skill is developed than not to record enough information. Stuart (1997) makes no distinction between a log and diary, believing that the emphasis should be on the opportunity for exploration and reflection, which the record makes possible.

LEARNING ENVIRONMENT

A good learning environment is one that fosters personal growth and development in a safe and supportive climate. The structure of the organization in which one works has the power to impede or encourage learning. Stress and insecurity often prevent practitioners from challenging their own or other people's practice. All members of a team contribute to the learning environment; therefore each has a responsibility

to foster a culture where learning is normal and valued. This should be an environment where experimentation of ideas and practice is supported by peers and managers, where practices can be challenged without retribution. Those who do not share the same philosophy may be antagonistic towards those who value reflective practice, thus creating barriers in the workplace. Where human resources are inadequate in comparison to the workload, priority is often given to accomplishing tasks, with very little or no time to review experience in a meaningful way. The longer the interval between the event and the reflective process, the greater is the likelihood of inaccurate recall of the event. The ENB (1994) states that a learning organization should have, among other attributes, a reflection of the needs of patients and clients at the core of their policies. Collaboration between educationists, service providers and practitioners is essential in the planning and management of work-based learning.

LEARNING OPPORTUNITIES

To be in the position to provide the expected high quality, client-centred care, continuing professional development is imperative (DoH 1994, ENB 1995). Universities offer a wide range of health-related programmes at certificate, diploma, degree and postgraduate levels, but not all will be specifically focused on developing midwifery practice. The ENB framework and higher award provide a flexible and practice-focused vehicle for practitioners to continue their education following registration. There can be selection from a menu of options within the framework, or the practitioner can follow a path leading to the ENB higher award and higher education honours degree. Accreditation of prior learning may be required in order to access the higher award, this will be discussed later. Although midwives have always been required to attend refresher courses every 5 years, post-registration education and practice (PREP) now requires midwives, nurses and health visitors not only to embark on post-registration education on a 3 year cycle, but to take responsibility for the type of programme they attend. They have to determine how their practice will be enhanced by the new learning. PREP often causes anxiety to practitioners, and some regard these four letters with suspicion (Voulsden 1998). Its intention is to protect the public by encouraging practitioners to maintain high professional standards. The PREP recommendations are only a slight variation from what midwives have always been required to do; as follows:

• *Notifying their intentions to practise*—however, in addition to midwives giving this notification to the supervisor of midwives in March each year, midwives, nurses and health visitors who are in current practice will have to complete a notification of practice form when they renew their registration every 3 years.

• *Periodic refreshment*—this has been a statutory requirement since 1936. The 5 year refreshment for midwives will continue until year 2000. From April 2001, all midwives will have to fulfil the PREP requirement, which is the equivalent of at least 5 days of relevant study every 3 years.

• *Return to practice refresher courses*—nurses and health visitors now fall into line with midwives who have always been required to undertake a specified length of refresher course before returning to practice, if they have been out of practice for at least 5 years.

Apart from the statutory refresher courses, many midwives have always engaged in other forms of continuing education both locally and nationally. They are now being encouraged to record such events and provide evidence of what learning took place. The emphasis is not so much on the education activities that the midwife has undertaken, but what was gained from the activities and how they will be used to inform practice.

PREP offers a more flexible way of maintaining professional development. Periodic refreshment can be undertaken in a variety of ways ranging from academic courses, attendance at half or full study days, visiting another unit, or privately exploring a topic of interest. The key issue is that the study must be relevant to the practitioner's professional practice. The choice of study has to be justified, and the manager has to be convinced that the needs of the practitioner, the establishment and the profession will be met and that the objectives set are realistic and achievable, as resources in terms of time and finance will be invested in the event. A good case therefore has to be thoughtfully prepared before attempting to negotiate study leave or funding. The UKCC has identified five broad categories to assist practitioners in the planning of their study activities. These are:

1. *patient, client, and colleague support*—which can include counselling skills
2. *care enhancement*—which may incorporate new approaches to care
3. *practice development*—this can be a relevant visit outside one's normal place of work, to enhance practice
4. *reducing risk*—this can include health promotion
5. *education development*—which can take the form of personal research.

The 10 key characteristics identified by the ENB (see Box 12.1) complement the above categories, giving practitioners a wide scope so that they can plan the most appropriate post-registration education to equip themselves to function effectively, and be able to review their practice. If the needs of society are changing, it follows that the educational needs of practitioners must also change. It is no longer enough to be competent only in the physical care of mothers. All aspects of care have to be considered; the sociological and psychological care are just as important and midwives have to be in the position to give holistic care to all mothers, taking into account their cultural, ethnic, religious and sexual orientation. It may be necessary to shop around in order to get the type of education that is appropriate and offers value for money. Distance learning may have to be considered by those who are restricted by domestic or other commitments; this, however, will not meet the needs of those for whom group interaction and peer support are important.

The practitioner should be clear about:

• the relevance of the event to current practice and career development

1. *Accountability*—ability to exercise professional accountability and responsibility in all spheres of practice, demonstrating sound knowledge and skills.
2. *Clinical skills*—possessing relevant specialist expertise to meet the specific needs of the client group being card for.
3. *Use of research*—ability to improve care by appropriate use of research to plan, implement and evaluate care.
4. *Team work*—ability to function within a multidisciplinary team in a flexible way to accommodate changing needs of clients and team members.
5. *Innovation*—ability to respond to the needs of clients' and employer's goals in an innovative and flexible manner.
6. *Health promotion*—appropriate use of health promotion strategies.
7. *Staff development*—active participation in the professional development of other staff members including learners.
8. *Resource management*—ability to utilize relevant information to allocate resources to benefit every client.
9. *Quality of care*—ability to evaluate standards set on an ongoing basis.
10. *Management of change*—ability to initiate, manage and evaluate change in practice.

Adapted from ENB (1991).

- the learning outcomes
- personal objectives
- how the event will be evaluated.

Until practitioners become confident in planning their own refreshment, guidance from supervisors of midwives, managers or educators will be required. Peer teaching and support should not be underestimated as a lot can be learnt from the experiences of other colleagues either on a one to one basis or in a group.

CREDIT ACCUMULATION AND TRANSFER SCHEME (CATS)

Education establishments in general, and midwifery education in particular, have had to adjust very quickly to many changes in the last few years. This has created much uncertainty for many practitioners and educationalists alike. One of the positive outcomes of this is the acknowledgement that repetitious learning is not only unnecessary but also uneconomic in more ways than one, and that learning takes place in a variety of settings for which credit can be given. The ENB framework provides the mechanism for achieving the UKCC standards of post–registration education in a structured but flexible way (Brown 1995). This makes it possible for practitioners to maintain their professional development in a variety of ways, and receive recognition and credit for the same. This is done through the CATS system, which makes it possible for academic credits to be awarded for learning provided it can be assessed (Hull & Redfern 1996, SEEC 1995). The flexibility of this system makes access to higher education possible for many who would not have otherwise had the opportunity to study at a higher level.

The Council for National Academic Awards (CNAA) which was responsible for validating awards in higher education institutions, such as polytechnics, recognized the need for flexibility in education attainment, acknowledging that learning occurs not only in formal settings but also in informal settings both intentionally and unintentionally, with some repetition of information. In the mid 1980s it introduced a system whereby previous learning can be recognized and given credits. The Open University Validation Service replaced CNAA in 1994. The ENB-validated programmes undertaken as part of the framework or the higher award are normally based on this system. CATS comprises of three elements: credit accumulation, credit transfer and credit exemption.

- *Credit accumulation*—credits can be accumulated or collected from a range of learning experiences to form part of the total credits required for a qualification.
- *Credit transfer*—credits gained in the past can be transferred from one programme to another either within the same institution or between institutions.
- *Credit exemption*—the recognition of previous learning makes it possible for exemption to be granted from a section of a course to avoid unnecessary repetition.

As Fox et al (1992) testify, the system can be complex and protracted as there has to be ample evidence to establish the quality and extent of the learning that had taken place, and that it equates to the learning outcomes of the programme from which exemption is sought. The education establishment has to justify the exemption or different entry point to a programme. Although the possibility of transferring relevant learning between programmes and institutions exists, the lack of central coordination of the scheme creates limitations. Lack of understanding between institutions with regards to standards and the desire of institutions to preserve their own standards often restrict the easy transfer of credits, and they may be reluctant to accept credits from other institutions. This necessitates some form of assessment of prior learning to enable the institution to award credits that can then be transferred to the programme of study or used to seek exemption. Unfortunately, lack of standardization causes frustration for some claimants whose credits from one institution may not be accepted by another.

What exactly are credits?

Credits are numerical values assigned to a specified learning experience that demonstrates that a particular level has been achieved. General credits are awarded for previous unaccredited learning, both certificated and non-certificated, when the claimant's learning has been assessed. The credits are unrelated to a specific module or course of study. These will have to be matched against the outcomes of a particular programme of study if credit transfer or exemption is required. Specific credits are obtained by matching the claimant's previous learning against the learning outcomes of the respective module or programme to be accessed. The credits awarded will be directly related to the programme in question.

The credit system works on the basis that 360 credits are required to obtain an honours degree, 240 credits for a diploma and 120 for a certificate course.

Level 1 (120 credits). This is equivalent to the standard of a certificate level course or 1st year of a degree course. Acquisition and understanding of knowledge, skills and attitude are demonstrated and applied to professional practice.

Level 2 (120 credits). This equates to a diploma level course, or 2nd year of a degree course. The learner is expected to be able to analyse critically, and be selective in the use of knowledge to inform practice.

Level 3 (120 credits). This is the standard of study of the third year of a degree course. This higher level of study requires creativity and the ability to synthesize, evaluate and select relevant knowledge appropriately to inform practice in a variety of settings.

Accreditation of prior learning (APL)

This is the recognition and the award of academic credits for learning that has been achieved through a formal course that was not credit rated. This includes courses offered at certificate level. The value of the credits assigned to a particular programme of study is determined by the institution offering the programme. One institution can, for example, offer 20 level 2 credits for the ENB Course 997, while another institution may offer 40 level 2 credits for the same course. This partly explains why some institutions are reluctant to accept credits from others without verification of their standards.

Accreditation of prior experiential learning (APEL)

It is now possible for credits to be awarded for learning that has taken place in non-formal settings that was not formally assessed, but for which the learner can provide evidence that learning did take place (SEEC 1995). This learning may have been achieved through life experiences in general, often unintentionally, during paid or unpaid work or study that was not formally certified. For prior learning to be accredited, it should be meaningful and relevant, and the onus is on the claimant to prove the extent of the learning that had taken place and identify the change in knowledge, skills and attitude that has resulted.

APEL places the emphasis on learning rather than teaching or learning opportunities, and practitioners are required to be in the position to articulate the learning that has taken place (see Ch. 2). It makes it possible for those who, for a variety of reasons, have not undertaken any formal course of study following registration, but have continued to learn from their experiences, to gain academic credits. The author has experience of midwives who undervalue their clinical experience and expertise and feel threatened by student midwives who are studying at a higher level. This is supported by Houston, Hoover & Beer (1997), who found that practitioners placed more value on previous educational experiences and were less able to draw on clinical experiences. Although often unintentional and informal, learning from experience is equally as important as formal learning as long as it can be articulated in a way that makes assessment possible (Garbett 1997).

Making a claim

For many practitioners, this will be a new experience which requires patience and good time management as it can be time consuming (Houston, Hoover & Beer 1997). To make a successful claim, the ability to reflect and identify and articulate learning experiences in a way that appropriate assessment could be made is imperative. Self-awareness and analytical skills are required for this complex process (Fox et al 1992). A well-kept reflective diary will prove to be an invaluable tool. The following points are likely to be applicable across universities.

The claimant has to decide on the value and level of credits required (specific or general) and be in a position to provide evidence to support the claim. If you intend to make a claim, you will be wise to allow yourself ample time between submitting the claim and the commencement of the intended programme of study.

It is not the responsibility of the assessor to search for the evidence in a mass of information provided, it is up to the claimant to identify clearly the appropriate evidence. Application is made using an approved form, and a fee is normally charged, which the appropriate education establishment determines. In some cases, this can be quite costly.

An advisor has been found to be helpful to guide applicants and ensure suitable submission is made that will be acceptable to the assessors. This will include advice on how to present the evidence to attract the required credits. If there is a shortfall, advice will be given as to how the deficits can be made up, which might take the form of a written or an oral assessment.

The number of hours an advisor will give per claim will vary between institutions, this should be clarified at the start of the process (SEEC 1995). The advisors are familiar with the criteria used by the assessors to award credits and are therefore well placed to advise and support claimants. It is good practice to ensure that the evidence provided is scrutinized by at least two assessors before the claims approval board approves credits. APL claims for courses longer than 5 years may necessitate evidence of the claimant's application of the acquired knowledge to practise. The use of profiling is invaluable when making a claim especially a claim for experiential learning. Though relatively new in midwifery, profiling has been in use in other spheres for many years (Price 1994).

PORTFOLIO OR PROFILE? WHAT IS THE DIFFERENCE?

The often interchangeable use of these two terms can be confusing. The UKCC often refers to 'personal professional profile', while the ENB publishes a 'professional portfolio' folder for use when accessing the higher award. Brown (1995) offers a distinction between the two, which many will find helpful. She considers portfolio to be a comprehensive compilation of evidence of one's achievement and development covering every facet of one's life. This could include voluntary work, paid employment, professional development and personal attributes and interests. Evidence to support these achievements could be presented in a variety of forms, including audio tapes, diaries, certificates, letter of commendation, photographs, or in any way that demonstrates creativity and innovation. It should reflect not only past achievements, but also current activities and future projections. Because of the nature of its content, a portfolio is private and personal with access restricted to the owner.

A personal profile on the other hand, is deliberately compiled for a particular purpose and for a particular audience. It is extrapolated from one's portfolio and is confined to a specific aspect of one's achievement. A professional profile will therefore contain evidence of development in the professional sphere and will include professional qualifications, critical incident analysis, evidence of attendance and evaluations of study days and conferences attended, personal publications and so on. For instance, a profile constructed to support an application for the post of a play group leader, will contain evidence such as experience of caring for children formally or informally, knowledge of child protection issues and so on. The fact that the information is designed for a particular purpose differentiates it from a portfolio. It is therefore no longer private to the owner alone but can be open to scrutiny by the identified audience—for example, members of an interview panel. For this reason, it is understandable that Brown (1995) advocates caution with regards to confidentiality and ethical considerations when recording incidents in the profile. If the distinction between profile and portfolio is acceptable, most midwives will be more concerned with compiling a professional profile than a portfolio.

Functions of a profile

Although the main function of compiling a profile is to meet one of the UKCC requirement for maintaining registration, there are other benefits not only to the midwife herself but to the managers. For the practitioner, it encourages reflection and makes her value her achievements, especially experiential learning. This will boost self-esteem and confidence and put her in a better bargaining position when negotiating support for professional development activities. Learning needs can be identified and appropriate plans made to meet those needs. The

manager will be able to assess the calibre of the midwife with less difficulty especially if working conditions are such that the opportunity to assess staff in practice is limited.

A professional profile can be used for a variety of reasons. Hull & Redfern (1996) warn that this should be considered when compiling one so that the relevant intentions will be conveyed to the selected audience, especially if those scrutinizing the evidence are not midwives and therefore cannot be expected to be familiar with midwifery culture and priorities. Many midwives, nurses and health visitors regard this exercise as unattractive, partly because of the compulsory nature of the UKCC requirement. However, this document can be used for a variety of reasons including those listed below and summarized in Box 12.2.

- to support a job application
- to claim academic credits though the APL/APEL system
- to identify learning needs and plan future goals
- to justify or reject career change.

Box 12.2 **Functions of a professional profile**
• **Promote** self-awareness
• **Review** performance
• **Opportunity** for negotiation
• **Foster** personal and professional development
• **Interviews** for job
• **Learning** needs identification
• **Experiential** learning is valued.

Compiling a profile therefore entails taking stock of yourself, consider where you are now, and how you got there. Is this where you would like to be? If not where would you like to be? Having decided where you would like to be, decide how you are going to get there, the help you might need to achieve this and the timescale.

Compiling a profile

It is worth remembering that a profile is more than a record of educational events attended. A comprehensive profile will include evidence of personal and professional development, and formulation of an action plan for the future. Kelly (1998) stressed that reflection is imperative if this is to be achieved. There is no wrong or right way of setting about this; the uniqueness of individuals and individual needs make it unhelpful to be prescriptive about the format or content. The perception and utilization of learning opportunities will vary between individuals and will to some extent influence the content and style of this document. The volume of information contained in the profile may be extensive; therefore a concise recording will make access easier. A half-hearted profile is of little use, therefore a lot of thought has to go into the planning.

A common question that midwives ask, is: where to start? The best place to start is where you feel most comfortable, where reflection and self-awareness are possible. You might find it helpful to start with a curriculum vitae (CV), and then expand on it, though it should not be seen as a mini version of the profile. Box 12.3 gives an example of headings for a CV.

Box 12.3 Information that could be included in a curriculum vitae

Personal details to include
Name
Address
Telephone number
Date of birth
Education
Pre 16 years
Post 16 years
Further education
Professional qualifications
Employment history (starting with the most recent)
Midwifery
Non-midwifery
Achievements
Awards
Scholarships
Innovations
Publications
Interests
Membership of professional organizations
Names of two referees

There are many profiles on the market, varying in cost and user friendliness. Buying a ready-made profile may be attractive to those who find the prescribed format helpful. A home-made one using a ring binder and dividers can be just as good, however, with some thought and creativity. Mitchell's (1997) critical review of a selection of commercially produced profiles supports Hull & Redfern (1996) in their call for careful thought and consideration before deciding which one to buy. Price (1994) warns that having a well–presented document does not necessarily mean that it will serve the intended purpose. It should, however, be comprehensive, coherent, accessible and flexible. The UKCC (1996) suggest, as a guide, three stages that could be considered:

1. review of past experience
2. self-appraisal
3. formulation of action plan.

1. *Review of past experience*—it is a matter of personal preference how far back this should be taken. Not all experience will be relevant, therefore you will have to be selective. Experience gained in other spheres such as voluntary work may be relevant to your professional development, especially areas that have enhanced leadership or interpersonal skills. Reflect on areas of professional practice where you have excelled, and where you have made a difference, however small. Also consider your disappointments, and what you have learnt from them. There may be areas where you feel uncomfortable and wish to improve. Collect all available evidence such as statements of attendance at study days. This is likely to take time; it will be wise to allow yourself plenty of time and set realistic deadlines.

2. Self-appraisal—this involves the ability to identify your strengths and weaknesses and formulate future plans. Give yourself credit where it is due and formulate plans to convert weakness into strength. An honest soul-searching exercise will be required. The ENB 10 key characteristics (see Box 12.1, p. 207) may be a useful guide to appraise your personal growth and development. You might find using the SWOT analysis (Box 12.4) helpful. This allows you to

---

Box 12.4 **Example of SWOT analysis**

Strengths
I enjoy supporting learners and newly registered practitioners, and many midwives value my experience. Having completed a course in counselling, I work as a volunteer counsellor at the women's centre.

Weaknesses
My time management is not always good, which leaves me little time for reading. My professional journals therefore remain in their wrappers for a long time before I make time to browse through them.

Opportunities
Our team leader is very enthusiastic and encourages midwives to utilize every opportunity that is available. Our link midwife teacher is supportive and always willing to offer help.

Threats
Many of my colleagues are studying for degrees. Although I undertake single modules that are of interest to me, I do not feel that I can commit myself to studying for a degree. I feel threatened that soon I will be one of the few who are not graduates. All midwives in our unit may be required to rotate into the community. I cannot drive, and I fear that my job might be at stake.

---

try to identify your strengths and weaknesses, the opportunities available to you and the factors that may be threatening to you.

For your strengths, be positive about yourself. Kelly (1998) believes that there is sometimes a tendency to overlook positive qualities and underestimate ourselves, while negative feedback dominates our conscious minds.

For your weaknesses, these may be ones that you have identified yourself or ones that other people such as colleagues, students or managers have brought to your notice. You can afford to be honest as only you can convert them into positive attributes.

For your opportunities, there are many resources that can be utilized to reach your goal. These may include colleagues, libraries and distance-learning packs.

For the perceived threats, in the present climate, you may identity a number of factors that may be deemed threatening. There have been and continue to be changes in the NHS, which will have direct or indirect impact at local level. Your biggest threat may, alternatively, be a particular individual within your work environment.

3. *Formulation of action plan*—having critically examined yourself, and identified your strengths and weaknesses, you will be in a position to identify areas that require attention and where you would like to develop. Consider a realistic action plan, maybe in consultation with a trusted colleague, setting yourself a realistic timescale. Review the action plan periodically and update as necessary.

Because this exercise is learner centred, it should empower midwives to take responsibility for their own professional development, and place more value on their experience and achievements. Carol Bates (1996) advocates planned learning skills exercises for those who have not studied recently and are now required to study at a higher level. This she believes will give the practitioners confidence and a positive mental attitude to embark on studying.

In the author's experience, midwives often cite time as an inhibiting factor to professional development. With work and family commitments, they complain that there appears to be little time for anything else. It is true that we can always fill whatever time we have, in the same way we can always make time for things that we deem important. By utilizing the available time more efficiently, it can be surprising how much can be achieved. It might be worth considering some form of time management strategy.

TIME MANAGEMENT

A useful starting point is to appraise how your time is spent currently, and try to justify the amount of time that is spent on each activity. You can either reflect on your activities during the past 2 weeks or, if this is difficult, start keeping a diary for the next 2 weeks. Two weeks is the minimum time; a month will provide a better and more realistic picture. Record every single activity, including watching television, telephone calls, shopping and going to the school concert. Try to justify the activities and the times spent on each of them and make necessary adjustment. You might find it useful to list all the activities in order of priority, which will make it easier to eliminate those that you can do without. You will need to make allowances for unexpected or infrequent demands on your time such as unexpected babysitting for your neighbour, a friend dropping in for coffee and a chat, or finding a note in your child's pocket about a parents' meeting that day. Try using one sheet of paper for each day to give yourself plenty of space to write as much as you need to. It is useful to remember that work, family commitment and social activities are all important and should be given due consideration. This exercise should be reviewed periodically as commitments and demands on your time change.

Summary

Learning is a lifelong event. A rapidly changing profession such as midwifery demands professionals who are prepared to accept learning as an ongoing process, in order to meet the demands of employers and clients. As a practice-based profession, there are many potential learning opportunities available which midwives can make use of with the right type of support. Employers expect employees to maintain a high standard and take responsibility for learning and to keep abreast of the ever-changing NHS.

Brookfield (1986) believes that the adult's life experience is an important learning resources and it has been shown how valuable this can be. For those who have not engaged in formal learning for a long time, or whose last study was at certificate level, lifelong learning and continuing education present a challenge. Learning empowers midwives, who in turn will empower the women they care for. Adults are stimulated to learn when the environment is conducive. Recognizing your dominant learning style will help you to get the most out of available learning experience. The ability to reflect also aids experiential learning.

This chapter shows how midwives can keep themselves updated and the value of taking responsibility for this. It has shown how past experience can be used to gain academic awards, as academic credits can be gained for both formal and experiential learning, and how compilation of professional profile can be used in a variety of ways to provide evidence of learning. All practitioners are required to maintain a professional profile.

With the various demands on the time of practitioners, good time management is imperative if all responsibilities are to be met, including professional, domestic and personal commitments. Midwives who are in control of their own education and practice are more likely to empower the women they care for to exercise choice and take control of their care.

Maintaining a comprehensive and flexible professional profile serves not only as a requirement of the UKCC but will also help to promote self-awareness, help the practitioner to identify appropriate learning needs and take steps to meet them.

REFERENCES

Bates C 1996 Study skills, fears, the future and the feel-good factor. Midwives October 109 (1305):272

Boud D, Walker D 1991 Experience and learning: reflection at work. Deakin, Geelong

Boud D, Keogh R, Walker D (eds) 1985 Reflection: turning experience into learning. Kogan Page, London

Brennan J, Little B 1996 A review of work-based learning in higher education. Department for Education and Employment, London

Brookfield S D 1986 Understanding and facilitating adult learning. Open University, Milton Keynes

Brown R A 1995 Portfolio development and profiling for nurses, 2nd edn. Quay Books, Salisbury

Clarke J B, Warr J 1997 Academic validation of prior and experiential learning: evaluation of the process. Journal of Advanced Nursing 26:1235–1242

DoH (Department of Health) 1993 Changing childbirth: report of the expert maternity group. HMSO, London

DoH (Department of Health) 1994 Nursing, midwifery and health visiting education: a statement of strategic intent.

Nursing, Midwifery and Health Visitor Education Forum, London

ENB (English National Board) 1991 Framework for continuing professional education for nurses midwives and health visitors. ENB, London

ENB (English National Board) 1994 Creating lifelong learners. Partnerships for Care. ENB, London

ENB (English National Board) 1995 Midwifery factfile continuing professional development. ENB, London

ENB (English National Board) 1998 Guidelines for pre-registration midwifery programmes of education. ENB, London

Evans N 1994 Experiential teaching for all, Cassell. London

Fox J, Nyatanga L, Ringer C, Greaves L 1992 APL: a corporate strategy. Nurse Education Today 12(3):221–226

Garbett R 1997 What's the point of APL/APEL. Nursing Times Learning Curve 1(2):15

Gibbs G 1992 Improving the quality of student learning. Technical and Education, Bristol

HMSO 1936 Midwives Act. HMSO, London

Honey P, Mumford A 1986 The manual of learning styles. Maidenhead. In: Bolt E, Powell J (eds) 1993 Becoming reflective. South Bank University, London, p 20

Houston L Y, Hoover J, Beer E 1997 Accreditation of prior learning: is it worth it? An evaluation of a pilot scheme. Nurse Education Today 17(3):184–191

Hull C, Redfern L 1996 Profiles and portfolios. A guide for nurses and midwives. Macmillan, London

Javis P 1983 Professional education. New partners of learning. Croom Helm, London

Javis P 1985 The sociology of adult and continuing education. Croom Helm, London

Kelly E S 1998 Self-awareness and development of your professional portfolio. RCM Midwives Journal (mid-month suppl) March:4–5

Kirkham M 1997 Reflection in midwifery: professional narcissism or seeing with women? British Journal of Midwifery 5(5):259–262

Knapper C K, Cropley A J 1985 Lifelong learning in higher education. Croom Helm, London

Knowles M 1980 The modern practice of adult education: from pedagogy to andragogy. Adult Education Co, New York

Kolb D A 1984 Experiential learning. Experience as a source of learning and development. Prentice Hall, Englewood Cliffs, N J

Laurillard D 1979 The process of student learning. Higher Education 8:395–409

Laurillard D 1994 Rethinking university teaching. Routledge, London

Mezirow J 1981 A critical theory of adult learning and education. Adult Education 32(1):3–24

Mezirow J 1991 Transformative dimensions in adult learning. Jossey Bass, San Francisco

Miller C, Tomlinson A, Jones M 1994 Learning styles and facilitating reflection. Researching professional education, research report series. ENB, London

Mitchell, M 1997 A critical review of published portfolios. British Journal of Midwifery 5(12):744–747

Price A 1994 Midwifery portfolios: making reflective records. Modern Midwife 14(1):35–38

Schön D 1991 The reflective practitioner, 2nd edn. Jossey Bass, San Francisco

SEEC (South East England Consortium) 1995 SEEC code of practice for the assessment of prior experiential learning. SEEC, Brentwood

Steele R 1998 Reflection as a way of gathering evidence for your portfolios. RCM Midwives Journal (mid-month suppl) May, 4–5

Stuart C C 1997 Reflective journals as a teaching/learning strategy: a literature review. British Journal of Midwifery 5(7):434–438

UKCC 1996 PREP and profiling. Register 17(Summer):7–10

Vousden M 1998 Who's afraid of PREP? Nursing Times Learning Curve 2(1):2–3

13 Influencing the future

Diane M Fraser

This chapter aims to:

- **Engender a thirst for new knowledge and the more effective use of evidence in practice**
- **Stimulate reflection and critical debate on policy and practices in midwifery**
- **Challenge the reader to initiate and capitalize on opportunities to become actively involved in influencing the maternity services.**

INTRODUCTION

At the beginning of the 1990s midwives in Britain gave an enthusiastic response to the Government's Select Committee report on the maternity services; known as the 'Winterton Report' as it concluded that women expect a better, less interventionist service (House of Commons 1992). In particular the report noted that the way in which the maternity services were organized frustrated rather than offered women the choices they wanted. Subsequent government responses in each of the four countries in the United Kingdom, of which Changing Childbirth (DoH 1993) is perhaps best known, became the catalyst for providers of the maternity services to review their practices.

Whilst it might be assumed that all those involved in some way in providing or using the maternity services would have been united in working towards common goals, this was not always evident. For example, according to Dunlop (1993) the medical profession saw

Changing Childbirth as a threat to obstetric practice and a charter for home births. Midwives, on the other hand, saw it as providing opportunities for greater autonomy for their profession and new schemes were implemented to address requests from women for greater continuity of care and carer. Whilst many of these schemes received a high profile (Flint 1993, Page 1995), a study undertaken by the Institute of Manpower Studies (Wraight et al 1993) found that the concept of continuity of care and carer was difficult to understand and to implement. The first half of the 1990s therefore failed to see as dramatic a change in the maternity services as had been hoped for. Not only had interprofessional friction been evident but there had also been friction within the midwifery profession itself. Reasons for conflict within the midwifery profession could be due to a number of factors such as:

- different views about teams, group or one to one practice
- 3 year versus shortened pre-registration programmes
- certificate, diploma or degree registration
- the move of education from NHS to higher education
- the prevailing competitive nature of the NHS
- salary grading differentials
- the value placed on hospital versus community practice.

If midwives pull in different directions, then progress in achieving better choice, control and continuity of care for all childbearing women is unlikely to be achieved. The aim of this chapter is to consider the pivotal role of midwives in influencing the future of the maternity services. To assist in this, 14 very different stakeholders have been asked to share their vision for the future of the maternity services. These visions are intermeshed with relevant research and evidence from the literature, as well as the author's personal reflections. Whilst the contributors to this chapter have been selected because of the influence they, or their organization, have had on the maternity services, it is hoped that their visions will challenge all readers to play a part in influencing maternity care locally, nationally or internationally.

The challenges

It will be seen that the 14 contributors share, in the main, a vision for all members of maternity service teams to work together to provide women-centred care. However, it is suggested that unless a critical mass supports that vision, it is unlikely to come to fruition. Dr Luke Zander, a GP, believes that midwives face many challenges if the ideals of midwifery-led care are to be realized (see Box 13.1). These challenges, which include the education of midwives, midwifery-based evaluation and research, and the organization of the service, form the framework for this chapter. A final section looks at leadership and the potential consequences of midwives failing to rise to the challenge in the next millennium.

Box 13.1 Dr Luke Zander, Department of General Practice, UMDS of Guys and St Thomas Hospitals

Exciting developments are taking place with regard to the delivery of maternity care. Many of these emanate directly from the Cumberlege Report 'Changing Childbirth', which had, as its basic tenet, the objective of establishing a more women-centred approach to maternity care. It underlined the need to stress the normal in pregnancy and labour and to find ways of enhancing the experiential dimension of pregnancy and birth. A direct result of this orientation has been to bring midwifery into the centre stage and to identify midwives as pivotal players in the multidisciplinary maternity care team.

In fulfilling this role, midwifery faces many challenges. How is midwifery-led care to be organized? How can it most effectively be integrated with that provided by general practice and the specialist obstetric services? What is to be the relationship between midwifery and the newly developing primary care groups? What form of educational programmes will most effectively prepare midwives to take on their increasing responsibilities? How can midwifery-based evaluation and research be developed and contribute effectively to decision making?

If successful in this endeavour, great benefit will be derived both by the midwifery profession and by women using the maternity services in this country.

THE EDUCATION OF MIDWIVES

The last decade of the 20th century has seen fundamental changes in the education of the future generation of midwives. Not everyone supported the move from the shortened pre-registration midwifery programme for registered nurses to the widespread introduction of the 3 year 'direct entry' programmes. Interestingly, it was not normally the midwives who worked alongside these direct entrant students who demonstrated prejudice towards their programme, but senior midwives who responded negatively when hearing anecdotal comments about them (Downe 1986, Fraser, unpublished work, 1994, Fraser 1996). Others expressed scepticism about the higher academic level of these new pre-registration programmes, believing they would favour intellectual at the expense of practical abilities.

Evaluation of pre-registration midwifery programmes

The definition and assessment of higher level skills and attributes within professional education and training is an issue that is attracting increasing attention (Eraut & Cole 1993). Society functions on the assumption that qualified professionals are competent to perform their professional tasks, but the whole notion of professional competence is increasingly seen as complex and multifaceted. Just what does it mean to be professionally competent? Can competence be adequately defined and within what range of difficult contexts can it be supposed to apply?

Those involved in professional education often subscribe to the idea of professional competence being at the heart of their assessment procedures. It is, however, difficult to ascertain exactly what is meant by professional competence in different professions and clearly stated explicit statements outlining professional competence are few and far between. Expert assessors assume they are clear about what they are assessing, but cannot easily explain the detail of

what is involved to others. There is also some evidence of the stress involved in failing students in professional education programmes if standards are left to individual subjective judgement and the profession involved has a 'caring' philosophy (Ilott, unpublished work, 1993). In the absence of explicit statements of assessment standards it is difficult to maintain high levels of confidence in the uniformity of professional education and training, especially when a different preparation for practice is introduced.

In order to evaluate the effectiveness of the new diploma and degree 3 year routes into midwifery in England, the ENB commissioned an evaluation study. This study, known as the EME (Effectiveness of Midwifery Education) project (Fraser, Murphy & Worth-Butler 1997), sought to establish some benchmark statements, allowing a distinction to be made between competence and incompetence to practise as a midwife (Worth-Butler, Murphy & Fraser 1994, 1995). During the study it became evident that there was no commonly shared definition of a competent midwife at the point of registration. There were some who expected the new midwife to manage a large antenatal/postnatal ward as soon as qualified. Others even expected a level of dexterity for certain skills that were not even evident in all new midwives trained via the shortened route. Thus a major challenge for the EME project team was to attempt to create a model of competence against which to judge student midwives who were about to complete their programme.

Midwifery has shared with many other professions a healthy scepticism for models of competence that can trivialize or compartmentalize what is a complex set of skills and abilities. However, in an autonomous profession such as midwifery it was vital that an acceptable way was found to make explicit the qualities and characteristics that should be discernible among competent practitioners. The views and opinions of interested parties and stakeholders were sought and from a synthesis of data a tentative model of competence emerged. The model was intended to demonstrate the holistic nature of midwifery competence through its three closely interlinked dimensions of competence:

- the ability to be autonomous and professional but 'with woman' (the professional/friend approach)
- the ability to provide individualized care (the individual approach)
- a sound knowledge base and appropriate skills for the provision of midwifery care (clinical competence).

The competent, newly qualified midwife should therefore be one who could integrate, with appropriate emphases according to context, all of these dimensions. The professional/friend dimension appeared from the study to be the most difficult aspect to teach and assess. It also proved difficult for some midwives when relating to students. It might be argued that, if a midwife becomes too friendly with a student, it might be more difficult to tell the student that she is not achieving a satisfactory standard. On the contrary, evidence from students and midwives locally would suggest that when the relationship is good then constructive criticism is more likely to be accepted and responded to positively. A major challenge arising from the EME study was the difficulty in assessing students in practice. If this challenge is not grasped effectively then the category of 'borderline' students will continue and as new midwives they will remain unprepared for contemporary midwifery practice (Fraser, Murphy & Worth-Butler 1997 Ch. 9).

Critics of the new programmes frequently complained about students' lack of psychomotor skills and expertise in caring for women if the latter become ill (Fraser, unpublished work 1994, Fraser, Murphy & Worth-Butler 1997). However, most midwives will lose their dexterity for some skills if opportunities to practise are limited. An assessment matrix was another important outcome of the EME study. This sought to provide an indication of key skills and capabilities necessary for registration whilst making it clear that others could be learned post-registration. The new diploma and degree programmes provide students with a greater depth and breadth of knowledge and ability to critique practice than

was the norm for 18 month certificate level programmes. It is suggested that it is more important for midwives to be knowledgeable and seek out someone with the appropriate skills when beyond their own expertise than to attempt, through inadequate knowledge of the potential consequences, a skill themselves or even enlist the assistance of an equally unskilled doctor.

Rather than being critical of new programmes there should be ongoing curriculum evaluation and improvement. In particular, there needs to be an emphasis on problem-based learning and opportunities for development of essential skills as well as comprehensive, valid and reliable assessment strategies (Fraser, unpublished work, 1998).

Collaboration between education and service

Meryl Thomas, from her wealth of experience as director of midwifery education and practice at the ENB, says in her personal vision that: 'those midwives in education' must 'work collaboratively with those in service' to 'equip midwives to work with greater flexibility across a variety of contexts of care and move strategically towards an all graduate profession' (see Box 13.2). An important challenge in this statement is for collaboration between education and service. The move to higher education has meant for many midwife teachers a relocation of base well away from maternity units and immersion in a culture which fails to prioritize the practice-based curriculum.

Concern for the effectiveness of the practice-based curriculum resulted in the ENB commissioning a study, known as the ROLE project, to investigate the role of midwife and nurse teachers or lecturers in practice (Day, Fraser & Mallik 1998). The picture that emerged from the case study sites was depressing, although less so for midwife than for nurse lecturers. Whilst lecturers, students, practitioners, managers and education consortia representatives agreed that the role of the lecturer in practice was important, it was found that very few lecturers achieved the 20% of time in practice recommended by the

Box 13.2 **Meryl Thomas, Director, Midwifery Education and Practice, ENB**

In the maternity service of the future, there will be more than lip-service to the role of the midwife as 'autonomous practitioner'. Activities focused on the needs of women will be strengthened by interprofessional and organizational collaboration. Different models and frameworks for delivering midwifery care should emerge within the reformed health service, supported by informed and appropriate educational opportunities. Midwives must rise to the challenge of making effective contributions in planning, purchasing and in delivery of quality woman-centred care, within the finite resources of the health service. Each midwife will be increasingly responsible and accountable for their individual contribution to the quality and standards of care. Midwives' effectiveness in forging alliances, collaborating and practising across the primary and secondary sectors will be key to their impact and value within the new NHS.

There will be no one to take us by the hand through this challenge. Midwifery leaders must emerge to recognize and grasp the opportunities inherent within the white paper 'The new NHS: modern—dependable' and the many papers which have followed relating to the government's implementation of their strategic vision. Successful initiatives will be those which support rather than undermine the government strategy. There is no blueprint for maternity services; we can influence as never before the development of services woman want.

Family friendly employment policies offering midwives equity and flexibility will be equally important if the vision is to be achieved. This will be more easily implemented outside of the secondary sector in supportive group practices where traditional organizational constraints do not exist.

The 1998 SNMAC report 'Midwifery: delivering our future' offers a lever to the profession to negotiate for change. It will be fundamental to success that those midwives in education work collaboratively with those in service. Collectively they must ensure the educational programmes equip midwives to work with greater flexibility across a variety of contexts of care and move strategically towards an all graduate profession.

The practice of midwives will be increasingly evidence based. In turn both practice and education will be developed and supported through effective, meaningful clinical governance into which statutory midwifery supervision will be linked as part of the NHS quality enhancement framework.

References:
HMSO: The new NHS: modern—dependable (December 1997); NHSE: Better health and better healthcare HSC (February 1998); HMSO: Our healthier nation—a contract for health; HMSO: The new NHS—modern and dependable HSC (April 1998); DoH: SNMAC report Midwifery: delivering our future (February 1998).

ENB. It is suggested that, unless lecturers are regularly visible in practice and some at least undertake a 'hands-on' role, not only will their support of students and practitioners be inadequate but their teaching will soon become outdated. Evidence from the study also stressed the importance of support from lecturers for practitioners in making assessment judgements.

An all-graduate profession?

A second challenge arising from Meryl Thomas' vision is to move towards an all-graduate profession. Not everyone would agree, although the midwife's role of autonomous practitioner who also works collaboratively with doctors and other professional groups requires high level intellectual abilities. Midwives need to have the capabilities to be able to recognize rapidly, to interpret and to act appropriately and quickly on some occasions, but on others to act following a period of reflection or deliberative analysis.

A potential difficulty in moving to an all-graduate profession is twofold. First, the entry requirement for degree programmes could deter a number of mature applicants who have the motivation and ability to succeed but lack conventional qualifications and academic writing skills. The second is the emphasis placed by universities on examinations, essays, written material, etc. Experience and research would suggest that a number of students, especially those with dependants, find it difficult to achieve in 3 years the requirements for competent midwifery practice and the written evidence for a good honours degree alongside the demands of home life (Fraser, unpublished work, 1998, Fraser, Murphy & Worth-Butler, 1997).

Striving for an all-graduate profession, whilst continuing to encourage mature as well as school leaver candidates, provides two particular challenges for the midwife educationalist. The first is a consideration of the length of the programme alongside demands for cost effectiveness. Midwifery, like nursing, appears to be pressurized to offer 3 year degree programmes, yet other university courses with practice or language components are frequently longer. The assumption that students from a broad entry gate can be prepared in 3 years to be fit for professional practice, fit for their employer's purposes and fit for the university's honours degree needs to be challenged.

The second challenge is the value placed on teaching and assessment by academic rather than health service staff and hence the way in which academic credits are awarded. The concerns of higher education in determining standards for academic awards within and between universities (HEQC 1995, 1996) makes the task of achieving credits for practice-based assessment even more difficult. Midwife teachers and lecturers will need to use evidence from all relevant reports, research and guidelines (e.g. ENB 1998) to ensure they take control of midwifery education programmes to equip students with the capabilities for contemporary midwifery practice as well as their university's academic award.

Learning and working together in higher education

A multiprofessional approach might be a more powerful way of investigating issues which are applicable across vocational programmes. Collaboration with medical colleagues in higher education could be a particularly powerful allegiance. The norm for obstetricians and general practitioners in medical schools has been to retain a practice case load alongside lecturing and undertaking research. Dr Lindsay Smith, a frequent spokesperson for the Royal College of General Practitioners, has as his personal vision a belief that interdisciplinary education, starting at undergraduate level, will reap benefits for all those involved in maternity care (see Box 13.3). The conference, 'Learning together' cited in Dr Smith's vision for the maternity services, acted as the catalyst for an innovative development at the University of Nottingham. In this university the academic division of midwifery made the unique move from being part of a school of nursing and midwifery to join with obstetrics and gynaecology to become a department of obstetrics, midwifery and gynaecology (Fraser

1997). Like Dr Smith's vision, it is hoped that this initiative will bring about benefits 'in terms of understanding, continuity and respect'. In particular, working together should stop the distress caused to women by overhearing interprofessional conflict like the following extract from a longitudinal study of the perceptions of childbearing women, 'I was aware of a conversation between doctor and midwives and this was inappropriate as I could hear their disagreement' (Fraser, 1999 p. 103).

Box 13.3 Dr Lindsay Smith, Ilchester Research GP Practice, Somerset

Using the research evidence, teamwork, access, education, organizational framework and involving women should all influence the quality of care that women receive.

Midwives need to: access the evidence base, critique it and inform women on relevant, valid evidence upon which to base their care; work as committed integrated team members to ensure continuity of care and carer (RCGP 1995); have unimpeded access to secondary care investigations; and work equally with GPs as the primary maternity care team (Smith 1996), to share the burden and joy of looking after pregnant women.

Such integrated team care should be based on inter-disciplinary education (Zungolo 1994), from undergraduate through vocational training to accredited professional development. Such education will reap benefits in terms of understanding, continuity and respect (NHS Executive 1997).

Carers must challenge accepted 'sacred cows' to level quality up, not down e.g. the assumption that midwife only care is best for low risk women, that two qualified midwives must attend a home birth and that all postnatal care needs a qualified midwife.

Finally, women need to be involved in not only clinical decisions, but also in defining the organizational structure, research priorities and rationing decisions.

References:
RCGP (Royal College of General Practitioners) 1995. The role of general practice in maternity care. Occasional paper 72. RCGP, London
Smith 1996. Should general practitioners have any role in maternity care in the future? British Journal of General Practice 46:243–247
Zungolo E 1994 Interdisciplinary education in pimary care: the challenge. Nursing and Health Care 15: 288–292
NHSE 1997 Learning together: professional education for maternity care. NHS Executive, London

MIDWIFERY-BASED EVALUATION AND RESEARCH

Emerging from the EME study was evidence that students were knowledgeable about research and able to critique studies rather than accept findings unreservedly. They were well able to question time-honoured practices or, as Dr Smith exhorts, 'challenge accepted sacred cows' (Box 13.3). This became more difficult once students left the security of a supportive peer group as, although the pre-registration programmes were effective in preparing them for a 'Changing Childbirth' maternity service, a number of new midwives became disillusioned when experiencing the realities of midwifery practice (Fraser, Murphy & Worth-Butler 1997). Why then do highly motivated new midwives become disillusioned or fail to act as change agents? Maybe it is partly a consequence of a short-staffed service with little time for critical reflection. It could alternatively be due to the lack of higher education opportunities for midwives in the past. Tricia Murphy-Black, Professor of Midwifery in Scotland, welcomes the recent increase in the broad areas of study in master's degrees available for midwives (see Box 13.4). This she suggests is essential at a time of 'ever-expanding information overload'. It will not be possible, nor necessary, for all midwives to study for higher degrees but those that have, Professor Murphy-Black argues, must be seen as offering a benefit to their colleagues and not perceived as being a threat. These colleagues should be used as a resource to assist all midwives to base their practice on sound research and best available evidence. The need for evidence-based practice is a recurring theme from all contributors to this chapter.

Professor Murphy-Black also emphasizes the need for research to be focused on the needs of mothers and babies. This is likely to involve midwives working collaboratively with other midwives and also interprofessional initiatives for health services research. However, midwives should consider becoming involved in perhaps less specifically focused research as well, as far-reaching scientific discoveries can sometimes be

Box 13.4 **Professor Tricia Murphy-Black, Department of Nursing and Midwifery Studies, University of Stirling**

The maternity services should combine two main aims—the safety and well-being of the mother and baby with meeting the wishes of the parents concerning childbirth. If the physiological model (i.e. that pregnancy and childbirth are a normal life event) is the basis for service provision, then there will be emphasis on the needs of the mothers. The focus of midwives, their education, the research base of practice, and the organization of midwifery care must be on mother and baby. The extent or limits of midwifery care should not be decided by the needs of others (e.g. taking on additional tasks or roles should only be agreed if it is to the benefit of mothers and babies).

There are three essentials for the future of midwifery:

- *Diversity in education*—while there has to be a certain number of core skills which all midwives will need to learn, we should encourage as much diversity as possible in the continuing education of midwives. One welcome development is the range of broad area of study in master's courses. The skills of critical thinking and analysis are needed, but diversity in the education of midwives can only help in this time of ever-expanding information overload. This will lead to midwives becoming specialists in certain areas, but this should not be seen as a threat but a benefit.
- *Effectiveness in practice*—midwives should know what to do, how to do it, when to do it and why it should be done. Wherever possible there should be a research base for practice, and if there is not research evidence that a certain practice, method or organization provides positive benefit for mothers and babies then it should be questioned. Midwives should have the autonomy to decide the policy for midwifery care.
- *Accountability for practice*—midwives should be accountable to the mother and baby. If a midwife's practice is negligent or dangerous, then the midwife must take the consequences. If policy is both effective and research based, then policy in itself should not be a source of conflict for midwifery practice or compromise the physical or psychological well-being of mother and baby.

serendipitous. Meg Goodman, in her vision on behalf of the Maternity Alliance, alludes to the unimaginable challenges that will face midwives as scientists have become able 'to manipulate human development and reproduction' (see Box 13.5). The cloning of Dolly the sheep in the latter part of the 20th century is one such example of the extraordinary advances of modern science. A challenge for midwives must therefore be to ask questions that childbearing women would want asking and to be knowledgeable and assertive enough to halt unethical research, whilst not impeding ethically acceptable scientific discovery (see Ch. 5). Perhaps the time has come to ask what we should do rather than what we can do.

As scientific advancement brings with it a host of possibilities, it will be even more important to retain sight of childbirth as a normal physiological life event which midwives and doctors can effect positively or negatively by their actions or omissions. Meg Goodman (Box 13.5) reminds us that women will be healthier in the future and will therefore need less medical intervention. However, the expectations of families are likely to increase, creating more demands on the NHS. The reporting of a debate about caesarean births on demand is one example of health professionals and user groups disagreeing about levels of choice for women and intervention by doctors (Carter 1998). In the debate, it is suggested that the risk to the baby is greater in conventional than caesarean deliveries. Midwives should surely be challenging the evidence for such a statement given the absence of a randomized controlled trial. A further question must also concern cost effectiveness and the need to target choice and research for those who are most in need rather than those who are most articulate. The less glamorous as well as the scientifically exciting aspects of the maternity services need investigating if we really are to become a 'healthier nation'.

Ann Thomson, editor of Midwifery, believes in her vision that midwives have a much greater role to play than at present in meeting the needs of families. She argues for midwives to be involved more in family planning and to support families for up to 6 weeks following delivery (see Box 13.6). By doing so there could be reductions in unwanted pregnancies, healthier lifestyles before conception as well as during

---

Box 13.5 Meg Goodman, Health Policy Officer, the Maternity Alliance

On the cusp of the 21st century, it is appropriate that the maternity services should look for their inspiration both back to their past and forward to scientific and professional possibilities of extraordinary magnitude. Community involvement, partnership with women, professional autonomy and expertise, continuity of care and carer are all strengths dating back to the earliest days of midwifery and now re-emerging as essential to maternity care for the future. At the same time, the seemingly exponential growth in our knowledge about and ability to manipulate human development and reproduction means that midwives will face challenges unimaginable only a few years ago.

Users of maternity services will also both resemble those of earlier generations and present new difficulties and opportunities. Economic and social divisions in this country and beyond will maintain the old poverty-related problems, even bringing back diseases and conditions we thought were beaten. Most women will, however, be healthier, more knowledgeable, less acquiescent and need less medical intervention than in the past. Maternity services will have to be more innovative, flexible, politically savvy and socially responsible than ever to meet all the demands that will be made of them.

Box 13.6 Ann M Thomson, Senior Lecturer in Midwifery, School of Nursing, Midwifery and Health Visiting, University of Manchester

A maternity service should be based in the community, utilizing primary health care principles, funded so that the funds provide the maternity services and do not subsidize other services. The services would meet the needs of women for family planning (not just contraception), antenatal care, care in labour and for birth, postnatal care for mother and baby, and in particular the promotion of breast feeding. These services would be available for those comtemplating pregnancy and until the baby was at least 6 weeks old. The woman and her family would be the centre of the service and services could be accessed from whoever the woman wished—midwife, GP or obstetrician.

Services, including the necessary social support services, would be provided where required by the individual and on a geographical basis. That means adequate support for all those wishing for a home birth, and adequate midwifery care from community to hospital and back to the community for those who have a hospital birth. Since the publication of the Peel Report (DHSS 1970) women have lost the confidence to have a home birth. Strategies would be employed to encourage appropriate women to redevelop this confidence.

The midwife would be provided with a salary that allowed her to work in a flexible manner to meet the needs of women and their families, but still meet her own family and social responsibilities.

DHSS (Department of Health and Social Security) 1970 Domiciliary midwifery and maternity bed needs, HMSO, London

pregnancy improved success in breast feeding. All these areas provide challenges for midwives to research their practice and that of others involved in providing a service to women at these times.

The differences midwives make to the childbirth experience often go unnoticed, as midwives have not always published their achievements in the past. Joan Walker, former secretary-general of the International Confederation of Midwives, emphasizes the difference midwives make 'in reducing, mortality and morbidity of mothers and babies' (see Box 13.7). She also stresses the importance of the midwife's role in enabling women to make safe choices. This can only be possible if midwives are knowledgeable about best evidence and regularly evaluate their practice. It can also be challenging for midwives to

encourage women in Western cultures to make safe choices when the rights of the individual are paramount and litigation is ever increasing (see Chs 5, 6 and 9). Midwives must also guard against being sucked into defensive practice. It is suggested that women are more likely to make safe choices if midwives develop the special 'friend' relationship referred to earlier in this chapter. Mary Newburn, speaking on behalf of the National Childbirth Trust, endorses this view. Her vision is for a maternity service where all women 'can speak of "my midwife" meaning a midwife whom they can get to know and trust, someone they feel confident to go to for sound research-based information or advice' (see Box 13.8). The challenge must be for midwives to be confident, knowledgeable and competent because if women are aware that midwives' practice is not based on best evidence then trust will be unlikely and fear might cause women to make unsafe choices for their care.

Box 13.7 Joan Walker, former Secretary-general, International Confederation of Midwives

Evidence shows that midwives are effective in reducing mortality and morbidity of mothers and babies. Therefore, midwives are symbolically placed to address the situation of 581 000 women who die each year around the world as a result of pregnancy or childbirth. On a global scale most midwives are women, therefore they must seek to achieve empowerment of women thus enabling a respect for their own profession and for each other. Midwives who evaluate their practice and keep abreast of change are founts of knowledge and expertise. They are in an ideal position to work with women during their reproductive health years, particularly around the time of pregnancy, delivery and during the postnatal period when care of the newborn is also an essential component of care. In enabling women to make the right choices for safe motherhood the midwifery partnership with other health care professionals is integral. At all times midwives must be politically astute and have a comprehension of other influences upon the lives of women, babies and families for whom they care. Where these influences are detrimental to safe motherhood then midwives must take a stance to bring about change.

The midwife/woman partnership can become a force for good in seeking of safe birth for all.

Note: The Code for ethics for midwives (reproduced in Ch. 5) is available from the ICM, Eisenhowerlaan 138, 2517 KN Den Haag, The Netherlands. The code also has explanatory notes and glossary.

Box 13.8 Mary Newburn, Head of Policy, the National Childbirth Trust

I have a vision of maternity care in which all women can speak of 'my midwife' meaning a midwife whom they can get to know and trust; someone they feel confident to go to for sound, research-based information or advice, someone they feel comfortable with and can really talk to. A woman's midwife would aim to provide the majority of care personally during pregnancy, at the birth and during the postnatal period, and ensure that a midwife colleague known to the woman was available at times s/he could not be.

As many midwives have children themselves or have other care commitments, being on-call for long periods and working irregular hours can be demanding. However, the benefits of flexible working and greater control over one's work seem likely to outweigh the demands provided that the case load is not too heavy and provided that midwives with young children are able to make flexible childcare arrangements. Sandall (1997) found that midwives working as part of a team experienced more stress than those who carried their own case load. The importance of not burdening midwives with an unreasonably large case load cannot be overemphasized. Midwives who wish to work part time should be able to carry a smaller case load. Employers should consult midwives about their childcare needs and help meet routine needs. In addition they should consider innovative ways of providing back-up to routine arrangements.

Box 13.8 **Continued**

In rural areas there are real challenges to achieving this degree of continuity of carer, particularly if births are centralized in large district general hospitals. I would like to see small and medium-sized maternity units retained and strengthened so that babies can be born in their local community or close to it, enabling families to be together around the time of birth and not separated, as many are now forced to be. This will mean finding innovative ways of providing obstetric, anaesthetic and paediatric back-up. Anecdotal evidence suggests that, when women are forced to travel long distances to give birth, there is a tendency for more births to be induced and for a higher caesarean section rate.

References:
Sandall J (1997) Midwives burnout and continuity of care. British Journal of Midwifery 5(2):106–111

Clinical effectiveness

Chapter 11 outlines ways to ensure quality in the maternity services and Chapter 1 provides guidance on accessing information. Unfortunately the well-researched 'Informed choice' leaflets (MIDIRS & NHS Centre for Reviews and Dissemination 1997) have not been purchased by many NHS trusts and an evaluation of their effectiveness is in progress at the time of writing this book. It is hoped that all midwives are at least aware of their existence and have access to them for reference purposes. In order to assist nurses, midwives and health visitors improve their clinical effectiveness, the NHS Executive (1998) has produced a 10 part resource pack with the following titles:

1. Clinical effectiveness—what it's all about
2. Clinical effectiveness—finding out more
3. Searching the literature
4. Critically appraising literature
5. Designing and carrying out a clinical audit
6. Preparing a proposal for clinical audit
7. Changing clinical practice
8. Designing a research study
9. Preparing a proposal for research
10. Writing and publishing on clinically effective practice.

With all the demands made upon a midwife's time both at home and at work a further challenge

is to develop a strategy to collaborate with colleagues to search the literature to check out their practices. Action research is an invaluable research approach for practitioners to collaborate and improve their practice together. However, before embarking upon any research, and action research in particular, support of managers is essential so that actions can be carried out not blocked. (The Further reading list at the end of this chapter provides some useful texts on research generally and action research in particular.)

THE ORGANIZATION OF A MIDWIFERY-LED SERVICE

Louise Silverton sums up the RCM vision for the future of the maternity services in Box 13.9. She picks up the themes of informed choice, continuity of care and clinical effectiveness discussed earlier. When it comes to leading the planning and commissioning of maternity care, she believes that midwives should be the lead professionals, in consultation with women, for the

Box 13.9 **Louise Silverton, Deputy General Secretary, the Royal College of Midwives**

For most women, pregnancy is a normal life event—not an illness. Maternity care must start from this point, supporting the woman as an active partner in her own health care, and responding to each individual's physical, emotional and social needs. Maternity services should be primarily rooted in the community, offering a full continuum of care to women near to where they live and work. This care must 'follow the woman' across professional and sectoral boundaries; it must be based on the principles of informed choice, continuity of care, clinical effectiveness, responsiveness and accessibility. Midwives should lead the planning and commissioning of maternity care, in close consultation with service users. While midwives should act as lead professional in the care of most women (healthy women with normal pregnancies), they will work in partnership with other professionals, in an environment of professional autonomy, equality and mutual respect. There is scope for a wide range of models of maternity care—midwifery group practices, community birth centres, and hospital care too for those women who need it or want it. Midwives, and women, should be involved in the development, monitoring and reform of maternity care at all levels.

majority of the service as childbirth is a normal physiological process. She also emphasizes the importance of midwives working with others in an environment of professional autonomy. This apparent juxtaposition of personal autonomy together with teamwork has been discussed more fully in Chapter 8. In the past, interprofessional tribalism has perhaps detracted from effective organization of the maternity services.

Jean Duerden, LSA midwifery officer, echoes the vision of the RCM as she also sees midwives taking a lead role in the planning and delivery of the maternity services (see Box 13.10). In particular she emphasizes the need for midwives to play a key role in the primary care groups (PCGs) of the new NHS. The members of PCGs have not necessarily considered the role midwives might play. An important challenge for

the profession will be to ensure they impact upon these PCGs whilst ensuring an integrated midwifery service is preserved. Like Meryl Thomas (see Box 13.2), Jean Duerden urges action not apathy from midwives to respond to Government reports, white and green papers. Midwifery, with its strength in statutory supervision, interprofessional teamwork and its community emphasis, has a lot of expertise to feed into health improvement plans, clinical governance and corporate governance. However, although the government's emphasis on primary care is to be welcomed, it is essential that the relationship between the primary care sector and acute sector is seamless. This is particularly important given that most women deliver in hospital and those with complicated pregnancies need continuity of midwifery care even more than those with unproblematic pregnancies.

Cathy Warwick, a midwife and general manager for women and children's services, emphasizes the importance of targeting resources in a cost-effective way, 'to ensure each woman and baby is discharged from the maternity services in optimum physical and emotional health' (see Box 13.11). All government ministers make demands on the nation's resources and difficult

---

Box 13.10 Jean Duerden, LSA Midwifery Officer, Leeds Health Authority

My vision for the future of maternity services sees midwives playing a key role in the primary care groups, some holding posts on commissioning groups and others working closely with all the primary care givers to ensure that all women of childbearing age are offered a full package of care, from pre-conception until the completion of 28 post natal days. The community midwife, based within the primary care group, will be the key player throughout. All antenatal and postnatal care will be provided in the locality at a 'one stop shop' which has ultrasound, laboratory and clinical facilities. A midwife will be available each day at this clinic for advice, parentcraft education, antenatal clinics and antenatal day care. Intrapartum care will be given in the maternity hospital, which the woman will have visited during her pregnancy with her partner to meet staff and orientate herself with the environment and entrances to the unit. The community midwife will also provide a home birth service and liaise closely with the core staff in the maternity unit, visiting the women on her case load each time she is in the maternity unit. All midwives will have an opportunity to work in each environment, perhaps 1 year out, 1 year in.

Whilst I would love there to be a more holistic approach of one midwife offering continuity of carer throughout, I am too much of a realist to think this could be a service for all women. Midwives have their own lives to lead and the more team members there are the more care becomes fragmented. My vision retains the key named midwife but intrapartum care, unless a home birth, is likely to be provided by another expert midwife.

Box 13.11 Cathy Warwick, General Manager, Women and Children's Services, King's Healthcare

Resources will be specifically targeted to ensure each woman and baby is discharged from the maternity services in optimum physical and emotional health. Patterns of care will be modelled on local population need. Services provided will be evidence based and cost effective.

Services will usually be provided in the community. Home birth will be a real choice. Professionals may be employed in a variety of ways but will have open access to secondary services. Care will be based on guidelines agreed by all parties regardless of professional background, place of work or employment status. Standards and outcomes will be monitored across the local maternity service.

Professionals will be deployed appropriately and effectively. Midwives will care for most women. Some women will receive care, or a proportion of it, from their family doctor or an obstetrician. At times a multidisciplinary team will be involved.

Box 13.11　Continued

Women will always be treated with kindness and respect and be able to communicate openly with care givers. Information will be readily accessible. Women will often know the professionals looking after them. Leaders in the service will aim to ensure a competent, stable and motivated workforce which meets the needs of women.

Flexible, imaginative and effective use of available resources to ensure a healthier population will be paramount.

---

decisions are always being made about how resources are allocated. Midwives will be challenged to develop business plans for a midwifery-led service that balances financial and quality issues and recognizes realism while still striving for idealism.

James Drife, professor of obstetrics and gynaecology at the University of Leeds, recognizes that, when childbirth is normal, the midwife is the most appropriate lead carer (see Box 13.12). He also stresses the importance of access to

---

Box 13.12　James Drife, Professor of Obstetrics and Gynaecology, Leeds University

Future antenatal care will be given mainly outside hospitals by midwives and general practitioners. The obstetrician's antenatal role will be in the care of high risk pregnancy and for advice if abnormality is suspected—particularly on ultrasound, when special expertise may be required. In labour, all women will be looked after by midwives, usually in hospital, but in future a midwife who requests medical aid will consult a senior obstetrician, not a trainee with a few months' experience. The Royal College of Midwives and the Royal College of Obstetricians and Gynaecologists have together published guidelines on minimum standards of care in labour, which specify consultant involvement—including some night work—in the delivery suites of the future. The aim is not to increase medical involvement in normal labour but to improve training and to support midwives and junior doctors when intervention is needed.

Confidential enquiries into intrapartum stillbirths show that although these tragedies are rare, over 75% are avoidable. Complaints and litigation are increasing and in future women will be still less willing to tolerate mistakes from doctors or midwives. Regular updates, teamwork and practice drills will make future intrapartum care even safer for babies and women, and more fulfilling for professionals.

---

someone with the appropriate expertise should complications arise. It would seem that he is suggesting that consultant care is inappropriate and too expensive in normal situations but essential in high risk pregnancies and for advice when needed. A challenge for midwives and obstetricians when organizing the maternity service must be to enable midwives retain and develop expertise in supporting women and obstetricians in cases of difficulty or complications and ensure obstetricians retain a normality perspective, for the majority of childbearing women. Professor Drife also believes that 'in future women will be still less willing to tolerate mistakes from doctors or midwives' and consequently health care professionals will not only need to keep themselves updated but also alert managers to those who fail to use best evidence in their practice. The new emphasis on quality in the NHS under 'New Labour' is unlikely to tolerate further scandals such as those in Bristol, Kent and Canterbury in 1997/1998. Midwives and doctors will need to engage in 'regular updates, teamwork and practice drills' (Box 13.12) to bring avoidable deaths to zero and live up to public expectations.

Continuity of carer remains a key challenge for midwives when oganizing a midwifery-led service. Ishbel Kargar, in writing her vision on behalf of the ARM, says that midwives must also provide continuity of midwifery care when women 'require the services of an obstetrician in hospital' (see Box 13.13). Over the years there

---

Box 13.13　Ishbel Kargar, Admin Secretary, ARM

In 1986 after 18 months consultation with health professionals and users of the service, ARM published a document which has influenced many beneficial changes in the last 12 years (ARM 1986).

The basic principles were (and still are) that maternity care should be based in the community, accessed by direct application to the community midwifery services rather than via a doctor, i.e. 'midwife-led'.

Each woman should have care individually tailored to her needs, and the opportunity to get to know and trust her midwives, i.e. 'woman-centred' care. Thus ideally, she would be attended by a small number of midwives (not more than four), providing continuity, which has been shown to be more effective than care from many different health professionals.

Box 13.13 **Continued**

This standard of continuity of midwife care should also be available to those women who require the services of an obstetrician in hospital, or who choose hospital for their childbirth care.

Midwives should be the recognized lead professional for maternity care, consulting with medical colleagues where necessary, with the consent of the client.

Reference:
ARM 1986 The vision, proposals for the future of the maternity services, available from ARM, 62 Greetby Hill, Ormskirk, Lancashire L39 2DT, price £1.00.

has been a tendency for midwives to work mainly in the community or mainly in hospital. Given that midwifery has a clearly defined sphere of practice (EC 1980, 1989) it is reasonable to expect midwives to offer care for the whole spectrum of the childbirth process. General practitioners who retain an interest in obstetrics are expected to function equally effectively in hospital and community settings, but for some midwives this appears problematic.

Supporting and trusting each other

Perhaps one reason why midwives are reluctant to work in less familiar contexts is the failure of midwives to support each other, to share expertise and differences in practice and to trust each other. A study to evaluate the impact of the supervision of midwives found that: 'two conflicting discourses ran through the data: the first concerned midwives' need for support, the second concerned the issue of trust' (Stapleton, Duerden & Kirkham 1998 p. 2). If midwives fail to receive support from each other, as well as their supervisor, and are distrustful then initiatives for a midwifery-led, seamless service are less likely to succeed. Pre-registration student midwives have in some instances also failed to receive the support they need to develop competence and confidence in their first post as midwives (Fraser, Murphy & Worth-Butler 1997). The same might also be true for community-based midwives when attempting to provide continuity of carer for women in labour.

Anecdotal comments have been made suggesting that clinical grading anomalies might influence the support offered by an E grade hospital-based midwife to a G grade community-based midwife. The challenge must be for midwives to support each other according to contextual expertise, not salary differential.

Continuity of carer

One midwife providing continuity of carer throughout pregnancy, labour and the postnatal period has remained an ideal for most women and many midwives but has remained difficult to manage. Schemes such as one to one midwifery practice (McCourt & Page 1996) would appear to be successful but Jean Duerden would argue that 'midwives have their own lives to lead' (Box 13.10). Ishbel Kargar offers a compromise by suggesting a maximum of four midwives to provide continuity jointly (see Box 13.13) but this could prove inadequate if members of the team become ill or have maternity leave. Mary Newburn's suggestion of smaller case loads for part-time staff (see Box 13.8) would also be affected by these eventualities.

When considering ways to organize better continuity of care and carer, job satisfaction for core hospital midwives will also be an important factor. If small teams of community-based midwives provide continuity of carer throughout, hospital-based midwives could end up only providing high tech support. Therefore ways need to be found to ensure all midwives have opportunities to undertake the full role of the midwife, necessary also to maintain registration, whilst ensuring 24 hour support from midwives skilled in using modern technology. Jean Duerden's suggestion (see Box 13.10) is for community-based midwives to provide minimal intrapartum care and for all midwives to spend time in both hospital and community environments. Given that this is the normal rotation pattern for pre-registration student midwives it could be one feasible way of organizing the service.

Intrapartum care seems to cause most dissension amongst midwives in relation to continuity of carer. Whilst most women, if asked, would prefer a known carer in labour, studies that have been carried out to elicit the perceptions of childbearing women have found that women do not necessarily expect to have 'their' community midwife providing care in labour (Fraser, 1999, Green, Coupland & Kitzinger 1998). What seems important is to develop a relationship with a midwife early in labour and for that midwife to stay throughout. Once labour has become well established women do not like a different midwife taking over their care. There was also evidence that, for a small number of women, an unknown carer was preferable in case they embarrassed themselves (Fraser, 1999). However, there are other women for whom a known carer seems to be high priority and perhaps these should be targeted specifically. They might include women who are particularly fearful of hospitals, those whose labours are more likely to be problematic, teenagers and women who have no birth partner, or women such as the one described in Case study 3.1 (p. 56)

Not all midwifery-led services are likely to be organized in the same way and trying to do so could account for floundering of team midwifery (Wraight et al 1993). Instead, the challenge must be to work with all interested parties locally, especially maternity service liaison committees, to work out the best way to provide a quality but realistic cost effective, woman-centred service.

LEADERS AND VISIONARIES

This chapter has sought to present a vision for the future of the maternity services from the perspectives of users of the service, midwives, obstetricians and general practitioners. As well as these visionaries, each local service and education department needs midwives with vision and leadership qualities to grasp every opportunity to develop a really woman-centred service and enhance midwifery research and practice.

Midwives might initially have been disappointed that the Government's 1998 green paper, 'Our healthier nation—a contract for health' (see Further Reading, p. 230) did not include the maternity services as one of the four priority

areas to be targeted (i.e. heart disease and stroke, accidents, cancer and suicides). However, as midwives play a key role in public health they should use the Government's acknowledgement that social and economic factors and the environment are key influences on public health to develop initiatives that will improve birth and parenting outcomes for socially and economically deprived families. There is also scope for midwives to take a lead in priority areas, such as teenage pregnancies, in health improvement programmes.

Meg Goodman (Box 13.5) reminds us to look to the lessons that can be learned from the past as well as looking to the future. Many midwives today will know of the driving energy of Zepherina Veitch (subsequently Mrs Henry Smith) and Dame Rosalind Paget in their fight for legislation for midwives in order to ensure all women were attended by a trained midwife in childbirth (Cowell & Wainwright 1981). The world of midwifery is a very different one a century later but it still needs strong leadership if the ideals of 'Changing Childbirth' are to be realized. Beverley Beech, speaking on behalf of AIMS, has some harsh words to say in her vision for the future of the maternity services (see Box 13.14). She believes we are heading towards an almost Aldous Huxley type of 'brave new world'. Whilst her pessimistic vision of the future might anger some readers, her cautionary tale should engender action not apathy. The

---

Box 13.14 **Beverley Beech, Honorary Chair, AIMS**

A vision of a 'brave new world'
The Winteron Report, Changing Childbirth, innumerable research papers, the Confidential Enquiries into Maternal and Infant Death, all gave clear direction for improving maternity care, and all are ignored by the majority of professionals. For those who perceive childbirth as the ideal opportunity to exercise power and control, albeit often unconsciously, the idea that midwives should act as the mother's servant is anathema. Many obstetricians, blinkered by their training and a love of machinery, continue to promote more technology and more fascinating developments— vaginal probe ultrasound, 3D ultrasound, new electronic fetal monitors, triple, quadriple and a test for everything is promoted.

Box 13.14 Continued

General practitioners have a budget and purchase care, home birth is marginalized and midwives are required to work to the GPs' rules and regulations, rather than those of the obstetricians. Small GP and midwifery units are closed so that maternity care is centralized in ever larger baby factories where women are monitored from conception to birth. Ultrasound examinations are carried out to establish that conception has taken place, and the mother will be required to have a monthly scan—just to check that the baby is developing properly. At 39 weeks she will be admitted for induction or a caesarean section, which will have increased to over 50% and will be promoted vigorously *as* 'protecting the woman's vagina', and as the method of first choice for most sensible women.

Independent midwives, as a result of lack of support from the Royal College and NHS midwives, will stop practising. Midwifery tutors, separated from practice, will train academically sharp graduates who have little or no understanding of the normal birth process, and will rarely see one before qualification, or afterwards.

The media will promote caesarean section as the ideal means of avoiding the pain of labour, and articles will continue to undermine women's confidence in their ability to give birth. The few women who still believe that childbirth is a normal physiological event will be harassed throughout their pregnancies, and many of them will have their babies taken into care on the grounds that they are irresponsible women who are not concerned about the welfare of their babies. For a very small minority, the only place to labour unhurried and without harassment will be in the woman's own home.

Unless every midwife acknowledges how far removed from normality hospital birth has become, formulates a strategy with parents, and actively works to address the overmedicalization of birth and their lack of power and influence, a 'brave new world' will continue to develop unchecked.

Winterton Report (House of Commons 1992) was the beginning of a charter for midwives to take a lead in childbirth and work in partnership with women and doctors to provide greater choice, control and continuity of care.

The collaborative work between the RCM and RCOG (see Box 13.12) is a positive example of midwives and obstetricians working together for the benefit of women rather professional autonomy. The new programme for the preparation of supervisors of midwives in England supports an empowering rather than a controlling philosophy in the maternity services (ENB 1997). New opportunities exist for midwives to study at diploma, degree and higher degree levels to equip them for leadership and the challenges of the future. The number of professors of midwifery is increasing, which enables midwifery to be recognized as a credible academic field in higher education.

The establishment of the National Institute for Clinical Effectiveness (NICE) by the Government provides midwives with the opportunity to demonstrate their expertise in the field of standard setting, clinical guidelines and audit by influencing the work of NICE as it pulls together guidelines work and develops national standards. Leaders are needed from midwifery to influence all aspects of the health service if midwifery is not to fall off the political agenda and the fears of Beverley Beech are not to be realized.

THE CHALLENGE OF THE BRAVE NEW WORLD

To conclude therefore, what 'brave new world' of the 21st century will you be entering and whose vision do you share? Can you remain where you are, assuming all is well with your professional development and the maternity services? Are you content to let others take action while you follow passively?

Will your 'brave new world' be like Huxley's 'insane utopia' where life is stable, conditioned and emotion free? Alternatively do you need to take action in order to ensure a 'Winterton world' where women's choice, control, satisfaction and individual care are as important as scientific progress? Or are you somewhere in between, responding to exciting scientific developments made possible by advanced technology but preferring to bury your head in the sand rather than take risks to help develop a woman-centred, midwifery-led service? It is suggested that the challenge of the 'brave new world' of the 21st century needs to be taken up by all midwives; apathy or the status quo has no place in a midwifery-led service. As an Australian midwife said at the International Congress of Midwives congress in Ontario, 'We have been given a window of opportunity ... we must capitalise on it and not rest on our laurels, we have to keep at it and use incremental steps, the priorities in health care will soon begin to shift once again

and the pendulum could very easily swing back the other way' (Robinson 1993 p. 1585).

REFERENCES

Carter H 1998 Call for caesarean births on demand. The Guardian 14-08-98:4

Cowell B, Wainwright D 1981 Behind the blue door, the history of the Royal College of Midwives 1881–1981. Ballière Tindall, London

Day C, Fraser D, Mallik M 1998 The role of the teacher/lecturer in practice (the ROLE project). ENB, London

DoH (Department of Health) 1993 Changing childbirth: report of the Expert Maternity Group. HMSO, London

Downe S 1986 Summary of recent survey assessing midwifery training schools attitudes to direct entry midwifery training. In: MIDIRS Information Pack no. 1, March 1986

Dunlop W 1993 Changing childbirth, commentary 2. British Journal of Obstetrics and Gynaecology 100:1072

EC (European Community) 1980 Midwives directives. EC Council Directive 80/155/EEC Article 4. Official Journal of the European Communities, Brussels

EC (European Community) 1989 Midwives directives. EC Council Directive 89/594/EEC Article 27, Ch. 5. Official Journal of the European Communities, Number L341/28, Brussels

ENB (English National Board) 1997 Preparation of supervisors of midwives. ENB, London

ENB (English National Board) 1998 Guidelines for pre-registration midwifery programmes of education. ENB, London

Eraut M, Cole G 1993 Assessing competence in the professions. Employment Departments' Methods Strategy Unit, Research development series, report no. 14:1

Flint C 1993 Midwifery teams and caseloads. Butterworth-Heineman, London

Fraser D M 1996 Pre-registration midwifery programmes: a case study evaluation of the non-midwifery placements. Midwifery 12:16–22

Fraser D M 1997 Change for whose benefit? The merger of midwifery and obstetrics in the University of Nottingham. MIDIRS Midwifery Digest 7(4):425–426

Fraser D M 1999 Women's perceptions of midwifery care: A longitudinal study to shape curriculum development. Birth 26(2):99–107

Fraser D, Murphy R, Worth-Butler M 1997 An outcome evaluation of the effectiveness of pre-registration midwifery programmes of education (the EME project). ENB, London

Green J, Coupland V, Kitzinger J 1998 Great expectations: a prospective study of women's expectations and experiences of childbirth, 2nd edn. Books for Midwives, Hale

HEQC (Higher Education Quality Council) 1995 Graduate standard programme. Executive summary. HEQC, London

HEQC (Higher Education Quality Council) 1996 Graduate standards programme: Academic standards in the approval review and classification of awards. HEQC, London

House of Commons Health Committee 1992 Second report, maternity services, vol 1. HMSO, London

McCourt C, Page L 1996 Report on the evaluation of one-to-one midwifery. TVU, London

MIDIRS & The NHS Centre for Reviews and Disseminations 1997 Informed choice in maternity care. MIDIRS, Bristol

NHS Executive 1998 Achieving effective practice: a cinical effectiveness and research information pack for nurses, midwives and health visitors. DoH, Leeds

Page L (ed) 1995 Effective group practice in midwifery. Blackwell Science, Oxford

Robinson K 1993 Professional autonomy—the view of midwives. In: ICM 23rd International Congress [abstract] ICM, Vancouver, Canada

Stapleton H, Duerden J, Kirkham M 1998 Evaluation of the impact of the supervision of midwives on midwifery practice and the quality of the midwifery care. ENB, London

Worth-Butler M, Murphy R J L, Fraser D M 1994 Towards an integrated model of competence in midwifery. Midwifery 10(4):225–231

Worth-Butler M, Murphy R, Fraser D 1995 Recognising competence in midwifery. British Journal of Midwifery 3(5):259–262

Wraight A, Ball J, Seccombe I, Stock J 1993. Mapping team midwifery: a report to the Department of Health. IMS report series 242. Institute of Manpower Studies, Brighton

FURTHER READING

Government reports on the health of the nation and the organization of the NHS make essential reading. Summaries can be a useful way to acquire an overview of the main points. An example is Healthcare Parliamentary Monitor (HPM) February 16, 1998 which summarizes the green paper: Our healthier nation—a contract for health.

HPM is published fortnightly while Parliament sits (tel. 0171 582 8350).

Altichter H, Posch P, Somekh B 1993 Teachers investigate their work: an introduction to the methods of action research. Routledge, London

Some books on action research can be quite complicated but this makes for clear reading and understanding. Along with John Elliott and others, Professor Bridget Somekh is one of the editors of the journal Educational Action Research.

Audit Commission 1997 First class delivery: improving maternity services in England and Wales. Audit Commission, Abingdon, Oxon

Denzin N K, Lincoln Y S 1994 Handbook of qualitative research. Sage, Thousand Oaks, CA
Not a book to read from cover to cover but has very helpful sections for the novice and experienced qualitative researcher.

Elliott J 1995 What is good action research? Some criteria. Action Researcher no 2, January 1995. Hyde Publications
In this short paper Professor John Elliott states the main features of good educational action research. These principles can equally well be applied to professional practice. Professor Elliott has immense expertise in the field of action research and has supervised nurses and midwives undertaking research to improve their practice. Most of his books and papers are worth reading.

ENB (English National Board) 1995 The challenge of Changing childbirth: midwifery educational resource pack. ENB, London
As the title indicates this is a resource pack to help midwives face the challenges of contemporary practice. It contains a number of activities, articles and original papers from known experts in their field of practice.

Hart E, Bond M 1995 Action research for health and social care: a guide to practice. Open University, Milton Keynes
Neither of the authors are midwives but some interesting case studies are presented from which principles can equally well apply in midwifery. Their typology does not in my view aid understanding and enable use of an action research approach.

Hicks C M 1996 Undertaking midwifery research, a basic guide to design and analysis. Churchill Livingstone, New York.
This is a useful text to help midwives refresh their memories of mathematics to help in the design and analysis of experimental and other quantitative research studies.

McNiff J, Lomax P, Whitehead J 1996 You and your action research project. Routledge, London
A different approach to action research from that adopted by Elliott and Altrichter et al. The reader will need to make their own judgements about appropriateness of the different schools of thought to their own purposes.

Miles M B, Huterman A M 1994. Qualitative data analysis, an expanded sourcebook, 2nd edn. Sage, Thousand Oaks, CA
A useful guide for those undertaking a qualitative research project. It should aid rigour in data analysis.

Polit D, Hungler B 1995 Nursing research, principals and methods, 5th edn. J P Lippincott, Philadelphia
A popular book amongst student midwives and nurses but it requires considerable time to digest.

Index